CASE STUD

Public Health Preparedness and Response to Disasters

Edited by

Linda Young Landesman, DrPH, MSW
Consultant and Visiting Lecturer
School of Public Health
University of Massachusetts, Amherst

Isaac B. Weisfuse, MD, MPH
Associate Professor of Clinical Public Health
Department of Epidemiology
Mailman School of Public Health
Columbia University

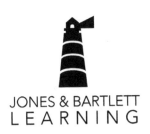

JONES & BARTLETT
L E A R N I N G

World Headquarters
Jones & Bartlett Learning
5 Wall Street
Burlington, MA 01803
978-443-5000
info@jblearning.com
www.jblearning.com

Jones & Bartlett Learning books and products are available through most bookstores and online book-sellers. To contact Jones & Bartlett Learning directly, call 800-832-0034, fax 978-443-8000, or visit our website, www.jblearning.com.

Substantial discounts on bulk quantities of Jones & Bartlett Learning publications are available to corporations, professional associations, and other qualified organizations. For details and specific discount information, contact the special sales department at Jones & Bartlett Learning via the above contact information or send an email to specialsales@jblearning.com.

Production Credits:
Executive Publisher: William Brottmiller
Publisher: Michael Brown
Managing Editor: Maro Gartside
Editorial Assistant: Kayla Dos Santos
Editorial Assistant: Chloe Falivene
Production Assistant: Alyssa Lawrence
Senior Marketing Manager: Sophie Fleck Teague
Manufacturing and Inventory Control
  Supervisor: Amy Bacus
Composition: Aptara®, Inc.
Cover Design: Scott Moden
Cover Image: © John Foxx/Stockbyte/Thinkstock
Printing and Binding: Edwards Brothers Malloy
Cover Printing: Edwards Brothers Malloy

To order this product, use ISBN: 978-1-284-05702-7

Library of Congress Cataloging-in-Publication Data
Landesman, Linda Young.
  Case studies in public health preparedness and response to disasters / Linda Landesman and Issac Weisfuse.
    p. ; cm.
  Includes bibliographical references and index.
  ISBN 978-1-4496-4519-9 (pbk.)—ISBN 1-4496-4519-4 (pbk.)
  I. Weisfuse, Issac. II. Title.
  [DNLM: 1. Disaster Planning—Case Reports. 2. Disasters—Case Reports. 3. Public Health Administration—Case Reports. WA 295]
  RA645.5
  362.18—dc23
                                                                    2013008471
  6048
Printed in the United States of America
17 16 15 14   10 9 8 7 6 5 4 3 2

Dedication

• • •

Dedicated to Morrie Young and Evelyn Miriam Horn Weisfuse

• • •

Table of Contents

Section

I

Case

1

The Great East Japan Earthquake
of March 11, 2011

Case

9 **Planning for the Republican National Convention 2004: Findings from the New York City Department of Health and Mental Hygiene**
Shadi Chamany. **195**

Case

10 **World Trade Center Attack on September 11, 2001**
Robyn Gershon. **209**

Case

11

Addressing the Mental Well-Being of New Yorkers in the Aftermath of the 9/11 and Bioterror Attacks

Section

III

Foreword

At a time when disaster and catastrophic events are escalating in scale globally with increasingly profound consequences, this book, *Case Studies in Public Health Preparedness and Response to Disasters*, edited by Linda Young Landesman and Isaac Weisfuse, is an exceptional resource. This book is designed to highlight, through a presentation of 16 cases, the responsibility of reducing preventable public health threats to life, the environment, social systems, and the economy. As reported in the Trust for America's Health 2012 Report, *Ready or Not? Protecting the Public's Health From Diseases, Disasters and Bioterrorism*, the public's health must be protected from emergency and disaster events, including extreme weather events such as Superstorm Sandy, man-made events such as threats of bioterrorism, and emerging infections such as the H1N1 pandemic flu. Drs. Landesman and Weisfuse and the case study authors provide a critical resource for public health, health care, and other preparedness partners to better prepare for and respond to all hazard emergencies and events.

Linda Landesman, DrPH, MSW, has once again applied, as she did in authoring the complementary book, *Public Health Management of Disasters: The Practice Guide*, her extensive professional experience as a clinician, administrator, educator, policymaker, and author in the realm of public health, health care, and emergency management to provide the field another essential textbook. Her service as assistant vice president for the New York City Health and Hospitals Corporation honed her leadership in the field of public health practice and administration. Dr. Landesman is a pioneer in clarifying the role of public health leadership and professional practice in multi-sector emergency management. Her work has been pivotal, along with support from the American Public Health Association, Association of Schools of Public Health, and Centers for Disease Control and Prevention (CDC), to create competencies and curriculum for formalized public health training in disaster preparedness and response. Dr. Landesman's research has tracked advancements in the field of public health preparedness, including policy, foundational principles, and roles and responsibilities of the public health workforce in relation to the organization of local and federal emergency management response systems and capabilities. Before the 2001 publication of both the first preparedness curriculum for schools of public health edited by Dr. Landesman and *Public Health Management of Disasters: The Practice Guide,* and now this text, professionals preparing the public health workforce faced a scarcity of adequate teaching resources and curriculum materials.

Isaac Weisfuse, MD, MPH, is an Associate Professor of Clinical Public Health in the Department of Epidemiology at Columbia University's Mailman School of Public Health. He is also Vice President for Science Policy at SIGA Technologies and was formerly a Deputy Commissioner at the New York City Department of Health and Mental Hygiene. His extensive experience and contribution to the field of public health infectious disease epidemiology, public health preparedness, and emergency management is an essential compliment to the editorial role with Dr. Landesman. Dr. Weisfuse's background in infectious disease control includes epidemiology and public health training through the Epidemic Intelligence Service (EIS) of the Centers for Disease Control and specific responsibilities for the control of Sexually Transmitted Diseases, Tuberculosis, HIV, Hepatitis, Vaccine Preventable Diseases, and other communicable diseases, including those caused by bioterrorism. His public health leadership and emergency operations management expertise derives from his oversight of NYC's Public Health Laboratory and direction of his agency's emergency preparedness activities. He served as an agency incident commander for all agency emergency responses from 2000–2012, which included the response to the World Trade Center Disaster, as well as pandemic influenza. Dr. Weisfuse's publications, including his role as a contributing author of *Terrorism and Public Health,* as well as his experience on the faculty of the Mailman School of Public Health at Columbia University, provided insight to this approach to educating both the present and future public health workforce. He was named after his great-grandfather who was a victim in the Ukraine of the mega-disaster 1918 flu pandemic.

This book is a critical must read, not only for those engaged in public health practice, but for all multi-sector response personnel. That is because all emergency and catastrophic events fundamentally pose a threat to the health, safety, and resilience of the populations involved. In *Case Studies in Public Health Preparedness and Response to Disasters,* Drs. Landesman and Weisfuse provide an essential textbook to advance the knowledge, skills, and abilities needed to create a prepared workforce. The text provides 16 competence-based and retrospective scenarios of an array of emergency events, many of which were previously considered unthinkable due to inadequate assumptions about what was possible.

This case study format is both descriptive and explanatory; it presents an analysis of developmental factors critical to the understanding of the context, evolution, and principles underlying each of the events. Each case highlights key features about the emergency and the significance of transformational leadership, command and control operations, management decisions, and strategies used as the events unfolded. This is important to the book's design and purpose because elucidation of causation provides a lens through which inquiry and systemic analysis help to clarify the underlying principles involved. This format also demonstrates the capability and competence required in the broad scale and in unique elements of each case. The cases help to clarify the inherent multi-disciplinary, cross-sector, and inter-organizational nature of public health and emergency management, the profound contributions of competent transactional leadership, and the challenges that leaders face in preparing for normal to unthinkable incidents. The process of studying these cases will enhance our professional competence in systems and critical thinking thereby increasing our capabilities in all phases of emergency preparedness and response.

There is much to learn from the competence-based case studies through analysis of critical issues, challenges, lessons learned, and the application of principles of public health and emergency management. This process is enhanced by the use of discussion questions provided at the end of each case that support inquiry and dialogue about the roles and responsibilities in preparing for escalating public health threats. A substantial resource that grounds the learning experience is the instructor's guide that ties competencies demonstrated in each case study to expected competence for daily performance on the job, as well as crisis driven performance capacity and capability.

This book is being published at a critical moment. Public health threats and diseases are on the rise internationally and in the United States. For the first time in recorded history, as reported in the United Nation's Office for Disaster Risk Reduction's 2012 Report on Natural Disaster in the World, there were 3 consecutive years of economic losses due to weather and climate related disasters that surpassed $100 billion, with the highest in 2011 exceeding $371 billion. Between 2002 and 2011 on average, over 245 thousand individuals were affected and over 106 million deaths were caused by natural disasters. In the United States, 2012 was an historic year for extreme weather, including Superstorm Sandy, Hurricane Isaac, and tornadoes impacting Texas, the Great Plains, the southeast, and the Ohio Valley. Climate change and warmer seasonal extremes are threatening environmental sustainability, economic and civic viability, and increasing loss of life and health impacts on survivors. In addition, with the 2011 CDC Framework for Preventing Infectious Diseases, the CDC warned of the need to control severe and emerging health threats associated with infectious disease outbreaks, the leading cause of death globally. The emergence of new infections, such as the novel 2009 H1N1 influenza virus, risks becoming "hard to control" global pandemics.

These unthinkable events pose serious threats to the United States and global resilience and security, and continue to challenge the adequacy of public health and emergency response system capabilities. The publication of this book, *Case Studies in Public Health Preparedness and Response to Disasters*, is a critical resource at this time to help increase competence and improve performance in the specialized preparation and education of present and future public health, emergency management, and other multi-disciplinary response personnel.

Kate Wright, EdD, MPH
Heartland Center for Public Health Preparedness
Saint Louis University School for Public Health and Social Justice

Preface

WHY THIS BOOK

Effective public health response following disasters received heightened national attention with the establishment of the National Health Security Strategy and the passage of the Pandemic and All Hazards Preparedness Act (PAHPA) of 2006 (reauthorized in 2013). Specialized training is needed to meet the requirement for a prepared workforce because the responsibilities are more complicated than in daily public health practice. Notably, as public health preparedness is still a fledging discipline, few materials are available that illustrate the actual tasks in responding to these specialized needs. Whether preparing an academic course or on-the-job training, faculty often have to hunt for teaching materials in numerous locations and from a variety of sources. This book facilitates that task by bringing together cases that demonstrate the core disciplines of public health practice. In addition, the material in these cases relates across occupations and is easily translatable to all disciplines involved in emergency management.

The 16 cases in this text depict a broad range of public health scenarios likely to be encountered and are instructional in how emergency preparedness happens in the field. The goal of each case is to provide sufficient material so that even those unfamiliar with the events would have a good understanding of the issues and implications and be able to apply the principles of their field to the case. The cases demonstrate the application of competencies established by the Association of Schools of Public Health. By studying these cases, students can build a foundation to understand the principles and practice of both emergency management and public health.

Just as significant is the fact that emergency preparedness and response is a multi-disciplinary undertaking. While demonstrating competencies developed for public health professionals, this collection of cases links the instructional aims of many disciplines because of the cross organizational nature of emergency response. To be effective, health and allied health professionals, emergency managers, first responders, and public administrators must also understand how to respond to emergencies with public health implications. This compilation of cases can be used to better prepare all involved in preparedness because the content is relatable to the breadth of responders.

TYPES OF CASES

Many of the contemporary issues facing emergency management and public health are presented in these cases. The incidents reported are examples of the strategies used to manage major issues encountered during emergencies. Each case reflects the perspective and opinions of the authors, many of whom were directly involved in the events described. Given the range of potential emergencies, the cases in this book are not representative of every possible scenario, but rather how to approach an emergency. Because emergencies require a cross-organizational response, many of the case studies are multi-faceted but can be grouped by key issues.

Three cases explore state level responses. The North Carolina flood following Hurricane Floyd is a personal look by Dennis McBride, then State Health Commissioner, at the challenges of managing an environmental disaster that evolved and deepened. Two cases involving public health laboratories demonstrate the complexity of surveillance and management. Amy Terry, Chris Atchison, and Michael Pentella examine the role of the Iowa state lab in communicating, educating, and managing specimens during a pandemic. In the second study, Chris Mangal, Chris Bean and Scott Becker tell us how science drove policy amid a multi-state investigation of an anthrax case.

The populations considered vulnerable during and following a disaster were broadly defined in the Pandemic and All Hazards Preparedness Act (PAHPA). The story of the Southern California wildfires explores the problems encountered in communicating to culturally and linguistically diverse populations during crisis situations, as told by Nadia Siddiqui, Dennis Andrulis, and Guadalupe Pacheco. Included are the need for community collaboration and coordination with public authorities. The theme of community coordination has a different focus with vulnerable patients at a residential facility in Pennsylvania described by Tamar Klaiman and Sylvia Twersky-Bumgardner.

The Gulf Coast of the United States was still recovering from Hurricane Katrina when the Deepwater Horizon Oil Spill struck in 2010. The long-standing environmental impact of this oil spill caused health problems for humans and wildlife, extensive damage to marine and wildlife habitats, and severely interrupted the way of life. James Diaz explores the scientific controversy and the public-private sector interaction in managing these complex events.

Four cases highlight national coordination, a hallmark in the most complex emergencies. Two focus on the 2001 attacks and subsequent collapse of the towers at the World Trade Center, which reshaped emergency preparedness in the United States. Robyn Gershon tells the behind-the-scenes story of evacuating the towers. Neal Cohen recalls his time as Commissioner of Health during the attacks and his task of meeting the mental health needs of the community in the days and months that followed. When the Republican National Convention was scheduled for New York City less than 3 years later, the Department of Health and Mental Hygiene was on alert. Shadi Chamany writes of the interdisciplinary efforts to prepare for and respond to that high security, national event. Finally, Michael Jhung tells a personal story of conducting national surveillance for pandemic influenza at the Centers for Disease Control and Prevention.

Healthcare systems present a specialized set of concerns. Doris Varlese and Kevin Chason provide a view of the local implementation of state regulations involving multiple stakeholders, including unions. They explore the intersection between law, healthcare delivery, and institutional policy making. Melissa Higdon and Michael Stoto's story about the Martha's Vineyard response to H1N1 portrays the challenges of organizing a system approach to public health preparedness. It explores how a healthcare system intersects with state and federal agencies. Joseph Marcellino relates the massive challenge of evacuating, shuttering, and reopening a 375-bed acute care public hospital within several days before and after a hurricane.

The three international cases span eight years. The most current is the 2012 Japanese earthquake, tsunami, and radiation catastrophe. Eric Noji provides the framework for the Tomodachi international response, which demonstrates the intersection between natural and technological disasters. Given the flooding in the northeastern United States following Superstorm Sandy (2013), the Tomodachi case provides lessons not learned by the Japanese. In Japan, survivors of previous tsunamis warned future generations of the risk by marking stones to document previous record tsunami levels, but future generations disregarded the warnings and built below the markers. Annette Ramírez de Arellano weaves the story of the prolonged events during the 2010 mine collapse in Chile. This multi-disciplinary tale demonstrates this extraordinary international response, and deals with the physical and emotional needs of both victims and families over an extensive period. Finally, Pietro Marghella and Isaac Ashkenazi discuss the healthcare response to a mass casualty terrorism event following the Madrid train bombings in 2004—a case that has new meaning following the Boston marathon bombings in 2013.

USE OF CASES

The cases in this book are based on actual events and provide real-world application of public health and emergency management principles. As a group, they describe what is involved in a public health response beyond what is reported in trade magazines, peer reviewed literature, or the *Morbidity and Mortality Weekly Report*. The cases bring realism to courses with an emphasis on functioning in multi-disciplinary settings. Such cases provide guidance to those who have not encountered these problems before by offering comprehensive information about what happened, how things were managed, and why decisions were made a certain way.

These case studies can be used both in the classroom and in online courses. The content includes a description of the events and an understanding of the issues and challenges, as well as a description of the process for handling these challenges. Each scenario is followed by discussion questions that can be easily incorporated into the classroom setting for an open dialogue between students. Questions are designed to stimulate both a review of the material and foundational principles. In some cases, the answer to a problem or the path to manage it is not evident. Some readers might think of handling the scenario differently. When finding one's own solution, it helps to know what others did in similar circumstances.

The cases are crafted so that they can be taught as a unified course with the theme of preparedness, or as a single session where specific themes are embodied in one case. Given the cross-disciplinary nature of emergency preparedness and response, instructors might want to teach these cases from a cross discipline perspective. Case seminars could be organized through inter-school coordinating committees so that students and practitioners alike are trained with other sectors involved in emergency response—public health, public administration, emergency management, social work and psychology, healthcare professionals, engineering, and others.

Acknowledgments

A book is a labor of love for everyone involved in transforming an idea into reality. Without the patience and dedication of each of the contributors, this casebook would not have been possible. Each case embodies the passion of the professionals who wrote it and we thank them for sharing their important stories.

The idea for this book started with a conversation that Mike Brown and Linda had in the exhibit hall during an APHA annual meeting. Mike's vision and encouragement have been much appreciated throughout the process. We are grateful for the support of our publisher at Jones & Bartlett Learning, Bill Brottmiller. His team—Chloe Falivene, Alyssa Lawrence, Kayla Dos Santos, Maro Gartside, and Sophie Teague—have been a delight to work with. We value their professionalism, their advice, and their hard work in this lengthy process.

The Association of Schools of Public Health (ASPH) has been a leader in preparing the public health workforce to carry out their role during emergencies. The ability to build cases that demonstrate various components of the ASPH competency model has strengthened the collection and will be an important stepping-stone in understanding the lessons related in these stories. Many thanks also go to Elizabeth Weist for her tireless efforts with the Appendix for this book.

In working with the contributors to finalize the cases, I had the pleasure of speaking with Elizabeth Talbot, the chief epidemiologist in the anthrax case, and truly appreciate her taking the time to share details about the investigation that she led.

For many years, Kate Wright has been a nationally recognized champion of preparing a competent workforce for the challenges of public health practice, especially in preparedness. We are honored to have her support for this work.

Finally, the end product is always better because of input from reviewers. We were fortunate to receive valuable feedback from professionals with a broad perspective and their views helped us refine the cases. Much thanks to:

- **Daniel Hahn**
- **Brian P. Pasquale**, *Trappe Fire Co. No. 1*
- **David M. Claborn**

- **Sheila Seed,** *Massachusetts College of Pharmacy and Health Sciences—Worcester/Manchester*
- **Charles C. Lewis,** *College of Health Care Sciences*
- **Elizabeth N. Austin,** *Towson University*
- **Enid Sisskin,** *University of West Florida*
- **Lenore Killam,** *University of Illinois Springfield*
- **Christopher J. Woolverton,** *Center for Public Health Preparedness, Kent State University*
- **Hans Schmalzried,** *Bowling Green State University*

Given the dramatic increase in catastrophic disasters in recent memory, it is crucial that everyone involved in preparedness and response understand the public health issues and work collectively to ensure that public health needs are met. We hope that these cases spur lively discussion and trigger universal preparation.

Linda Young Landesman and Isaac Weisfuse

About the Editors

LINDA YOUNG LANDESMAN, DRPH, MSW

Dr. Landesman has a long and distinguished career in public health working as a clinician, administrator, educator, policy maker, and author. In 2012, Linda retired from her work as the assistant vice president at the Office of Professional Services and Affiliations at the New York City Health and Hospitals Corporation (HHC), a position she held since 1996. At the HHC, she was responsible for over $870 million in workforce contracts between HHC and medical schools and professional medical groups. Linda has been responsible for the oversight, restructuring, negotiation, implementation, monitoring, and evaluation of these affiliation contracts. While at the HHC, Dr. Landesman was recognized for her innovative work when she received an award for business process improvement from the Technology Managers Forum.

Dr. Landesman began her career practicing clinical social work in academic medical centers in Southern California. Linda worked with women with alcoholism, children who had cystic fibrosis and their families, women with high-risk pregnancies, and families whose babies required care in the neonatal intensive care unit. Dr. Landesman was the principal investigator for the first national curriculum on the public health management of disasters, developed through a cooperative agreement with the Association of Schools of Public Health and sponsored by the Centers for Disease Control and Prevention. She also developed national standards for emergency services response.

Dr. Landesman has been appointed and served on numerous committees and community boards, including the Westchester Children's Association; New York City Metro Regional Advisory Committee for the New York State Health Benefit Exchange; School of Public Service Leadership Advisory Council, Capella University; Masters of Public Health Program Community Advisory Board at Long Island University; New York State Regional Advisory Committee for the Health Care Commission for the Twenty-First Century; Commissioners' Advisory Committee, New York City Department of Health and Mental Hygiene; Advisory Committee,

World Trade Center Evacuation Study; WMD Advisory Council, New York City Department of Public Health; Emergency Preparedness Council, New York City Health and Hospitals Corporation; Research Subcommittee, Advisory Group Subcommittee, OEM Subcommittee, Curriculum Subcommittee, and WTC Subcommittee, Center for Public Health Preparedness, Mailman School of Public Health of Columbia University; Violence Prevention Subcommittee, Albert Einstein College of Medicine; Environmental Subcommittee, New York Academy of Medicine; F30 accelerated writing groups and content expert, ASTM; and the Disabled in Disaster Advisory Group, Orange County, California.

Dr. Landesman is a member of the Public Health Association of New York City, New York State Public Health Association, and Herman Biggs Society, and a Fellow at the New York Academy of Medicine. She has edited and/or authored eight books, including the landmark book, *Public Health Management of Disasters: The Practice Guide*, now in its third edition. She has written dozens of journal articles and book chapters. Dr. Landesman earned her BA and MSW degrees from the University of Michigan. She received her DrPH in health policy and management from the Columbia University Mailman School of Public Health. Her doctoral dissertation focused on hospital preparedness for chemical accidents and won the Doctoral Dissertation Award from the Health Services Improvement Fund in 1990. She is currently on faculty of the Public Health Practice Program at the University of Massachusetts—Amherst where she teaches research methods and public health emergency management online.

ISAAC B. WEISFUSE, MD, MPH

Dr. Weisfuse is an associate professor of clinical public health in the Department of Epidemiology at the Mailman School of Public Health at Columbia University and is vice president of science policy for SIGA Technologies. He served in the New York City Department of Health and Mental Hygiene and retired in 2012 after a 24-year career. His last position was deputy commissioner of the Office of Emergency Preparedness and Response, which helps New York City prepare and respond to the health aspect of emergencies.

Dr. Weisfuse trained in internal medicine and served as an epidemic intelligence service officer at the Centers for Disease Control and Prevention (CDC) in the hepatitis branch. He joined the New York City Department of Health and Mental Hygiene (DOHMH) in 1987 as a medical epidemiologist, working on HIV/AIDS issues. During his tenure he was in charge of or supervised a wide variety of programs, including programs for sexually transmitted diseases, HIV, tuberculosis, communicable diseases, lead-poisoning prevention, vital statistics, public health laboratories, emergency management, and immunization.

Dr. Weisfuse twice received awards from DOHMH for his work: the Public Health Achievement Award for work on sexually transmitted diseases, and the Public Health Award for Excellence for his role in the 9/11 response. He was also awarded the Master Teacher Award in Preventive Medicine from the State University of New York at Downstate. He taught infectious disease epidemiology at Columbia University's Mailman School of Public Health for 10 years, wrote numerous articles and book chapters, and mentored seven CDC preventive medicine residents. He served as incident commander for all emergency activations since 2000 including 9/11, the 2003 blackout, inhalational anthrax in a drummer, the Republican National Convention, H1N1 influenza pandemic, and Hurricane Irene, as well as being a liaison to the National Broadcasting Company during the 2001 anthrax attack. He was asked by the CDC to lead their H1N1 vaccine task force, which he did from mid-December 2009 until April 2010. Dr. Weisfuse served on 'Team B,' which provided expert advice to the CDC during the 2009 influenza pandemic. He has extensive experience in countermeasure distribution and evaluation of hospital capacity to respond to large-scale emergencies.

Contributors

Elizabeth Ablah, PhD, MPH
Associate Professor
Department of Preventive Medicine and Public Health
Program Director, Emergency Preparedness
University of Kansas School of Medicine—Wichita
Wichita, Kansas

Dennis Andrulis, PhD, MPH
Senior Research Scientist
Texas Health Institute
Associate Professor
University of Texas School of Public Health
Austin, Texas

Isaac Ashkenazi, MD, MSc, MPA, MNS
Retired Colonel
Israeli Defense Forces
International Expert for Crisis Management & Leadership
Faculty of Health Sciences
Ben-Gurion University of the Negev
Director
Urban Terrorism Preparedness
National Preparedness Leadership Initiative
Harvard University
Boston, Massachusetts

Christopher G. Atchison, MPA
Director
State Hygienic Laboratory
University of Iowa
Coralville, Iowa

Christine L. Bean, PhD, MBA, MT (ASCP)
Laboratory Director
New Hampshire Public Laboratories
Concord, New Hampshire

Scott J. Becker, MS
Executive Director
Association of Public Health Laboratories
Silver Spring, Maryland

Laura A. Biesiadecki, MSPH, CPH
Director
Advanced Practice Centers Program
National Association of City and County Health Officials
Washington, DC

Shadi Chamany, MD, MPH
Director
Clinical and Scientific Affairs Unit
Bureau of Chronic Disease Prevention and Tobacco Control
New York City Department of Health and Mental Hygiene
Queens, New York

Kevin Chason, DO
Director
Emergency Management
The Mount Sinai Hospital
New York, New York

Neal L. Cohen, MD
Associate Provost for Health and Social Welfare
CUNY School of Public Health
Hunter College of the City of New York
New York, New York

James H. Diaz, MD, DrPH, FACPM, FACOEM, FACMT
Professor of Public Health and Preventive Medicine
    and Program Director
Head
Environmental and Occupational Health Sciences
School of Public Health
Professor of Anesthesiology
School of Medicine
Louisiana State University Health Sciences Center
New Orleans, Louisiana

Kristine M. Gebbie, DrPH, RN
Adjunct Professor
Faculty of Health Sciences
Flinders University School of Nursing and Midwivery
Adelaide, Australia

Robyn R. M. Gershon, MHS, PhD
Professor
Department of Epidemiology and Biostatistics

Philip R. Lee Institute for Health Policy Studies
School of Medicine
University of California, San Francisco
San Francisco, California

Audrey R. Gotsch, DrPH, MCHES
Professor
Department of Health Education and Behavioral Sciences
University of Medicine and Dentistry of New Jersey
School of Public Health
Piscataway, New Jersey

Melissa A. Higdon, MPH
Research Assistant
Harvard School of Public Health
Boston, Massachusetts

Michael A. Jhung, MD, MPH
Medical Epidemiologist
Influenza Division
Centers for Disease Control and Prevention
Atlanta, Georgia

C. William Keck, MD, MPH
Professor Emeritus
Department of Family and Community Medicine
Northeast Ohio Medical University
Rootstown, Ohio

Tamar Klaiman, PhD, MPH
Assistant Professor
University of the Sciences
Philadelphia, Pennsylvania

Chris N. Mangal, MPH
Director
Public Health Preparedness and Response
Association of Public Health Laboratories
Silver Spring, Maryland

Joseph A. Marcellino, EMT-P, MPH, FACHE
Director of Emergency Management
Coney Island Hospital
Brooklyn, New York

Pietro D. Marghella, DHSc, MSc, MA, CEM, FACCP
Professorial Lecturer
School of Public Health and Health Services
The George Washington University
Washington, DC
Adjunct Professor
Healthcare Emergency Preparedness Program
Boston University School of Medicine
Boston, Massachusetts

Andrew D. McBride, MD, MPH
Assistant Secretary and Health Director (former)
North Carolina Department of Health and Human Services
Raleigh, North Carolina

John E. McElligott, MPH, CPH
Public Health Policy Analyst
Association of Schools of Public Health
Washington, DC

Eric Noji, MD, MPH
Consulting Physician
Global Health Security
Medical Epidemiologist (retired)
Centers for Disease Control and Prevention
Atlanta, Georgia

Guadalupe Pacheco, MSW
Senior Health Advisor
Office of Minority Health
Office of the Secretary
U.S. Department of Health and Human Services
Rockville, Maryland

Michael Pentella, PhD
Associate Director
State Hygienic Laboratory
University of Iowa
Coralville, Iowa

Annette B. Ramírez de Arellano, DrPH
Independent scholar
Washington, DC

Nadia Siddiqui, MPH
Senior Health Policy Analyst
Texas Health Institute
Austin, Texas

Michael A. Stoto, PhD
Professor of Health Systems Administration and Population Health
Georgetown University
Washington, DC

Amy L. Terry, MS
Management and Administration Fellow
State Hygienic Laboratory
University of Iowa
Coralville, Iowa

Sylvia Twersky-Bumgardner, MPH
Clinical Instructor
Temple University
Department of Public Health
Philadelphia, Pennsylvania

Doris R. Varlese, JD
Varlese Legal and Consulting PLLC
Scarsdale, New York

Elizabeth McGean Weist, MA, MPH, CPH
Director
Special Projects
Association of Schools of Public Health
Washington, DC

Section

I

Natural Events

Case

1

The Great East Japan Earthquake of March 11, 2011

An example of the cascading crisis: earthquake, tsunami, with secondary nuclear reactor damage

Eric K. Noji

BACKGROUND

All disasters have multiple causes; there is never a disaster that has only one cause. On Friday, March 11, 2011, an earthquake that measured between 8.9 and 9.0 on the Richter scale rocked Japan. The epicenter of the earthquake was approximately 43 miles (69 kilometers) east of the Oshika Peninsula of Tohoku. It triggered a 32-foot (10-meter) tsunami that wiped out whole communities and caused explosions at two Japanese nuclear power facilities. The tsunami and subsequent radiation release devastated Japan, killing almost 16,000 people. This earthquake has been named the Tohoku earthquake, or the Great East Japan Earthquake.

Japan's social, technical, administrative, political, legal, healthcare, and economic systems were tested to their limits by the nature, degree, and extent of the socioeconomic impacts of the earthquake and tsunami, as well as by the possibility of a "nightmare nuclear disaster."[1]

THE SCIENCE OF EARTHQUAKES

The earth's outermost layer consists of the crust and upper mantle, known as the lithosphere. The lithosphere is divided into large rigid blocks, or plates, that are floating on semifluid rock. Japan lies approximately 250 miles from where these tectonic plates are colliding at their convergent borders, with one plate being dragged (subducted) beneath the other.[2] Japan, part of the volcanic belt known as the Pacific Ring of Fire, is particularly susceptible to subduction-zone earthquakes. This belt surrounds most of the Pacific Ocean and includes the western part of North and South America. The oceanic crust underlying the Pacific Ocean is spreading, and old crust is being subducted back into the earth's interior along the Ring of Fire. Because the oceanic crust rubs against the continental crust, most of the world's earthquakes happen in this setting.

On the day of the Tohoku earthquake, at 2:46 PM local time, at a point approximately 20 miles (32 kilometers) below sea level and 80 miles (129 kilometers) east of Sendai Japan, there was a slip in part of the subduction zone. The Philippine plate was subducted below the North American plate at an angle of about 15 degrees. This resulted in an earthquake, categorized as "great" on the Richter magnitude scale,[3] that ruptured a fault several hundred miles long, roughly parallel to the east coast of Japan.

THE SCIENCE OF TSUNAMIS

The word *tsunami* comes from the Japanese language and means "giant wave." It is a series of water waves caused by the displacement of a large volume of a body of water, which can be triggered by earthquakes, volcanic eruptions, and the like. The tsunami wavelength is much longer than normal sea waves, with a series of waves that can reach heights of 40 to 50 feet (12 to 15 meters) and be hundreds of miles long in large events.

Not all earthquakes generate a tsunami. To cause a tsunami, the precipitating event must result from an ocean-based earthquake and must also change the level of (raise or lower) the sea floor. If the level of the sea floor does not change, the earthquake will not generate a surface wave. If the level of the sea floor goes up or down, the earthquake generates a large water bulge, or water dimple, over the area where the sea floor has moved. When an earthquake generates a water bulge, the water moves outward in all directions—just like throwing a rock into a pond and watching it ripple. If this wave encounters shallow water, it will slow down and increase in amplitude, just as normal waves do at the shoreline. In other words, the wave will grow. The more shallow the water becomes, the higher the wave will be because all of the wave energy now builds wave height. With heights totaling 10 feet (3 meters) or more, a tsunami wave can overwhelm all low-lying structures when it strikes the coastline.

Following an earthquake, some buildings are already weakened or collapsed. Other buildings may be poorly constructed and are swept away when the waves hit. All of the debris—cars, pieces of buildings, shipping containers, boats, and the like—are carried along with the rushing water, smashing into anything in their path.[4]

How powerful was the tsunami that followed the earthquake in Japan? The tsunami following the Tohoku earthquake was 30 to 132 feet (10 to 40 meters) high. This wave was large and powerful enough to devastate miles of Japan's coast and inland.

THE SCIENCE OF NUCLEAR POWER

The facility producing nuclear power is similar to a coal-fired power plant, except that the heat source is a nuclear fission reaction instead of coal. In both types of plants, you need to make steam. Steam passes through a turbine and the turbine spins a generator, which makes electricity. Nuclear power plants are near bodies of water because they need a method of cooling, and the ocean is a very convenient source of large amounts of cool water.

How Nuclear Radiation Harms People

The type of nuclear radiation typically released from a damaged nuclear power reactor involves gamma radiation. Gamma rays have enough energy to break bonds between the nucleotides within human DNA when they strike them. During normal day-to-day living, our body can repair itself with enzymes that reattach the nucleotides that break loose. However, larger-scale damage overwhelms the repair mechanism, resulting in nucleotides being left out or added, or sections of DNA may be inappropriately joined. This may lead to altered protein synthesis and to the later development of various types of cancer.[5]

Types of Radioactivity Released from Damaged Reactors and Harm Caused

One common form of radioactivity released from damaged reactors is radioactive iodine. The human body then concentrates this radioactive iodine in the thyroid gland as it builds thyroid hormones. This concentration of radioactivity leads to more damage to the thyroid than to other areas of the body. Half of the radioactivity decays in 8 days, so the buildup does not last a long time. However, if a lot of radioactive iodine is released and blown over crops, humans or animals eating those crops will take in the iodine. Administering potassium iodide tablets helps block radioactive uptake.

Following the reactor damage at Chernobyl in 1986, the incidence of thyroid cancer rose up to 10 times in exposed children, the most susceptible group. The World Health Organization has estimated that up to 50,000 cases of thyroid cancer will be directly attributable to the Chernobyl radiation leak.[6] While it was believed that the damaged reactors in Japan would not release the amount of iodine that was released at Chernobyl, people living within several miles of the reactor site were evacuated as a precaution.

JAPAN'S NUCLEAR CONCERNS IMMEDIATELY FOLLOWING THE EARTHQUAKE

The Japanese nuclear power plants have backup generators to run the cooling water pumps when the electricity grid goes down. Those generators worked perfectly after the earthquake, but failed after the tsunami. The plants also had surge walls constructed in the ocean to protect the coastline in the event of a tsunami. However, the surge walls were insufficient because the tsunami was so large.

The tsunami flooded the generators and the backup pumps for the generators. When those backup pumps failed, pressure built up inside the reactors, and hydrogen was produced due to the high temperatures. The high hydrogen concentrations inside the reactors resulted in multiple explosions. On March 15, 2011, 4 days after the earthquake, there was a huge spike in radiation levels following a new explosion and fire at the Fukushima Daiichi plant in Okuma, Japan.

Fortunately, the problems surrounding the nuclear power plant did not result in a true disaster, as the entire plant remained intact following the massive earthquake. In a final measure to avert a crisis, the authorities flooded the problematic reactors with seawater. The effects of this last-ditch effort were twofold: a chance to avoid a nuclear meltdown and the destruction of the reactor. Flooding a plant disables the reactor, and it can never be used again. Although the authorities' goal was to keep enough seawater in the plant to avoid a meltdown, the end result was still uncertain. There were plenty of reasons for concern, and a disaster could have easily developed in the days, weeks, and months following the earthquake.

MEASURES OF EARTHQUAKE PREPAREDNESS

Japan has many measures in place to mitigate the damage caused by earthquakes, which spared the population from a far worse outcome following the Tohoku earthquake.[3] These preparations include the following:

- *Warning people, to minimize loss of life.* When an earthquake occurs, it initially sends out waves that travel through the earth, known as body waves. The fastest of these waves involve compression and are called P-waves or primary waves. Slightly slower waves, known as S-waves or secondary waves, are very destructive because they shake things from side to side. Because there is a time difference in the arrival and detection of the P-waves and the S-waves, once P-waves are detected, a warning system sounds, escalators in Japan are stopped, trains come to a halt, gas main valves are shut off, and people are encouraged to seek protective cover. This warning sound provides as much as a minute of warning time—enough to stop the trains and allow people to protect themselves—before the more destructive secondary waves arrive. This warning system is reinforced with regular drills.

- *Emergency drills.* From a young age, children are taught how to protect themselves if an earthquake occurs so they are prepared to take cover.
- *Emergency rations.* The Japanese people store emergency rations in their homes, enough for a couple of days in the event that they are without food or water for a period of time.
- *Building codes.* Houses and buildings are designed and built to sway with the back-and-forth motion of earthquake waves. The idea is to build things so that if the earthquake is very severe, rather than the building collapsing (as it would if it were made of brick or concrete), it will sway without breaking; if it sways too much, it will deform and bend, but still give people time to get out.

PROTECTION AGAINST TSUNAMIS

Advance warning and vertical evacuation are the keys to surviving a tsunami. Important life-saving principles include the following:

- Monitoring technologies and warning systems
- Knowing where, when, and why a tsunami occurs in order to notify populations to evacuate
- Knowing when to evacuate and where to go before a tsunami wave arrives

Japan has an extensive system of coastal barriers designed to prevent high waves from flooding areas where large populations live. Following the Tohoku earthquake, the resulting waves were higher than the Japanese had expected, and water poured over the barriers. As part of Japan's early warning system, when a big earthquake occurs, officials determine whether it might cause a tsunami. If they think it will, they quickly alert the population. However, people have to then be able to go somewhere safe (e.g., higher ground if they are on land in low-lying areas; out to deeper water if they are in a boat). If the warning time is too short, people will not have time to evacuate to a safer area.

Evacuation for a tsunami is complicated both by the short time between the earthquake and the arrival of the tsunami wave, and by the damage and loss of function to buildings and infrastructure caused by the earthquake and its aftershock sequence (see **Figure 1-1**). For those who choose not to evacuate or are unable to evacuate, the odds for survival are lower. It is nearly impossible to outrun or divert a 32-foot-high, debris-laden, ocean wave that arrives with a high velocity (i.e., 20 miles per hour or faster) and moves rapidly inland, covering 1 mile or more of land.

Figure 1-1

Causes of damage from a tsunami.

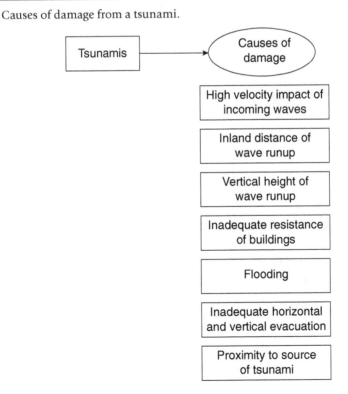

IMPACT OF CULTURE

The Japanese are an amazingly stoic and disciplined people. Japanese culture has always emphasized the importance of *gaman*, which means the ability to endure hardship with patience and without complaint. Furthermore, the Japanese are well aware that they live in a country subject to frequent earthquakes and tsunamis. Each community in Japan has developed emergency procedures to follow in the event of a serious tremor or a tsunami. There are periodic drills for people to practice how best to protect themselves in the event of a major earthquake or tsunami.

The Japanese are known as a people who are among the most disciplined and hard working in the world. They are used to rebuilding their homes and communities, whether after earthquakes, tsunamis, or the dropping of atomic bombs. The great earthquake in the Tokyo area in 1923 claimed the lives of nearly 130,000 people. In Yokohama, 90% of all homes were damaged or destroyed, while 350,000 homes in Tokyo met the same fate, leaving 60% of the city's population homeless. And the Japanese rebuilt. Because of their core values and history, the Japanese people met this unbelievable catastrophe with a calm, disciplined response.

Despite these strengths, there were cultural stumbling blocks that impaired acting decisively after the Tohoku earthquake. Japan's own preliminary investigation showed disagreement and confusion over who should be making the final decisions. As evidenced following the Kobe earthquake in 1995, this was partly cultural. The Japanese decision-making process, which emphasizes group rather than individual decision making, might have been a hindrance for dealing with an emergency situation. It is difficult to quantify, but it seems that making multi-billion-dollar decisions such as these is more difficult to do promptly in the Japanese culture than, for example, in the United States.[7]

EVENTS IN JAPAN

On March 11, 2011, a 9.0 earthquake with an epicenter approximately 80 miles east of Sendai, Japan, generated a tsunami that reached heights of up to 132 feet (40 meters) and, in the Sendai area, traveled up to 6 miles (9 kilometers) inland (see **Figure 1-2**). It was the fourth-largest recorded quake.[8]

The earthquake and tsunami destroyed or damaged over 125,000 buildings, with almost 20,000 individuals killed or injured. In addition, the events caused several nuclear accidents, including the

Figure 1-2

Map of Japan and epicenter of earthquake.

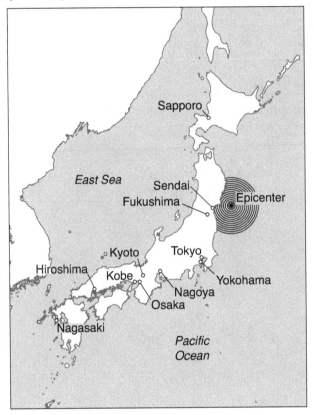

Source: Adapted from http://sertit.u-strasbg.fr/SITE_RMS/2011/05_rms_japan_2011/05_rms_
japan_2011.html

ongoing level 7 meltdowns at the Fukushima nuclear power plant complex. The earthquake and tsunami caused damage to much of Japan's infrastructure—destroying roads and railways, triggering numerous fires, and collapsing a dam. Over 4 million households were left without electricity, and 1.5 million were left without water. The earthquake moved the city of Honshu 1.4 miles to the east and shifted the earth on its axis by approximately 7 inches.[9]

During the initial response, Japan's Meteorological Agency issued earthquake and tsunami warnings. It only took seconds for the earthquake's P- and S-waves to do their damage. The tsunami reached Sendai only 15 minutes following the earthquake. Devastation was widespread. The aftermath included a 300-second shaking from the main shock and hundreds of powerful aftershocks, many at the magnitude of a strong earthquake (see **Figure 1-3**). The magnitude of this earthquake can be compared to the 1994 Northridge, California earthquake or the 1995 Kobe, Japan earthquake, which each had about 10 to 20 seconds of ground shaking. Coupled with the

Figure 1-3

Map showing intensity of shaking from earthquake on March 11, 2011.

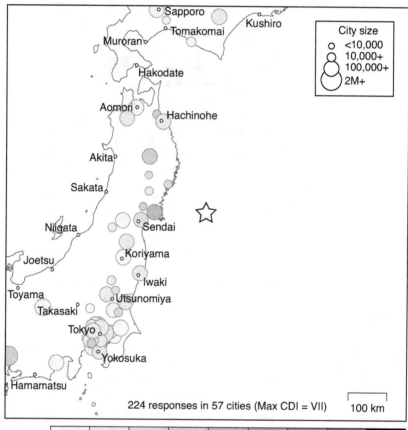

Intensity	I	II–III	IV	V	VI	VII	VII	VII	X+
Shaking	Not felt	Weak	Light	Moderate	Strong	Very strong	Severe	Violent	Extreme
Damage	None	None	None	Very light	Light	Moderate	Moderate/ heavy	Heavy	Very heavy

Source: http://earthquake.usgs.gov/earthquakes/dyfi/events/us/b0001r57/us/index.html

Figure 1-4

Aerial view of damage to Sukuiso, Japan.

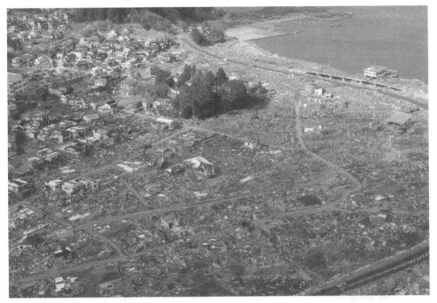

Source: McCord D., U.S. Navy from the National Geophysical Data Center, National Oceanic and Atmospheric Administration, U.S. Department of Commerce. Available at: http://www.ngdc.noaa.gov/.

tsunami, there was widespread damage to homes, buildings, essential facilities, nuclear facilities, and critical lifelines (e.g., transportation infrastructure). Together, the ground shaking and subsequent wave caused major damage in northern Japan (see **Figure 1-4**).

The earthquake and the aftershocks triggered widespread fires, including massive blazes at oil refineries. Four million households were left without electricity. The subways and trains shut down for almost 2 months.[4] This was all complicated by the damage to nuclear power plants, the effects of which continued well into the recovery phase.

Some of the nuclear power plants in the region shut down automatically, leading to an evacuation of several thousand people. All search, rescue, and relief operations; evacuations; and international humanitarian assistance efforts were conducted within the framework of possible significant radiation release and nuclear meltdown resulting from the fires and explosions at the Fukushima Daiichi nuclear facility. A week after the earthquake and tsunami, Japanese efforts focused on the pools used to store spent nuclear fuel, now dry or nearly so, because the consensus was that the dry rods could heat up and spew intense radiation. Subsequently, radioactive contamination of soil, coastal waters, and groundwater was detected, with radiation levels as high as 10,000 times the maximum government standards.

As a result of these developments, the U.S. Centers for Disease Control and Prevention (CDC), Food and Drug Administration (FDA), Environmental Protection Agency (EPA), and Customs and Border Protection (CBP) issued informational updates in the following areas:

- Screening procedures for elevated radiation levels for individuals returning from Japan
- Travel guidance for humanitarian volunteers
- Screening procedures for food products from Japan
- Environmental monitoring/potassium iodide
- Monitoring maritime and air traffic from Japan

RESPONSE

The major goal of the response was containment, especially to prevent a meltdown at the Fukushima nuclear facility, where the normal cooling system was compromised by the earthquake and tsunami. To that end, emergency workers tried helicopter water drops, heavy-duty fire trucks, and water cannons to cool down Japan's dangerously overheated nuclear reactors and spent fuel pools.

Coordination at the National Level

Immediately after the earthquake and tsunami, the Japanese government began implementing its postdisaster response plans in a highly charged environment with the constant threat of the possibility of significant radiation release and a nuclear meltdown. The fires and explosions in the Fukushima Daiichi nuclear facility and radiation levels that were 1,000 times the normal levels created a nightmare disaster response scenario for the government of Japan. Approximately 140,000 people living within a 20-mile radius of the plant were evacuated. The increased risk from radiation stymied search and rescue operations, which were already operating beyond the "golden window" where most lives can be saved, and slowed humanitarian assistance.

Search and rescue operations—an international effort—were organized within hours and continued for months. Approximately 50,000 members of Japan's Self Defense Forces were mobilized immediately to the hardest-hit areas. Tokushu Kyuunan Tai, the search and rescue unit of the Japan Coast Guard, was dispatched to accelerate search and rescue operations. The Japanese Red Cross dispatched 62 response teams within 24 hours of the earthquake.[3] The teams were primarily for medical relief and included 400 personnel—doctors, nurses, and support staff—who worked from mobile medical clinics.

During the crisis, between 300,000 and 350,000 people were evacuated. The tsunami and earthquake knocked out power supplies in addition to those supplied from the Fukushima power plant. Because the tsunami hit in the winter months, there was an immediate need to provide shelter against the cold and a need for clean water. There was difficulty with the evacuations and difficulty finding food, shelter, and especially water for those needing temporary housing (see **Figure 1-5**). Shortages, closed roads, and lack of fuel made it nearly impossible to meet survivors' basic needs. The aid needed most was provided by organizations such as the International Red Cross and the International Medical Corps. They supplied food, clean water, blankets, fuel, and medical supplies.[10]

During the response phase, responders worked to reduce secondary damage such as fires from broken gas lines and water contamination from broken water lines. Teams were organized to inspect the infrastructure of buildings and utilities. Through all of this, first responders were tasked with utilizing critical information to make rapid decisions in order to provide emergency assistance for victims of the earthquake. As soon as people were available to assist the first responders, the assignment of these personnel to various tasks, such as search and rescue teams, began. Utilizing geographic information systems (GIS), grid maps of collapsed buildings were produced. Mapping data allowed emergency responders to identify severely damaged areas; prioritize medical needs; map out areas that would be suitable for the distribution of food, water, and supplies; and locate emergency medical centers and emergency shelters.

International Humanitarian Assistance

In the recovery phase, Japan needed support in managing the incoming offers of assistance and donations. The entire international community participated in these efforts. Humanitarian assistance was pledged or dispatched to Japan by many countries to mitigate the

Figure 1-5

Rescuer following the earthquake/tsunami.

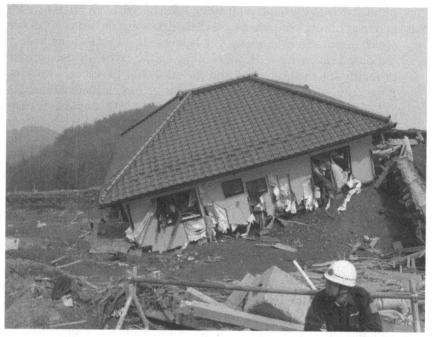

Source: NOAA/NGDC, Patrick Fuller, IFRC.

possibility of thousands of deaths and to provide specialized health care in light of possible waterborne diseases, the effects of high radiation levels, and a possible nuclear meltdown. Japan received offers of assistance from 116 countries and 28 international organizations.[11] Japan requested specific assistance from the United States, United Kingdom, Australia, and New Zealand, in addition to requesting the activation of the International Charter on Space and Major Disasters for readily available use of satellite imagery of affected areas.

The U.S. Agency for International Development deployed search and rescue missions at the request of the Japanese government. Ninety medical teams from Médecins Sans Frontières arrived on Sunday, March 14, and were deployed in the Miyagi prefecture. The USS Ronald Reagan was dispatched immediately to Japan and, at the request of the Japanese government, made helicopters available and began assisting in urgent search and rescue missions. U.S. marines were already stationed in the area and assisted in local search and rescue missions. Teams from Germany and China also arrived that Sunday to assist Japan's recovery.

THE FUTURE

This case study on the Great East Japan Earthquake of March 11, 2011 focused on appropriate leadership knowledge and skills required for effective performance during rapidly changing situations and crisis events within and external to most organizations. Despite best-laid plans, actual crises often require the ability to deal with the unexpected. Crisis events not only require flexibility, but also depend heavily on effective delegation and well-planned resource logistics. Health professionals planning or preparing for deployment to situations that are experiencing rapid change or crisis events need to be especially careful when considering what skills they require.

Long-term recovery from this disaster will take many years. Stakeholders must recognize the difference between meaningful short-term recovery and the ultimate long-term goal. Long-term recovery plans must consider the constraints of the predisaster social situation, including baseline economic characteristics and political conflicts that require the involvement of local people and political structure as the key central stakeholders. Major effort will be needed to rebuild schools, homes, hospitals, and roads; reestablish the sanitation infrastructure; recover from environmental damage; address long-term healthcare needs; and provide preventive care.

The recovery phase may also be an opportunity for the growth of policies that address pre-tsunami preparedness, such as enhancing the art and science of knowing when to evacuate and where to go before a tsunami wave arrives. Key stakeholders in the recovery include the people who are still homeless as a result of the earthquake and tsunami, the Japanese government, the organizations that were supporting Japan's efforts to disseminate aid to those people, and lastly, the international markets who were invested in Japan's economy. While this disaster left thousands of people homeless, it hit one of the most disaster-prepared countries in the world; Japan is very much in control of the recovery efforts and is able to provide the majority of necessary resources.

The fallout from the Fukushima power plant and the disruption to businesses affected stakeholders well beyond Japan's borders. Japan has the third-largest economy in the world. The closing of plants, highways, and ports caused disruption of production and investment flow that was felt worldwide. It was estimated that $287 billion in market capital was wiped out when stocks dropped just after the disaster. Japanese car manufacturers, electronics companies such as Sony, and other global companies such as GlaxoSmithKline all shut down due to the disaster. With so many lives at stake and the stability of the global market at risk, Japan needed to quickly assess the damage and begin the recovery process as efficiently as possible.

Returning to economic strength will require the same degree of national will and sacrifice that produced the "Japanese economic miracle" following the devastation of the Second World War. By 1945, nearly half the surface area of all Japanese cities had been reduced to rubble by American bombers. Still, the Japanese rebuilt their country to become the number two economy in the world only 4 decades later. In the Kobe earthquake of 1995, 5,000 people perished and more than 100,000 were left homeless. Today, Kobe is once again one of the loveliest and most prosperous cities in Japan. The Japanese will rebuild after this latest catastrophe, as they have always done—with calm patience and determination.

DISCUSSION QUESTIONS

1. Which competencies described in the Appendix does this case demonstrate?
2. Describe two examples of ways of mitigating the impact of such events using the following two preparedness strategies:
   • Disaster Vulnerability Assessment
   • Critical Infrastructure Protection of Health Care Delivery Systems
3. What is the difference between a tsunami and a tidal wave?
4. Give three examples of how you would lead when preparations are insufficient and when core values are threatened? How would you respond to unanticipated situations when time is of the essence, and planned approaches do not work?
5. "Reputations are made or lost in crises" is a core observation from almost all major past disasters. Please give three examples in recent history of natural or human-generated disasters where this was a particular outcome.
6. How might the nuclear reactor disaster have been prevented or repaired more quickly with proper planning and tools and more effective media relations? What is the meaning of the word "Tomodachi"?

REFERENCES

1. Fuse A, Yokota HJ. Lessons learned from the Japan earthquake and tsunami, 2011. *Nippon Med Sch.* 2012;79(4):312–315.
2. Sample I. Nuclear scare grows with an orange flash and a violent blast: health concerns as hydrogen explosion at Fukushima 1 nuclear power station injures 11 and destroys containment building. *The Guardian.* March 14, 2011. Available at: http://www.guardian.co.uk/world/2011/mar/14/fukushima-nuclear-power-plant-japan. Accessed March 3, 2013.
3. Aramaki S, Ui Y. Japan. In: Thorpe RS, ed. *Andesites: Orogenic Andesites and Related Rocks.* New York, NY: John Wiley & Sons; 1982:259–292.
4. Maegele M, Gregor S, Yuecei N, et al. One year ago not business as usual: wound management, infection and psychoemotional control during tertiary medical care following the 2004 tsunami disaster in southeast Asia. *Crit Care.* 2006;10:1–9.
5. Ohnishi T. The disaster at Japan's Fukushima Daiichi nuclear power plant after the March 11, 2011 earthquake and tsunami, and the resulting spread of radioisotope contamination. *Radiat Res.* 2012;177(1):1–14.
6. World Health Organization. CHERNOBYL at 25th anniversary: frequently asked questions, April 2011. Available at: http://www.who.int/ionizing_radiation/chernobyl/20110423_FAQs_Chernobyl.pdf. Accessed April 14, 2012.
7. Earthquake Engineering Research Institute. Learning from earthquakes: the March 11, 2011, great east Japan (Tohoku) earthquake and tsunami—societal dimensions. Oakland, CA: EERI; August 2011. Available at: http://www.eqclearinghouse.org/2011-03-11-sendai/files/2011/03/Japan-SocSci-Rpt-hirez-rev.pdf. Accessed March 22, 2013.
8. U.S. Geological Survey website. Japan: seismic hazard map. Available at: http://earthquake.usgs.gov/earthquakes/world/japan/gshap.php. Accessed March 3, 2013.
9. NOAA National Geophysical Data Center, World Data Service for Geophysics. March 11, 2011 Japan earthquake and tsunami. Available at: http://ngdc.noaa.gov/hazard/tsunami/pdf/2011_0311.pdf. Accessed March 2, 2013.
10. Sakai T. What have we learned from Japan's major earthquake, tsunami and nuclear incident? *World Hosp Health Serv.* 2011;47(4):10–12.
11. The U.S. Army Office of the Surgeon General (OTSG). Operation Tomodachi: proceedings of the after action review—medical issues and recommendations. San Antonio, TX; July 29–30, 2011. Available at: http://omicsgroup.org/journals/2167-0374/2167-0374-2-108.php?aid=7466. Accessed March 20, 2013.

2

Southern California Wildfires of 2007: Preparing and Responding to Culturally and Linguistically Diverse Communities

Nadia Siddiqui, Dennis Andrulis, and
Guadalupe Pacheco

BACKGROUND

In late October 2007, 23 wildfires ravaged Southern California, affecting 7 counties, including Riverside, San Diego, Santa Barbara, Ventura, San Bernardino, Orange, and Los Angeles. San Diego County, in particular, suffered its worst wildfires in history—in terms of intensity, size, and impact—disproportionately affecting its large culturally and linguistically diverse populations. Whereas one-third of San Diego County had a Hispanic and Latino population, nearly 70% of the burn area was inhabited by this group, including concentrations of immigrants and migrant farmworkers from Mexico.

Overall, the response of the federal, state, and local governments to the 2007 wildfires was applauded for being swift and coordinated. In addition, San Diego County faced its broadest evacuation effort. However, reports from advocacy and community-based organizations revealed serious barriers to and gaps in communication between federal, state, and local responders and culturally and linguistically diverse populations. Of particular concern were the large numbers of diverse people who did not evacuate—due to fear related to their immigration status, misinformation, or simply no information regarding evacuation—from areas under mandatory evacuation, jeopardizing their safety, health, and lives. Barriers to communication—including language, culture, and mistrust—also manifested in the immediate aftermath during sheltering, response, and relief. These barriers and challenges, in many cases, resulted in delayed response or little to no means of recovery for those facing immediate health concerns, loss of jobs and housing, and other damages.

This case presents the events that unfolded during and immediately following the Southern California wildfires in San Diego County in 2007, focusing on communication between key public health and emergency response players and diverse populations. For the purposes of this case, diverse populations refer to people of different racial, ethnic, cultural, or linguistic heritage. Diverse populations comprise people with limited English proficiency (LEP), recent immigrants from foreign countries (both documented and undocumented), migrant workers, and others from diverse racial, ethnic, or linguistic heritage. Given the concentration of the Hispanic and Latino population in San Diego County, this case primarily presents data, stories, and examples from this ethnic group.

THE SAN DIEGO FIRES

On the morning of October 21, 2007, San Diego County faced what would become the largest firestorm and evacuation in the county's history. At approximately 9:30 AM Pacific standard time, strong Santa Ana winds, sometimes called "Devil's Breath," combined with extreme heat and drought, created the perfect circumstances to ignite the Harris wildfire in the far south of San Diego County, near the U.S.–Mexico border. Shortly thereafter, the Witch Creek Canyon fire began in central San Diego County, and within the following 2 days, another 5 fires were ignited, together ravaging nearly 15% of the county (see **Figure 2-1**). The firestorms resulted in 93 firefighter injuries, 23 civilian injuries,

Figure 2-1
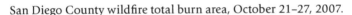

San Diego County wildfire total burn area, October 21–27, 2007.

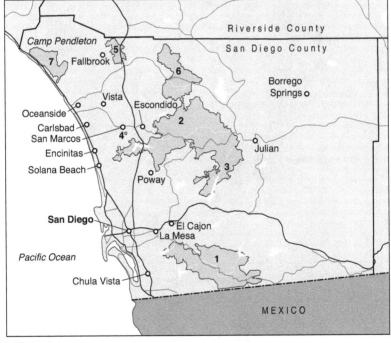

Firestorms

1. Harris Fire	3. McCoy Fire	5. Rice Canyon Fire	7. Horno Fire
2. Witch Creek Fire	4. Coronado Hills Fire	6. Poomacha Fire	

Source: Adapted from Wiegand D, Steckelberg A. *The San Diego Union-Tribune.* Available at: http://weblog.signonsandiego.com/multimedia/utmedia/071030fireweek/.

and 10 civilian deaths. Approximately 1,600 homes and structures were destroyed, and a total of 368,340 acres of land was burned, including rural farmlands. The fires were finally contained on November 9, 2007.[1] San Diego County is the fifth most populated county in the United States and the second most populated in California, with an estimated 3.1 million residents. **Figure 2-2** depicts the concentration of San Diego County's population in relation to the wildfire evacuation areas.

Figure 2-2

Population density and evacuations during San Diego County wildfires, October 21–27, 2007.

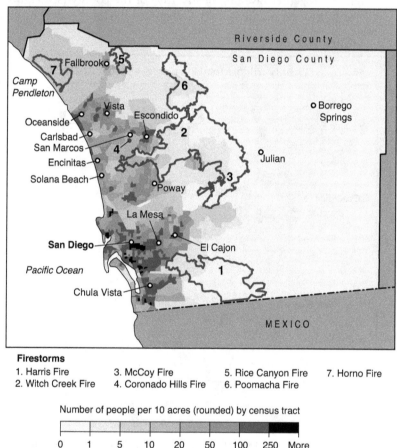

Firestorms

1. Harris Fire	3. McCoy Fire	5. Rice Canyon Fire	7. Horno Fire
2. Witch Creek Fire	4. Coronado Hills Fire	6. Poomacha Fire	

Number of people per 10 acres (rounded) by census tract

0   1   5   10   20   50   100   250   More than 600

Source: Adapted from Wiegand D, Steckelberg A. *The San Diego Union-Tribune.* Available at: http://weblog.signonsandiego.com/multimedia/utmedia/071030fireweek/.

Coinciding with general population growth since 2000, the county has experienced steep increases in racial and ethnic diversity. According to the 2010 U.S. Census, non-whites or racial/ethnic minorities compose more than half of San Diego County's population. Hispanics and Latinos represent the largest ethnic group—one-third of the county, or an estimated 991,348 residents. Approximately 11% of the population is Asian and 5% is black or African American. Whites only comprise 49% of the county's total population.[2] In addition, one-fourth of San Diego County is foreign born, and over one-third speaks a language other than English at home. An estimated 460,503 individuals have LEP or do not speak English very well.[3]

As the dominant ethnic group in the county, Hispanics and Latinos are highly concentrated (65%) in the southwestern region of San Diego County, including southeastern San Diego, National City, Chula Vista, and the border area of San Ysidro—communities not far from where the Harris fires blazed.[4] In recent years, however, the Hispanic and Latino population has grown dramatically in northern San Diego County, particularly with immigration of many indigenous Mexican families, including farmworkers. For example, in Escondido, a city close to the large Witch Creek and Coronado Hills fires, the Hispanic and Latino population grew from representing 23% of the city in 1990 to 39% in 2000 and 49% in 2010.[4] Similarly, other cities and towns near the fires, such as San Marcos and Fallbrook in North San Diego County, have large and growing Hispanic, Latino, and diverse populations (see **Table 2-1** and **Figure 2-3**).

San Diego County also has a unique population of immigrants from southern Mexico—such as the Mixtec community—who neither speak English nor Spanish; rather they communicate in a wide array of indigenous or native languages from their respective regions. Many of these immigrants work on the farms of San Diego.

It is estimated that there are approximately 24,570 immigrant or migrant farmworkers—primarily from Mexico—in San Diego County.[6] While commonly referred to as "migrant" farmworkers, many of these individuals are, in fact, a permanent part of the community given the year-round nature of the agricultural industry. Migrant farmworkers in San Diego contribute to the county's fourth largest and 1.4 billion dollar agricultural industry. However, they face significant socioeconomic and health disparities, along with anti-immigrant sentiments, making them considerably more vulnerable to public health emergency and disaster situations. Estimates indicate that nearly half of the migrant farmworker population is undocumented. In addition, many of these families are of mixed status; in other words, either one or both parents may

Table	
2-1	**Total Population and Percent Hispanic or Latino in Communities with Greatest Impact from the 2007 San Diego Wildfires[5]**

	Total Population	Percent Hispanic or Latino
Witch Creek Fire		
Escondido and San Pasqual River Valley	111,557	32%
Poway	48,104	10%
Ramona, Santa Ysabel, and Mesa Grande	34,505	17%
Rancho Bernardo	17,888	8%
Rancho Santa Fe	8,153	5%
Poomacha Fire		
Pauma Valley, Palomar Mountain, and Valley Center	17,561	23%
Harris Fire		
Jamul/Dulzura	9,092	20%
Taecate/Potrero	1,031	54%
Rice Fire		
Fallbrook/Rainbow	42,562	30%

Source: Data from San Diego Regional Disaster Fund. Community Needs Assessment Report: After-the-Fires Fund. San Diego, CA: The San Diego Foundation; 2007. http://www.sdfoundation.org/CivicLeadership/Programs/SanDiegoRegionalDisasterFund.aspx. Accessed March 21, 2013.

be undocumented, or some or all of their children may be U.S. citizens. Other data show that 70% of migrant farmworkers in California lack health insurance and their median income ranges between $7,500 and $10,000 per year.[6] In certain areas, such as Vista in San Diego County, migrant farmworkers have even lower socioeconomic status. For example, 96% of migrant farmworkers in Vista are uninsured, their median educational attainment generally ranges between fourth and sixth grade, and 87% of dwellings inhabited by this population are shared by two or more households.[6]

The wildfires impacted rural and farm communities, including Escondido, Fallbrook, Ramona, and Valley Center, devastating the livelihood of many migrant farmworkers. Several farmworker

Figure 2-3

Percentage of Hispanic or Latino population by census tract in the San Diego region, 2009.

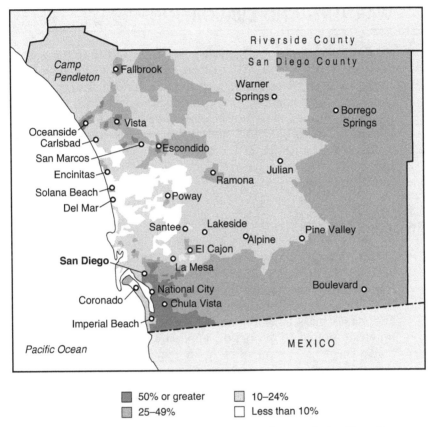

Source: Modified from U.S. Census Bureau, 2010 Decennial Census for San Diego County, California.

families lost their homes, their jobs, or both. In addition, many farmworkers continued to labor in fields during the fires due to lack of warning or information on evacuation procedures by their employers. This posed an imminent threat to the health of farmworkers who were unnecessarily exposed to dangerous air contaminants and faced a disproportionate burden of injuries.[6] For example, the Harris fires resulted in 19 burn victims who were admitted to a burn center, of which 11 were undocumented immigrants.

WARNING AND EVACUATION

As the fires began, the San Diego County Office of Emergency Services (OES), the San Diego County Sheriff's Department, and the City of San Diego issued warning notifications and evacuation orders. Multiple channels of communication were utilized, including computerized mass-notification systems, such as Reverse 911; television, radio, and internet; police and fire rescue sirens and loudspeakers; authorities and responders going door-to-door; and informal, face-to-face interactions, such as with neighbors and family members.[7,8]

Reverse 911 Calls

Designed with funding from the U.S. Department of Homeland Security, the Reverse 911 notification system was created to enhance regional disaster response capabilities.[9] The system uses geospatial mapping to identify residents living in areas vulnerable to a disaster and makes mass telephone calls for warning and evacuation communication. In a 1-hour period, approximately 240,000 calls can be made. The major advantage of this system is that it allows for timely, targeted, and consistent emergency communication to a wide population. In the San Diego wildfires, Reverse 911 was the dominant form of warning communication. Approximately 587,000 homes (almost half the county) were called using Reverse 911.[1] While helpful for directing residents to specific shelters, the system was also useful in pinpointing where to send and locate emergency and public health resources.

Despite the many advantages, however, Reverse 911 did not reach everyone. In fact, based on survey data, one study estimated that only 42% of households in the affected areas actually received a Reverse 911 call.[1] Families without landline telephones or registered cell phones were among those who did not receive a call. For example, many immigrant and farmworker communities in the Pala, Pauma, Rincon, and Rice Canyon regions of North San Diego County did not receive Reverse 911 calls. In addition, given that vital information and instruction was only provided in English, many non-English speaking populations in the region were also not reached through the system.[5]

Television, Radio, and Internet

While television and radio are typically common sources of emergency information in communities, postdisaster survey data revealed that only about 8% of residents affected by the fires received their first warning from these sources. This may be because media often does not provide specific information that is necessary for evacuation and other protective action. For individuals with LEP, this was another source of information that they could not make use of. As one woman stated, "I watched the English channels but it was hopeless because I can hardly understand it."[10] Many Spanish language television stations did not interrupt regular programming to provide information until many days into the fire.[10] In addition, while the Internet was used to obtain follow-up information on the wildfires, it was not a primary source for initial warnings.

Door-to-Door and Face-to-Face Interactions

Approximately 4% of residents received information from authorities who came directly to their homes, and another 4% from informal, face-to-face interactions. Information delivered by family, friends, neighbors, employers, and apartment managers was cited as being effective in ensuring compliance with mandatory and advisory evacuation orders. Door-to-door interactions with authorities, however, had mixed results. In some neighborhoods, such as those in Fallbrook, police officers going door-to-door were the primary source of warning, and many residents did comply. However, in other communities, such as Valley Center, preexisting tensions related to immigration status between authorities and immigrant and migrant families caused this method to be much less successful. This was in large part due to the fact that as border patrol traveled through neighborhoods with mandatory evacuation notices, they were also fulfilling their mandate to detain people who could not establish proper immigration status. This resulted in many immigrants, both documented and undocumented, staying back for fear of being detained or deported. The actions of other law enforcement agencies also reportedly contributed to sentiments of fear and intimidation, including the San Diego Sheriff's Department, San Diego Police Department, and U.S. Marshal.

No Communication

More than one-third of the county's residents reported receiving no warning communication at all.[1] For example, residents in Warner Springs in northeastern San Diego County, homes on Indian reservations, and those located in remote canyon or hillside areas were among the communities that did not receive any form of warning or communication. Individuals and families with LEP, in particular, faced difficulties obtaining information. The following is an account of the lack of communication received by vulnerable diverse communities.

> A young child living on the Indian reservation received no warning of approaching fire until he awoke during the night to a river of fire blazing toward his family's trailer. He quickly awoke his family and his and other families fled to seek safe shelter. Another family waited until the last possible minute to flee in fear of attracting the attention of the border patrol, whose vehicle was parked outside of their home during the fires.[4]

Migrant farmworkers of indigenous Mexican heritage—many of whom are undocumented—were among those physically as well as linguistically hard to reach with warning and evacuation orders.[11] Initially, until several days into the fires, no formal communication was reported to this group from officials. Many, such as the indigenous Mexican population of Mixtec, do not speak or understand English or Spanish, and generally are less likely to trust people unless they are approached speaking their language or dialect.[11]

SHELTER, RESPONSE, AND RELIEF

Approximately 515,000 residents of San Diego County evacuated in response to the warnings and evacuation orders. Forty-five shelters and evacuation centers were set up, including Qualcomm Stadium and Del Mar Fairgrounds, which were the largest, along with schools, civic centers, and churches. The evacuation sites were managed by the American Red Cross, including about 4,000 personnel and 800 volunteers who were supported by 70 Medical Reserve Corps (MRC) volunteers (composed of 48 nurses, 15 physicians, and 1 nurse practitioner, among other health providers) and 25 city emergency response personnel.[8]

Public Health and Emergency Response

A significant component of the successful coordinated response to the wildfires was preexisting relationships between the public health and emergency response systems. Existing ties between the local American Red Cross and the San Diego County Public Health Department facilitated direct communication and ready access to information for both entities. For example, a database of healthcare providers maintained by the county health department and shared with the American Red Cross allowed for timely mobilization of medical resources.[9] As such, the county health department was able to staff each evacuation center run by the American Red Cross with at least one public health nurse who monitored health needs and provided basic first aid.

Cooperation among the county, the Hospital Association of San Diego and Imperial Counties, and the San Diego County Medical Society also facilitated a strong, coordinated response effort.[12] For example, the county's Emergency Medical Services employed its geographic information systems (GIS) mapping capabilities to overlay and identify hospitals, nursing homes, and other healthcare facilities at risk from fires, as well as those that could serve as evacuation centers. Preexisting ties afforded the opportunity to obtain patient census and plan for possible facility evacuations in a timely manner, as well as to continue to monitor bed capacity and other resources.

Recovery Assistance

As the wildfires continued to ravage the region, a number of designated local assistance centers (LACs), later known as Disaster Assistance Centers, were established and served as one-stop shops for disaster relief services and recovery information. These centers assisted evacuees in filing for insurance claims, applying for financial assistance, and obtaining temporary housing.[13] Only some LACs provided on-site translators to assist Spanish-speaking individuals and families.

Language Services

Only modest amounts of on-site interpretation and translation services were provided during sheltering and response. Specifically, 10 American Red Cross teams were deployed from Mexico to assist in interpretation and translation at sheltering grounds.[8] Personnel from the San Diego Immigrant Rights Consortium (SDIRC)—a conglomerate of community, faith, labor, and legal organizations that support and preserve the rights of immigrants through service, advocacy, and education—played a key role in meeting this need. As Andrea Guerrero, chair of SDIRC in 2007, stated in an interview:

> The Immigrant Rights Consortium served as interpreters for FEMA [Federal Emergency Management Agency], Red Cross, city and county officials at the evacuation centers and at other locations. They did not come equipped with the language capacity needed, such as assisting the Spanish-speaking monolingual community. They have not distributed information in Spanish. The Spanish information that is available has been translated by us or by news agencies. It has not been made publicly available by the emergency response agencies themselves.[14]

Despite the language service resources, reports suggest that considerable gaps remained in meeting the need for language interpretation and translation at evacuation and local assistance centers, particularly for the Spanish-speaking monolingual community.

Law Enforcement

City officials invited U.S. Border Patrol to set up a tent at Qualcomm Stadium for informational purposes about the fire locations; however, their presence created immediate apprehension among both documented and undocumented immigrants.[14] The situation was further exacerbated when San Diego city police began checking for identification of evacuees to fulfill their mandate for enforcing the law and ensuring people had proper immigration status. One family, while encouraged by relief workers to take needed supplies back home, was accused of looting and was deported for not having appropriate identification and immigration documentation.[14] This created even more fear and intimidation among both documented and undocumented immigrants, who were reluctant to seek shelter at Qualcomm Stadium and other evacuation centers.

> During the San Diego wildfires in 2007, public employees asked evacuees to produce proof of identity and proof of residence from evacuated areas to enter the emergency shelter, access emergency

food and water, and speak to a relief worker. Families who had escaped the fires with only the clothes on their backs were turned away, despite no legal requirement for proof of identity or residence in order to establish eligibility for emergency shelter and assistance.[15]

Many undocumented immigrants did not seek aid because of lack of trust in rescue workers. In many cases, the risk of deportation was seen as far more dangerous than the fires themselves.[11] In fact, many recent immigrant and farmworker families endured much harsher conditions in attempts to enter the United States. For these individuals, avoiding being caught by U.S. Border Patrol or Immigration and Custom Enforcement agents was seen as a greater priority than escaping the fires.[11,16]

Community Services

Community-based organizations (CBOs), advocacy groups, churches, and other community coalitions played critical roles in filling gaps in response and relief to Hispanic or Latino immigrant and migrant farmworker populations.

Community-Based Organizations

Many Hispanic-serving CBOs were involved in the procurement and distribution of services, while also ensuring cultural sensitivity. The initial response of CBOs and Hispanic-serving agencies was based on the perceived needs of Hispanic and Latino immigrant communities. Their actions included creating ad hoc points of distribution for supplies (e.g., generators, food, water, face masks) that were advertised via local Spanish-language radio and television stations; utilizing community workers to collaborate with farmworker communities to directly deliver evacuation notices and supplies; offering transportation for evacuation; setting up Hispanic and Latino shelters (not run by or associated with the federal or state government); collaborating with the American Red Cross to provide translation; and playing a critical liaison role between government entities and officials and the diverse communities impacted. In essence, these trusted organizations played critical roles in providing needed services to vulnerable individuals and populations.

While many CBOs and Hispanic-serving organizations were swift to mobilize resources and services in response to the wildfires, some experienced serious delays and barriers to their efforts. Given the sheer size and magnitude of the fires, some CBOs and health clinics were closed in the initial days of the disaster either due to evacuation orders or inability of staff to travel to work. In some cases, this resulted in serious delays or lack of access to essential emergency and response services for the most vulnerable immigrant and LEP communities.

Advocacy Organizations

Advocacy-oriented CBOs, such as the American Friends Service Committee (AFSC), were swift to respond to complaints (via phone and radio) of the presence of border patrol and law enforcement and the detainment of undocumented immigrants. The AFSC investigated these complaints at Qualcomm Stadium, where a mass shelter was set up, as well as in other local communities. Other advocates documented the accounts of Hispanics and Latinos, and immigrants.

Churches

Many vulnerable immigrant communities, including those fearful of authorities, turned to faith-based organizations for assistance during the firestorms. A number of churches served as temporary shelters as well as collection and distribution sites for food, clothing, and other emergency supplies. As trusted entities, neighborhood churches particularly played a critical role in serving as liaisons between emergency responders and evacuees of immigrant origin. They were also able to offer information and resources in a more culturally sensitive and linguistically competent manner.

Community Coalitions

As media and advocacy organizations raised the awareness of the disproportionate impact of wildfires on immigrants and migrant farmworkers, coalitions of community organizations were swift to mobilize resources and fill gaps in response and relief for this group. In particular, San Diego's Farmworker CARE (Coordination/ Communication, Advocacy/Access, Research/Resources, Empowerment/ Education) Coalition—a collaboration of several government entities,

CBOs, and local emergency response agencies—came together to address the unmet needs of diverse communities. In particular, the group dispatched community health workers, or *lideres comunitarios*, to provide guidance to immigrants and migrant farmworkers on accessing shelters, clinics, and other relief resources.[17] In addition, the coalition sought to continue to provide services following the initial response and relief phases, particularly to communities reluctant to evacuate or access services and help from mainstream sources. For example, member agencies partnered with the American Red Cross to deliver food directly to community members in affected areas that did not evacuate (rather than holding food at a shelter). These organizations also worked to ensure that families were not forced to move to a shelter, but remained in safe, trusted, and comfortable community-based settings. The coalition also worked with Latino farmworker families to obtain food stamps and secure temporary housing, for example, by helping families file FEMA applications to receive funding for temporary housing.[18]

AFTER ACTION REPORTS AND LESSONS LEARNED

Postdisaster assessments and reports are critical to improving future preparedness, warning, response, and relief efforts. Following the containment of the fires, the city and county of San Diego developed After Action Reports to examine disaster response. These were extensive and conducted relatively swiftly, particularly in comparison to past disasters in California, such as the 2003 wildfires.

While organizations and agencies provided considerable documentation following the wildfires, there was little mention of the challenges, barriers, and treatment of diverse LEP populations. Hispanic-serving organizations were the primary resource for bringing these concerns and problems to the attention of state and local agencies and others. As a result, several reports emerged from these sources highlighting barriers and challenges:

- Inadequate culturally sensitive preparedness education
- Lack of established translation and interpretation services and tools
- Underutilization of ethnic media and native-language radio stations by city and county responders

- Little reassurance and information about issues related to immigrant eligibility for disaster assistance and emergency medical services

In addition, Hispanic- and immigrant-serving organizations acknowledged that they were unaware of local response players and were not involved in local preparedness planning, response, or relief activities. Agencies cited the importance of preexisting relationships and links to response players as critical for providing services to diverse populations.

CONCLUSION

The devastation wrought by the California wildfires affected millions across Southern California, but the burden of its consequences was acutely—and in some ways disproportionately—felt by both documented Hispanic and Latino families and undocumented immigrant families. Language and cultural needs, norms, and customs affecting communication were well served by many community groups, aid organizations, and some officials. But at the same time, other agencies and service-sector agendas sowed mistrust or provided inadequate or late information, whereas lack of coordination at times left these communities and populations on their own to sort through messages and to seek out trusted support sources.

The description of these events, subsequent response, and results in this case reinforce the vulnerability of diverse and, especially, immigrant populations during wildfires. The presence and commitment of critical organizations and other entities highlight the challenges and consequences to ensuring more effective integration of vulnerable individuals into plans and actions. However, it also emphasizes the value of identifying and fully involving community-based and community-accessible assets. These resources—many of which have considerable experience in addressing the needs of these populations—can both perform important functions and serve as an informational reference point for others who are less familiar with how to address such vulnerabilities. Finally, the lessons learned from the wildfires, cast in the context of developing and adapting services, programs, and policies, can work to minimize the ill effects on diverse populations in the future, both for areas in California and across the country.

DISCUSSION QUESTIONS

1. Which competencies described in the Appendix does this case demonstrate?
2. What communication issues do immigrant communities face (especially those with LEP) that can affect their response in emergencies?
3. Which actions do agencies or organizations take that can encumber effective communication and engagement of diverse populations during an emergency?
4. What are ways that organizations can coordinate messages during emergencies?
5. What roles do data and mapping of diverse population characteristics and community assets play in planning for and responding to wildfires and other emergency events?
6. What should be the public health responsibility in coordinating and facilitating communication response to wildfires affecting diverse communities?

REFERENCES

1. Sorensen JH, Sorensen BV, Smith A, Williams Z. *Results of an Investigation of the Effectiveness of Using Reverse Telephone Emergency Warning Systems in the October 2007 San Diego Wildfires, Prepared for the Department of Homeland Security, Federal Emergency Management Agency.* Oak Ridge, TN: Oak Ridge National Laboratory; 2009.
2. U.S. Census Bureau. Profile of general population and housing characteristics: 2010 demographic profile data, San Diego County, California. 2010. Available at: http://factfinder2.census.gov/faces/tableservices/jsf/pages /productview.xhtml?pid=DEC_10_DP_DPDP1&prodType=table
3. U.S. Census Bureau. Selected social characteristics in the United States: 2007–2011 American Community Survey 5-year estimates for San Diego County, California. 2011. Available at: http://factfinder2.census.gov/faces /nav/jsf/pages/searchresults.xhtml?refresh=t#none.
4. Reproduced from Nunez-Alvarez, A., Martinez, K. M., Gastelum, F., & Ramos, A. (2007). *San Diego Firestorm 2007 Report: Fire Impact on Farmworkers & Migrant Communities in North County.* San Marcos, California: National Latino Research Center.
5. San Diego Regional Disaster Fund. *Community Needs Assessment Report: After-the-Fires Fund.* San Diego, CA: The San Diego Foundation; 2007. Available at: http://www.sdfoundation.org/CivicLeadership/Programs/SanDiegoRegional DisasterFund.aspx. Accessed March 21, 2013.

6. Martinez KM, Hoff A, Nunez-Alvarez A. *Coming Out of the Dark: Emergency Preparedness Plan for Farmworker Communities in San Diego County.* San Marcos, CA: National Latino Research Center; 2009.

7. City of San Diego. After action report: October 2007 wildfires. 2007. Available at: http://legacy.utsandiego.com/news/metro/wildfires/images /080225afteraction.pdf. Accessed March 21, 2013.

8. Office of Emergency Services (OES). *2007 San Diego County Firestorms After Action Report.* San Diego, CA: County of San Diego; 2007.

9. Madoori S. 2007 San Diego county wildfire response: a lesson in disaster preparedness and collaboration. *Disaster Med Public Health Prep.* 2008;2(1):15–16.

10. Shore E. Ethnic media cover the fires. *New America Media.* October 25, 2007. Available at: http://news.newamericamedia.org/news/view_article .html?article_id=b5100c5213c00fe7203d2b065baa82ee. Accessed March 21, 2013.

11. Martinez A. The unseen victims of California's wildfires. *New America Media.* October 26, 2007. Available at: http://news.newamericamedia.org /news/view_article.html?article_id=d70074999a1b81cef632488c949812aa. Accessed March 21, 2013.

12. Haynes BE. San Diego county's 2007 wildfires. *San Diego County Medical Society.* 2008. Available at: http://sdcms.org/publications/san-diego-county% E2%80%99s-2007-wildfires. Accessed March 5, 2013.

13. Jenkins JL, Hsu EB, Sauer LM, Hsieh YH, Kirsch TD. Prevalence of unmet health care needs and description of health care–seeking behavior among displaced people after the 2007 california wildfires. *Disaster Med Public Health Prep.* 2009;23(2 suppl):S24–S28. Available at: http://www.jhsph.edu /bin/c/y/DMPHP_Kirsch.pdf. Accessed March 5, 2013.

14. Andrea Guerrero, Chair, San Diego Immigrant Rights Consortium Interview for *Democracy Now,* October 29, 2007.

15. American Civil Liberties Union. Governor signs important disaster victim protection bill. 2008. Available at: http://www.aclu.org/immigrants-rights /governor-signs-important-disaster-victim-protection-bill. Accessed March 5, 2013.

16. American Friends Service Committee. Preliminary report: the state of civil and human rights for migrant communities in San Diego county during the firestorms of October 2007. Available at: http://www.indybay.org /uploads/2007/12/30/afsc-preliminary-report-sd-fires-final.pdf. Accessed March 5, 2013.

17. National Latino Research Center. Farmworker preparedness during San Diego wildfires. *Public Health Practices.* Available at: http://www .publichealthpractices.org/practice/farmworker-preparedness-during -san-diego-wildfires. Accessed March 5, 2013.

18. Benitez S, Rodriguez E. *Averting Disaster: What the California Wildfires Can Teach Us About Reaching Latinos in Times of Crisis.* Washington, DC: National Council of La Raza; 2008.

Case

3

The 1999 North Carolina Floyd Flood

Andrew D. McBride

BACKGROUND

The 1999 flood following Hurricane Floyd was North Carolina's greatest natural disaster. It inundated almost one-quarter of the state's land mass. The unexpected flooding overwhelmed people, homes, towns, farms, utilities, communications, roads, and emergency response capabilities.

Almost the entire eastern coast of the United States—from the greater Miami, Florida, area to Plymouth, Massachusetts—was placed under a hurricane warning for Hurricane Floyd. While warnings for the southeastern Florida coast proved unnecessary, they were still prudent, given the uncertainty of the forecast and the time required to evacuate residents and take other precautions that are indicated in response to a large and potentially severe hurricane.[1]

Much the same as a tornado, a major flood abruptly rearranges the landscape. The flood waters lift cars and trucks and place them atop distant buildings. Skeletons of buildings that manage to survive the deluge often have their foundations irreparably damaged. The contents of homes are as equally ravaged as they would have been in a colossal fire.

The trauma of a major flood shocks its victims. Survivors have ongoing public health needs and may need long-term access to mental health services for cases of posttraumatic stress disorder (PTSD) and depression; they may also permanently lose their jobs and need assistance in acquiring employment and income. Many people are dislodged from their regular healthcare providers for extended periods of time. The flood after Hurricane Floyd triggered a cascade of human, social, and environmental events with long-lasting, if not permanent, health effects. The main distinction between the long-lasting effects and the permanent effects is that permanent effects could, and did, result in communities that were never wholly reestablished after the flood. To meet these challenges, public health professionals will be working long after first responders have hung up their gear.

First responders—firefighters, police, and National Guard personnel—typically operate under a command-and-control structure. In general, first responders are out in the midst of a disaster or crisis, are committed to saving lives, and take significant risks in their rescue efforts. Public health workers are accustomed to working in a more collaborative environment rather than a hierarchal one. Public health responders work in a much longer time frame than first responders.

The role of public health grows in importance in the aftermath of the disaster.

The work of public health professionals can last from hours during the onset of the disaster to days, weeks, months, and even years after initial events have passed. They are involved in ongoing issues such as finding shelter and housing; identifying available medical care (and sometimes providing direct care); and assuring the public's health by inspecting food and water operations, housing, schools, hospitals, and other public facilities. Public health is also expected to protect the people from environmental pollution and safety hazards. The Floyd flood occurred before the September 11, 2001, terrorist attack on the World Trade Center in New York City; however, it provided a valuable lesson in public health preparedness. As such, it may be especially applicable to rural or sparsely populated regions or other areas that have not developed more robust disaster preparedness and emergency response protocols.

Some aspects of disaster preparedness and emergency response must be tailored to a local area or particular state. Eastern North Carolina is rural and agricultural. Factory farming of chicken, turkey, and pork is the economic centerpiece. The flood caused over $2 billion in economic losses to the agriculture industry. The crop, building, and equipment losses were substantial. The loss of animal life was equally remarkable: 2 million chickens, 700,000 turkeys, and over 30,000 hogs.

North Carolina is one of the leading hog-farming states in the country;[2] the farming being a well-entrenched, significant, and highly profitable business. The processes by which the North Carolina hog industry operated (e.g., the use of open-pit lagoons for hog waste) posed well-known and controversial threats to the environment and the public's health.[3] Because it occurred in areas where hog farming was prevalent, the Floyd flood substantially jeopardized the health of both the people of North Carolina and its ecosystem.

North Carolina had a long history of family hog farms that had morphed into industrial hog operations over the previous years. During the 1990s, hog productivity rose more than fourfold to an estimated nine million hogs. During this decade, the political infrastructure had been embroiled in a controversy over the environmental pollution of hog waste. Concentrated animal feeding operations (CAFOs) were utilized by North Carolina's hog-farming industry. In CAFOs, large numbers of animals are kept in a small indoor area, called a parlor. The hog industry relied on archaic methods of animal waste disposal via the use of open cesspools. These pools, called lagoons, can be 3 to 5 acres and 20 feet deep in size. They service the thousands of animals confined in 2 to 5 parlors. When the lagoon becomes full, its content is sprayed as fertilizer on nearby fields.

As the state health director of North Carolina's Department of Public Health (DPH) during the Floyd flood, I had the opportunity to practice my public health skills during a major natural disaster. Wealthy communities were able to prepare, evacuate, and rebuild relatively quickly. Poor communities with inadequate resources in all areas (e.g., transportation, the availability of funds for mitigation efforts, and inadequate insurance for rebuilding) suffered exponentially. This scenario was most vividly repeated in the more recent disaster that occurred in New Orleans after its levee failures.

HURRICANES AND THE FLOYD FLOOD

The state of North Carolina knows hurricanes well. The Outer Banks of North Carolina is one of the most hurricane-vulnerable locations in the country.[4] North Carolina, having experienced over 400 hurricanes since 1851,[5] ranks fourth in the number of hurricanes in the United States, after Texas, Florida, and Louisiana.

On September 2, 1999, Floyd originated as a tropical wave that emerged from western Africa. The storm proceeded westward across the eastern tropical Atlantic, strengthened by the enhanced upper oceanic heat content along its track. (The upper oceanic heat content is the average temperature of the upper levels of the ocean. Scientists use depths ranging from 300 to 750 meters to determine this measurement.)

On September 13, 1999, Floyd was aimed at the central Bahamas when it turned toward the United States. The westward turn marked the beginning of a major strengthening of the storm. Maximum sustained winds increased from 95 knots to 135 knots. Floyd was at the highest intensity at Category 4 on the Saffir-Simpson Hurricane Scale.

From September 13 to 15, for environmental causes not well understood, the intensity of Floyd diminished. As Floyd neared the North Carolina coast, its maximum winds decreased below those experienced during a Category 3 storm. On September 16, downgraded to a Category 2 hurricane, Floyd made landfall near Cape Fear, North Carolina.[1]

In a short period of time, Floyd dumped 15 to 20 inches of rain on portions of eastern North Carolina and Virginia. In Wilmington, North Carolina, the total storm rainfall was record setting: 15 inches in a 24-hour period.[1] As a windstorm, Floyd was categorized as Category 2; however, as a rainstorm, Floyd caused as much destruction as a Category 5, the most destructive hurricane. The Saffir-Simpson Hurricane Wind Scale defines a Category 5 hurricane as:

> Catastrophic damage will occur: A high percentage of framed homes will be destroyed, with total roof failure and wall collapse. Fallen trees and power poles will isolate residential areas. Power outages will last for weeks to possibly months. Most of the area will be uninhabitable for weeks or months.[6]

The ground on North Carolina's coastal plain was already saturated; only weeks before, Hurricane Dennis had drenched the eastern part of the state. The cumulative record rainfall from Hurricanes Dennis and Floyd led to widespread and prolonged flooding in eastern North Carolina. With the exception of the Lumber River Basin, all of the major river basins in eastern North Carolina experienced flooding at the 500-year recurrence interval.[7]

Floyd was not a typical North Carolina hurricane (see **Table 3-1**). "Floyd didn't just swat the beaches. It brought a slow wave of destruction to the coast from inland areas, flooding anything and everything in its way."[8] It caught even the most veteran emergency responders by surprise.

> As the storm approached, Dan Summers, then emergency management director for New Hanover County, sent his wife "inland" to Greenville to be with their son. "That wasn't such a good thing in retrospect," he said. Pitt County wound up being one of the most heavily flooded and damaged areas in the state.[8]

NORTH CAROLINA'S RESPONSE STRUCTURE

To those of us in the Emergency Operations Center (EOC) in Raleigh, the beginning of the Floyd flood was both serious and exciting. On the day before Hurricane Floyd hit, the core emergency operation players were very confident, experienced, and prepared.

No stranger to hurricanes and flooding, the North Carolina Emergency Management System was well organized to respond to

Table	
3-1	**Floyd Facts**[4,9,10]
Storm Surges	15-foot storm surge at Long Beach, Oak Island.
	Other parts of the coast had storm surges around 10 feet.
Tornados and Tornado Warnings	National Weather Service averaged 2 tornado warnings per hour as Floyd approached.
Rainfall	Maximum rainfall between September 14 and 17 was 24.06 inches at Southport.
	Wilmington received more than 19 inches of rain in the same time period.
River Crestings	Tar River crested 22 feet above flood stage in Tarboro.
Wind Gusts	The peak wind gust was 138 mph recorded on a rooftop at Wrightsville Beach.
	Peak gust at Topsail Beach was 123 mph.
Evacuations	Triggered evacuation of 2.6 million people from 5 coastal states.
	Large numbers of evacuees moving north caused problems as Floyd moved up the coast.
	In Charleston, South Carolina, the average evacuee spent 9 hours traveling.
Deaths	57 deaths directly attributable to Floyd: 56 in the United States, 1 in the Grand Bahama Islands. 35 of the 57 occurred in North Carolina.
	Most were drowning deaths in fresh water.
Financial Losses	Total estimated losses in North Carolina were nearly $6 billion in 2008 dollars.
Agriculture Loss	An estimated 21,500 hogs, 753,000 turkeys, 2.1 million chickens, and 619 cattle died.
Housing	Complete destruction of 7,000 homes.
	17,000 homes uninhabitable.
	Another 56,000 homes damaged.
Rescues	1,500 people required rescue.
Utilities	Estimated 500,000 people without power.

Source: Data from East Carolina Regional Engagement Center, Hurricane Floyd, 1999. http://www.ecu.edu/renci/StormsToLife/Floyd/index.html. "Service Assessment. Hurricane Floyd Floods of September 1999." National Oceanic and Atmospheric Administration, National Weather Service. Silver Spring Maryland. http://www.nws.noaa.gov/os/assessments/pdfs/floyd.pdf; and Herring, D. University of North Carolina at Chapel Hill School of Education. LEARN NC "Hurricane Floyd's lasting legacy," http://www.learnnc.org/lp/editions/nchist-recent/6168.

hurricanes.[11] North Carolina has long-established protocols and procedures for dealing with hurricanes, from evacuation to cleanup in the aftermath. At the time, emergency management was housed in the Department of Crime Control and Public Safety (DCC&PS). The entire department was part of the state police structure. The North Carolina DCC&PS, established by state statute in 1977, was revamped in 1997 to adopt the national model for managing emergency operations, known as the incident command system (ICS).[12] The ICS began as a best practice for fighting forest fires and was implemented nationwide as the organizing structure for managing emergencies. At the core of the ICS, a single individual is in charge during an emergency. The incident commander at the state level can be the director of public safety, the head of the state police, or the emergency management director. The incident commander during Floyd was the state's Emergency Preparedness Coordinator. It is not a role that will usually be assumed by public health, as Incident Command Systems create a hierarchical, top-down structure, with a primary focus on managing the first responders. As such, public health was not always integrated into the state's response structure. At the time, it was only when the incident commander needed something from public health professionals that the Department of Health became involved.

ROLE OF PUBLIC HEALTH

Public health personnel, while not embraced during the immediate response to Floyd, were able to branch off and carry out the necessary protective activities in the aftermath of Floyd. There were few conflicts, primarily because the EOC was mainly oriented toward physically getting food and water to victims and searching for survivors. Public health was clearly welcome, but was not the lead nor directly involved in many of the first-responder activities. The public safety staff steered clear of issues surrounding trauma, food safety, and the provision of local public health services. Rather, the DPH focused on a variety of other activities:

- Facilitated continuity of medical care by reuniting people, particularly the elderly, with their providers
- Coordinated care for special needs populations, such as patients with acquired immunodeficiency syndrome and those with end-stage kidney disease
- Recruited area mental health practitioners to work with the victims

- Worked with the Federal Emergency Management Agency (FEMA) on issues regarding trailers that FEMA provided for temporary housing: (1) inspected trailers provided by FEMA, (2) responded to complaints about the siting of the FEMA trailers, (3) investigated concerns that there were environmental risks with the proposed sites, and (4) worked with the FEMA staff to make the trailers as habitable as possible
- Worked with the school system to link displaced children back to their home schools

State Department of Public Health Preparedness Response

In 1998, 1 year before Floyd, the North Carolina DPH established an interdepartmental antiterrorism task force to address the public health response to threats from bioterrorism. In addition to state employees from the DPH, this task force included members representing public safety within the state, the North Carolina Department of Environment and Natural Resources (DENR), and the state's Departments of Transportation and Tourism. This task force focused its activities on preparing for man-made disasters.

Before the Floyd flood, the state DPH played a limited role in most hurricane events. Previous federal funding to help states prepare for public health disasters was directed toward the state's public health laboratory. This public health funding was used to upgrade each state laboratory's capability to identify and handle chemicals and biologic agents during incidents involving terrorism. Although serious disasters had struck North Carolina previously (e.g., the high winds of Hurricane Hugo in September 1989), the state's director of public safety did not call for a major public health presence in hurricane preparedness, nor was there any formal structure within the DPH to respond.

Public Health Response for Floyd

Because Floyd had all the signs of a catastrophic hurricane, it was an "all hands on deck" situation. As health director, I approached North Carolina's secretary of health and human services, Dr. Bruton, and strongly recommended that public health have a formal role in the state's disaster preparedness and response. Dr. Bruton agreed that this was part of our mission and that the DPH clearly had an important role to play before, during, and after the flood. Given the severity of the storm, it would have been unlikely for any department that volunteered to have been denied participation.

With the governor's agreement, the DPH began preparations to deploy staff and establish a public health command center. This public health command center was separate and distinct from the EOC, which was established by the emergency response staff. It was physically located in the state's regular public health building. The establishment of the public health command center involved setting up computers, providing office and clerical supplies, stocking medical supplies for the nurses to use, and providing other supplies to the volunteer environmental staff from nonaffected regions. Skill sets of nonprofessional volunteers were vetted for potential assistance.

THE EMERGENCY OPERATIONS CENTER

Based on weather predictions, the state EOC initiated full operations about 10 days before Hurricane Floyd struck land, and the EOC ceased formal operations about 2 weeks after the major flooding occurred. Within a few days of the start of the flood, the EOC gradually reduced its activity level and its staffing, as the need for first responders decreased. However, the workload for public health personnel accelerated while this formal structure diminished. This was to be expected due to the remaining public health issues that were dealt with through the collaborative activities of public health. After all rescue and initial response work was completed by first responders, health department staff began its work.

The EOC was located in a governmental building in Raleigh, North Carolina. It was a large room that accommodated several hundred people. People were seated in an auditorium arrangement with the participants facing a podium. Each agency within the EOC had several seats behind its own expanded table with several phones. Each seat had a phone line, and the walls were lined with large monitors.

For most of the state-level public health players, it was their first experience working in the EOC. While a relatively small group within the DPH had experience with public health emergencies and first responders during other hurricane situations and environmental contamination events, the majority had never previously been involved in disaster response. Although health department staff lacked a history with the EOC, many had established collegial relationships with the emergency management personnel during the normal course of business. Nonetheless, most, if not all, members of the department intuitively felt that they had an important role to play because of the anticipated magnitude of Floyd. Once the EOC was activated, the entire public health staff appropriately, almost instinctively, blended into the EOC team.

Most did not know what to expect. As it turned out, they were not alone. Practically everyone in the EOC was caught off guard to some degree. Everyone was initially overwhelmed by the unusual confluence of events. Staff, who prepared for a typical strong hurricane, found themselves responding to a catastrophic flood situation. There were three distinct phases to the EOC operation: the prestorm period, the operations phase, and the wind-down phase.

The Prestorm Period

The meteorologist's report received by the EOC in the hours before Floyd made landfall was a curveball. Because the meteorologist informed the EOC staff that Floyd had been downgraded from a Category 4 to a Category 2, our expectations for the disaster were duly decreased. The meteorologist wrapped up his briefing with an opportunity to ask questions. Everyone in the EOC was concerned but confident about the situation given North Carolina's considerable experience responding to previous hurricanes. The room was very quiet. Almost seeming to try and put an end to the silence in the room, a person in the front of the briefing hall asked a question: "Is there going to be much rain associated with this hurricane?" Casually, the meteorologist said that there would be some heavy rains. Even this admonition appeared to be perfunctory; after all, aren't all hurricanes accompanied by "heavy rains"? Forgotten was the old adage among responders that "hurricanes are floods in disguise."[13] Even during the uncontrollable and massive rain and the subsequent flooding that slowly evolved, the emergency workers seemed to maintain their demeanor and confidence.

The Operations Phase

During the phase when the EOC was fully operational, the operations center was full of rumors, unexpected delays, miscommunication, disappointments, great and tragic news, knowledge gaps, and surprises. For approximately 2 weeks we learned of the locations where massive flooding occurred and experienced the relief that wind damage was much less than anticipated. First responders were screaming instructions back and forth, sending rescuers to people who did not need to be rescued or refused to be rescued. Prioritization in the handling of these communications fell to the incident commander. Rather than losing focus or panicking, most disaster responders became more rational as time elapsed. The EOC team was keenly aware of the chaos and danger they would encounter. They were single-minded in protecting and rescuing all people, animals, and property in harm's way. For the veterans of hurricanes, both in the EOC and out in the middle of the action, nothing seemed to surprise them.

When the flooding ended, a frantic call from an eastern North Carolina state legislator seemed to jar many in the EOC. In his county, a poultry farmer had called in a panic after he discovered his chickens had perished in the flood. This was one of the first calls from an elected official to the EOC. I, like the rest of my colleagues, was intensely involved in responding to the range of human problems: flooded roads were jammed with thousands of fleeing cars, sewage treatment plants were overflowing, and businesses, schools, and churches lacked power. People were making countless, frantic calls for help to 911 and to the local and the state EOCs. The EOC responded well to the concern over the dead chickens, though it took us by surprise.

The atmosphere of the EOC was calm and collegial. Rather than panicking, jumping to conclusions, or passing judgment on the information that flowed into the EOC, and without fretting over the "people, first; animals, second" dilemma, the EOC quickly triaged and disposed of problems or situations as they were presented. However, the state legislator's message heralded a change in the direction of the rescue team. *Hurricane Floyd* became *the Floyd Flood*. In the end, animals would play a much larger role in the disaster than I and others had initially imagined.

The Wind-Down Phase

Eventually, the EOC began the wind-down phase. For public health staff, this was a bit of a depressing period, where we left the EOC and returned to the public health command center and continued (and even increased) our efforts to assist the public. Public safety was basically done. Search and rescue was futile. Postmortems of emergency response activities were being held. First responders scheduled well-deserved vacations and time off. Public health, on the other hand, was busy providing counseling to traumatized victims, opening temporary food service facilities in school cafeterias, and arranging for immunizations for children who no longer resided in a community with a functioning local public health department.

ESTABLISHING A PUBLIC HEALTH COMMAND STRUCTURE WITHIN THE EOC

The DPH had three explicit responsibilities: (1) ensure the health of the population, (2) conduct public health surveillance, and (3) coordinate the infusion of federal, state, and local public health assets into the affected localities. The DPH had an implied responsibility to provide direct public health services in the absence or unavailability of such local services.

When drafting new players to a sporting enterprise, many professional or college athletic teams will recruit the best athletes, regardless of the prospect's background in playing a particular position. It was the same with the DPH staff in the command unit. I, along with my top deputies, identified key staff that would be needed in the EOC: the chief epidemiologist, the state environmental health director, the state's local public health coordinator, nursing staff, and social workers. The DPH established a round-the-clock presence in the EOC using senior public health department staff, chosen based on status and ranking within the department, regardless of job title. Most of these personnel were heads of departments. They were chosen for their known skills to communicate and their knowledge of public health practice and principles. In the end, almost all DPH department heads were selected for some duty in the EOC. These senior personnel supervised the key staff. Based on needs as they arose, additional DPH staff who either possessed desired skill sets (e.g., nursing), subject matter expertise (e.g., environmental health), or local knowledge (e.g., former or current residency within an affected area) were also recruited.

The DPH nursing coordinator was particularly effective in coordinating the public health nursing response due to her excellent organizational and communication skills, which were crucial in the chaotic EOC environment. One of her responsibilities involved recruiting skilled public health nurses from counties that had experienced limited or no impact to be deployed to heavily impacted areas.

Off-line DPH meetings of key staff (away from the EOC) were important. We met on an as-needed basis, often with senior public health staff, at the DPH headquarters in Raleigh in our public health command center. For the first 2 weeks or so these meetings were held 7 days a week, but they became less frequent over time. The agenda of the meetings included updates on the latest information. "How are we doing?" sessions were very important, as the staff felt they were literally in untested waters. These meetings functioned as a place to establish command and control of the public health response working within the main EOC. The public health command center worked in cooperation alongside the EOC, but was focused on its public health role, and was especially involved in working with the local public health departments to get them up and running by providing technical expertise and additional staff as needed.

At our first informal public health meeting, it was apparent that we were dealing with an overwhelming situation. The state EOC received feedback that local health departments were faced with a plethora of unmet community needs coupled with uneven capacity to meet those needs. There were reports that a number of municipal water systems had collapsed. There were reports, most of which were not readily confirmed, that people were isolated in a church. In Princeville, bodies from shallow graves floated through town. Prior to the flooding, the Neuse River keeper, Rick Dove, routinely flew over the Neuse River to monitor pollution. He continued that monitoring during the flooding and reported massive overflows of waste water from hog lagoons; however, we were unable to confirm contamination of drinking water from these overflows. While counties such as Rocky Mount were heavily flooded, some had a sound infrastructure for emergency management and were coping better than others. Other heavily impacted counties appeared to have sparse preparedness infrastructure and needed a hands-on approach from the state.

ESTABLISHMENT OF ZONE STRUCTURES

It became clear that the DPH had to get closer to the action in order to meet its responsibilities. During one off-site meeting, we devised our own zone approach to assist the affected counties. Each zone had different needs, and based on available information, the DPH postulated which needs it would address and in which order they would be taken. As best as could be determined by the state EOC and FEMA, 13 of the 66 affected counties were identified as having the most need. For administrative and management purposes, the DPH established 7 zones to cover these 13 counties. Each zone had a zone coordinator who was a senior experienced state DPH employee with a significant background in the practice of local public health. The zone coordinators were assigned to make on-the-ground contact with local health departments in their assigned zone.

Zone coordinators were directed primarily to assist or provide consultative services to the local health director. In instances where their assistance was not directly requested, the zone coordinator served as a liaison between the locality and the state DPH. The roles of the zone coordinators were as diverse as the localities they served. As agents of the DPH, zone coordinators conducted ground-level surveillance and reported back to the DPH. The zone coordinators observed the operation of first aid stations and shelters, local health department activities, and restoration projects, among other activities. One zone coordinator reworked a food service operation to increase safety and minimize the possibility of a foodborne outbreak. In one instance, a zone coordinator served as the interim health director in the absence of a permanent local health director.

The zone coordinators worked with the local health departments and facilitated the distribution of state and federal assets in various ways, such as providing assistance for testing of well water by the state laboratory. Zone coordinators, working with local authorities, helped organize students and faculty to conduct housing assessments. This assessment focused on housing safety and determined if the homes were fit for human habitation or if the residents needed temporary or permanent relocation. The zone coordinators also facilitated the integration of outside public health nurses and environmental health specialists.

In addition, the DPH assigned department staff to be coordinators for the regions. During these meetings, the zone coordinators reported back to the health director and a central director, Steve Cline, the director of the North Carolina DPH environmental health. Sometimes the coordinators were in the field and could not return to Raleigh. When telephone line communication was available, we received on-the-ground updates from the staff.

Health department staff deployed to the field were housed and fed by the local emergency response personnel. The staff in the field did not return to the DPH command center for meetings. They communicated through the local health directors/departments, and this communication was monitored by zone commanders, who attended the DPH command center meetings.

DROWNED HOGS

While not having enough information to make the best informed decisions, the DPH had to set priorities based on the most worthwhile information available. The interconnectivity of humans and animals would become more obvious as the disaster unfolded. The best example of this was the decision on what to do about the drowned hogs. We never anticipated that poultry and livestock issues would become a major focus for the DPH. The goal was to keep any negative outcomes as minimal as possible.

There were about two thousand lagoons in the flood area, and most of the lagoons and the parlors were supposed to have been built above the flood plain. In addition to the dead chickens, which we dealt with before the larger, more complicated hog issue was brought to our attention, local reports about breaches of numerous hog lagoons came into the EOC. The possibility of massive quantities of hog waste deluging flood victims and rescuers posed a huge communicable disease risk in the midst of a catastrophic flood. The breeched hog lagoons were a major threat that was compounded by other communicable disease threats: swamped sewage treatment plants and subsurface sewage systems, along with the disruption of municipal and private water supplies.

Prior to Floyd, there had been other major breakdowns of the hog lagoons that caused considerable contamination of waterways and drinking water. But Floyd promised to be a major assault on the system due to the massive amount of rain. In addition to the loss in livestock, thousands of pets (dogs, cats, birds, and reptiles) were killed or forever lost in the chaos of Floyd.

Breached Hog Lagoons

As many as 10 thousand hogs were kept closely confined in 3 or 4 large metal shed-like buildings, or parlors. Untreated waste from the parlors was channeled into the outdoor lagoons. A typical lagoon is a stagnant pool of recalculated water, open to the ambient air and saturated with excrement and other wastes from the parlors. The lagoons had long posed a risk of communicable disease to nearby communities due to various bacterial and viral pathogens and parasites. In addition, hog waste is known for containing endocrine disruptors, heavy metals, and high nitrate and phosphorus loads. The threat of a public health disease outbreak was of primary concern. In addition, the stench and soil, water, and air pollution were long time public health concerns.

Our starting point for containment of this risk began with the principle that all flood water should be considered polluted. This is well known by all public health personnel who have ever been involved with flooding situations. During his daily helicopter flights over the impacted area, Rick Dove observed conditions on the ground and alerted the DPH. He continued his fly-overs of locations where the lagoons appeared to be at imminent risk of overflowing. The DPH monitored sewage treatment facilities and tested drinking water, looking for evidence of contamination from the lagoons. Fortunately, the state DPH never found that any drinking water was contaminated by any breached lagoons, and we have no evidence that anyone was sickened by these situations.

Dead Hogs

A few days after the flood, several thousand pigs drowned at a remote farm. The incident commander requested direction on disposal of the carcasses. Again, there was no preexisting protocol, and we were faced with making decisions with only the information that we had. We all wrestled with the problem of disposal of the dead hogs. The first option considered was to simply bury the pig carcasses. However, many homes and neighboring farms were on private wells. Burying the carcasses in an area where many people were dependent on a shallow water table for drinking water was too risky. Knowing that the burial of massive numbers of hog carcasses could contaminate the groundwater, we discarded this option. Another option was to ship the carcasses to another location. This was also dismissed, as the logistics would have caused too long of a delay. We would have had to identify a site, identify a contractor to take the carcasses, and arrange for pickup and shipping in the middle of a flooded area with impassable roads, all complicated by the bureaucratic hurdles of arranging for bids, contracts, and the like.

Our best option was cremation, which was quickly adopted as the solution. But even with that solution, there was the risk of air pollution in a part of the state with a high prevalence of asthma. One of the first responders mentioned that shrub-burning machinery would work, and after confirming with the manufacturer of the equipment, we moved ahead. The protocol was initially developed by the emergency staff who first proposed burning the carcasses, primarily because they had located the shrub-burning equipment about 35 miles away. After the burning proposal was presented to the state DPH, we advised the first responders that we would be monitoring the burning. State agriculture and environmental staff finalized the methodology on the spot.

We recognized that we may have to exceed air standards at that point in time, and we wanted an idea of how much we would exceed them. We had no experience with the disposal of hog carcasses by burning utilizing shrub-burning machines. We explored the effects that this procedure would create. We retained an air pollution specialist, Vinny Anaje, from North Carolina State University, to monitor the burning operation. The DPH issued a press release. The media coverage that followed focused on the fate of the pigs and ignored the state's serious work in determining the optimal method of carcass disposal and overseeing and monitoring the actual cremation process.

COMMUNICATING RISK AND PROTECTIVE ACTIONS

It is almost a cliché to state that communication is the first function to be compromised in an emergency. Following Floyd, there was not a lack of communication but rather an abundance of information from the media, official sources, and the public. Rumors spread throughout the state. In our response, we first separated these accounts into serious rumors and scattered rumors. If we received numerous reports of the same rumor from different areas, it was prioritized higher. We responded to confirmed situations by sending formal notices out to local health directors and other involved agencies. We actually ignored some rumors (e.g., snakebites), as we determined that merely addressing the rumor could result in giving it legitimacy. We did not want people worrying about snakebites, when, in fact, there were only unconfirmed rumors of snakebites. With assistance from the Centers for Disease Control and Prevention (CDC) and from experts at the University of North Carolina School of Public Health and North Carolina State University, the DPH crafted a number of messages. Both the director of health and human services and the state health director participated in several press conferences. With this caliber of experts and the cooperation of the press, the DPH was able to effectively communicate with the public to the greatest extent possible. When necessary, press releases were sent out repeatedly.

VOLUNTEERS

From the first day of the disaster, citizen volunteers flocked to eastern North Carolina. Faith-based groups, colleges, and civic groups were eager to help. For many devastated individuals and families, these volunteers were invaluable. While unorganized and lacking a clear set of instructions, volunteers offered immediate support long before official help arrived. Although this support was helpful for the isolated flood victims, the volunteer work was at times counterproductive to recovery efforts. Some homes were prematurely "restored" without proper mold and mildew remediation. Improperly prepared and served food was provided. Unsanitary clothing and toys were donated.

As the response evolved and the number of volunteers grew, these well-meaning groups and individuals began to present problems for the professional staff assigned to field operations. Volunteers who were not part of the formal response did not always bring useful skills or resources. Many had little knowledge about the communities in which they found themselves. The flood had devastated a largely rural and impoverished section of the state. The flooded environments were hazardous, and the numerous volunteers were an added burden to the already overwhelmed first responders and rescuers. The flooded area was littered with walking hazards—broken glass, building debris, and toxic household and industrial materials and containers. Both local and state officials responded by providing the public with educational information and warnings of local environmental hazards. We issued press releases on many subjects, from common-sense advice such as washing hands to more complicated recommendations regarding how to avoid toxic materials.

To be efficient, the response needed manpower that would follow the direction of the incident commander. Zone coordinators and other DPH staff found that college students turned out to be our ideal army. The DPH approached the University of North Carolina School of Public Health and several Historically Black Colleges and Universities (HBCUs) and recruited volunteers with public health skill sets in environmental and community health education. In addition, many students from the HBCUs were residents from the flooded communities and knew people who had been displaced. Several hundred students volunteered. One task of these recruited volunteers was to help victims understand the FEMA assistance program. The students' mission was also to provide needed public health information to disaster victims and to conduct public health needs assessments.

JUST-IN-TIME TRAINING

Just-in-time training, or training right before staff or volunteers are deployed, provided the volunteers with information and instructions to ensure they were skillful in their assigned tasks. This training was performed by senior staff of the DPH and the Department of Environmental and Natural Resources (DENR). Just-in-time training was provided to three groups: (1) the volunteer college students, (2) public health nurses, and (3) local and state professional environmental specialists. The same training was provided to all to build cohesiveness and efficacy in the field. The environmental professionals were recruited to conduct inspections and provide direct services to the affected areas. They were particularly focused on residential health and food, water, and safety concerns. The students quickly adapted to the environment and the people. The disaster victims not only benefited from the information and education provided by the students, but also experienced boosts in morale and hopefulness generated by the students' energy and commitment.

THE ROLE OF THE UNIVERSITY OF NORTH CAROLINA SCHOOL OF PUBLIC HEALTH

Repeated rumors of possible communicable disease and other health risks from the flood spread rapidly. Stories of snakebites and toad-transmitted illnesses arose. The most persistent rumor was that everyone needed protection against tetanus. The DPH was perplexed by the rumors about tetanus immunization. We did not know if it was just a persistent rumor or if it was really needed. After consulting with the CDC, we were advised that concerns over tetanus fell into the rumor category, and we did not set up a tetanus immunization protocol or procedure.

In spite of official communications from the emergency medical and public health agencies, these medical and health rumors persisted. To combat the ongoing rumors about health issues, William Roper, dean of the University of North Carolina School of Public Health (SPH), offered the school's assistance. Along with the staff of the DPH, the faculty and staff of the SPH developed a video teleconference on the public health aspects of the flood. The teleconference was targeted at the local health departments. Utilizing experts, the SPH conducted this interactive teleconference with all of the local health departments. Its purpose was to answer frequently asked questions. Experts in epidemiology, communicable disease, and environmental health presented information on relevant topics such as mold and mildew identification, health effects and remediation, routine adult and child immunizations, and food and water safety. Local public health staff had the opportunity to ask questions of the experts.

Finally, because it was flu season, we also worked with local public health departments to start providing vaccination for influenza. These vaccinations were normally administered by local public health departments anyway, not by the state health department.

CONCLUSION

Directing the public health response during the Floyd flood was one of the most memorable events in my career in public health. Until I was personally on the scene during a flood, I, as many do, discounted the degree of trauma a flood inflicts, along with the amount of damage. It is no less than losing everything in a fire. Like many major disasters in the United States and throughout the world, the poorest communities were the hardest hit. During Floyd, the vast majority of those displaced were African Americans from rural areas with extremely low incomes.

Most of the industrial pork industry is located in the rural areas of eastern North Carolina. Duplin County, predominantly an African American, low-income population, is one of the largest pork growers, with a ratio of about 60 hogs to each resident. Today, North Carolina still has the lagoons. Despite the fear that groundwater and a significant number of wells could have been contaminated and that a serious disease outbreak could have occurred, the industry has not changed and the state has not mandated that it do so. The pork CAFO industry has never solved the problem of what to do with hog waste. The political dilemma is a classic one: residents and public health advocates opposed to the health risks battle the hog industry's economic contributions to the state and the hog industry owners' contributions to the elected politicians. However, the Floyd flood initiated a national discussion of the disposal of livestock carcasses. Since Floyd, much work has been done to establish protocols for the disposal of livestock carcasses during disasters.

On a more positive note, the response of the people of North Carolina was amazing. In Duplin County alone, hundreds of people came from all over to help in any way they could. There were students and carpenters and health aides and seniors. These volunteers did not want to leave, even during the times that we had to tell them that there was not really anything they could do and that staying was dangerous. Also, as a result of the effort with the universities and colleges, many follow-up academic projects were instituted. Most of the projects focused on issues around environmental health, nursing, social services, and community education in the affected communities.

The Floyd flood gave an opportunity for North Carolina leaders to showcase their training and talent at its best. In the public sector, not only did the first responders and public health and safety personnel step forward, but members of the private sector, such as insurance companies, industrial agricultural interests, and various business entities within the counties, also played important roles.

DISCUSSION QUESTIONS

1. Which competencies described in the Appendix does this case demonstrate?
2. During a disaster, those responding may not refer back to the details of their ready-made plans. Why does this happen? Did this happen during the response to Hurricane Floyd? If so, why spend time planning?
3. Initially, a natural or man-made disaster overwhelms resources, environmental checks and balances, and the ability of responders to function fully. What skills or attributes should an individual possess to meet these challenges?
4. What skills or strengths should individuals or organizations possess to respond to a prolonged disaster (weeks or months)?
5. What are the signs that a disaster has entered a recovery phase?
6. What role does mental health services play in disaster response and recovery?
7. What roles do art, philosophy, and religion play in disaster preparedness and response?
8. How does a community handle the loss of human or animal lives?
9. Are you personally (and your family) prepared for a disaster that might strike your community? A community that you may be visiting? What role does self-preparation play in mass disasters?

REFERENCES

1. Pasch RJ, Kimberlain TB, Stewart SR. Preliminary report: Hurricane Floyd, 7–17 September, 1999. *National Hurricane Center.* 1999. Available at: http://www.nhc.noaa.gov/1999floyd.html. Accessed March 7, 2013.

2. Duke University Markets & Management, North Carolina and the Global Economy Capstone Course website. Hog farming. 2004. Available at: http://www.duke.edu/web/mms190/hogfarming/. Accessed March 7, 2013.

3. Center on Globalization, Governance, and Competitiveness. North Carolina in the global economy: hog farming. 2007. Available at: http://www.soc.duke.edu/NC_GlobalEconomy/hog/overview.shtml. Accessed March 7, 2013.

4. U.S. Department of Commerce, National Oceanic and Atmospheric Administration, National Weather Service. Service assessment: Hurricane Floyd floods of September 1999. Available at: http://www.nws.noaa.gov/os/assessments/pdfs/floyd.pdf. Accessed March 22, 2013.

5. Atlantic Oceanographic and Meteorological Laboratory, Hurricane Research Division. Chronological list of all hurricanes which affected the continental United States: 1851–2007. February 2008. Available at: http://www.aoml.noaa.gov/hrd/hurdat/ushurrlist18512007.txt. Accessed March 7, 2013.

6. National Weather Service, National Hurricane Center. Saffir-Simpson hurricane wind scale. 2012. Available at: http://www.nhc.noaa.gov/aboutsshws.php

7. Bales JD, Oblinger CJ, Sallenger AH Jr. Two months of flooding in eastern North Carolina, September–October 1999: hydrologic water-quality, and geologic effects of Hurricanes Dennis, Floyd, and Irene. *Water-Resources Investigations Report 00-4093*. United States Geological Service. 2000. Available at: http://pubs.usgs.gov/wri/wri004093/flooding.html. Accessed March 7, 2013.

8. McGrath G. Ten years later: remembering hurricane Floyd's wave of destruction. University of North Carolina at Chapel Hill School of Education. Available at: http://www.learnnc.org/lp/editions/nchist-recent/6267. Accessed March 7, 2013.

9. East Carolina Regional Engagement Center. Hurricane Floyd, 1999. Available at: http://www.ecu.edu/renci/StormsToLife/Floyd/index.html. Accessed March 22, 2013.

10. Herring D, University of North Carolina at Chapel Hill School of Education. Hurricane Floyd's lasting legacy. *LEARN NC*. Available at: http://www.learnnc.org/lp/editions/nchist-recent/6168. Accessed March 22, 2013.

11. State Climate Office of North Carolina. Overview. Available at: http://www.nc-climate.ncsu.edu/climate/ncclimate.html. Accessed March 7, 2013.

12. North Carolina Department of Public Safety. Emergency management. Available at: https://www.nccrimecontrol.org/index2.cfm?a=000003,000010. Accessed March 7, 2013.

13. Orrock J. Wind, waves, rain and tornadoes. *Carolina Sky Watcher*. 2001;8(2):5. Available at: http://www.erh.noaa.gov/mhx/Newsletter/0601ltr/page5.html. Accessed March 20, 2013.

4

Residential Facilities and Functional Needs: Preparing for and Responding to Emergencies in Pennsylvania

Tamar Klaiman and
Sylvia Twersky-Bumgardner

BACKGROUND

Long-term care facilities that accept Medicare and Medicaid patients are required by federal law to be certified. Such certification includes the requirement that facilities have detailed emergency plans and that they train their employees to carry out the specifics of this plan.[1] This requirement essentially ensures that all long-term care facilities have an emergency plan in place, because the majority of nursing home patients receive Medicare or Medicaid insurance.[2] In addition, the interim final rule for Section 6113 of the Affordable Care Act (ACA), effective March 23, 2011, requires that long-term care facilities follow specific federally regulated notification and planning procedures prior to the closure of any long-term care facility. However, the temporary relocation of residents due to emergency conditions, such as the circumstances in this case, are specifically excluded from these rules under the ACA.[3]

States are responsible for licensing healthcare facilities and therefore for enforcing these federal codes. Often, states may have independent legislation that mirrors federal regulations. In Pennsylvania, long-term care facilities are required to

> have a comprehensive written disaster plan which shall be developed and maintained with the assistance of qualified fire, safety and other appropriate experts. It shall include procedures for prompt transfer of casualties and records, instructions regarding the location and use of alarm systems and signals and firefighting equipment, information regarding methods of containing fire, procedures for notification of appropriate persons and specifications of evacuation routes and procedures. The written plan shall be made available to and reviewed with personnel, and it shall be available at each nursing station and in each department. The plan shall be reviewed periodically to determine its effectiveness.[4]

PROVIDING FOR THOSE WITH FUNCTIONAL NEEDS

Emergency preparedness efforts to address functional needs occur on the national, state, regional, and local levels. The federal government has identified planning for functional needs in an emergency as a priority area, and the equitability and accessibility of emergency efforts are part of civil liberties as defined by federal statute, including the Americans with Disabilities Act.[5] These laws require equal access and nondiscrimination in the provision of emergency planning response and recovery. The Centers for Disease Control and Prevention's (CDC) realization of the National Health Security Strategy includes capabilities to meet functional needs during the entire emergency life cycle. To comply with federal mandates, preparedness activities are required so that individuals with functional needs can receive and act on emergency orders, which will protect them in an emergency situation.

Definition

Individuals with functional needs include those who have physical, medical, sensory, or cognitive disabilities or those who are vulnerable due to cultural, geographic, or socioeconomic factors. People with functional needs can be found in community residences living with or without assistance and in congregate facilities, such as assisted living facilities and group homes.

In addition, those with functional needs include individuals who need assistance with activities of daily living such as bathing, clothing, eating, grooming/personal hygiene, toileting/continence, and mobility. For example, individuals with hearing impairments may have difficulty receiving an evacuation order. There may be language barriers that impede an individual's ability to understand what is required by an emergency order. Individuals who do not have a car may have difficulty evacuating. Furthermore, an individual with mobility impairments may not have access to an adapted vehicle that would enable them to act on an evacuation order.

Acting on an order of evacuation has certain physical, mental, and social requirements. Because of the range and breadth of difficulties that those with functional needs might experience during an emergency, this group of individuals does not require the same assistance nor do they have the same needs. As such, "one-size planning" does not fit all. This is especially true in congregate facilities, where there are often individuals who are neurotypical with impaired mobility living in the same facility as individuals with cognitive impairments but normal mobility.

Many long-term care facilities serve clients with special needs who may need Functional Needs Support Services (FNSS) during an emergency. If these clients require evacuation to an emergency shelter, they are likely to need specialized support. FNSS provide

the assistance that enables individuals to maintain their independence in an emergency shelter for the general population.[6] FNSS
includes the following:

- Reasonable modification to policies, practices, and procedures
- Durable medical equipment (DME)
- Consumable medical supplies (CMS)
- Personal assistance services (PAS)
- Other goods and services as needed

Functional Needs in Pennsylvania

Based on planning guidance from the CDC,[7] the Pennsylvania
Department of Health (DOH) convened a workgroup in 2010 to prepare for the needs of special populations during an emergency. This
workgroup, with representatives from state agencies, nonprofit organizations, and consumer advocates, assisted the state in developing
a strategic action plan. The goal was to delineate action steps that
would strengthen the commonwealth's planning and response for
groups with functional needs during emergencies. The Pennsylvania
DOH also worked actively with the state's Emergency Medical
Services (EMS) council to identify appropriate structures that can be
used as special medical shelters for individuals with functional needs
who live independently in the community. In addition, many counties have established registries of individuals who would have special
needs during an emergency.

At the state level in Pennsylvania, preparing for populations with functional needs is part of the planning process for
the expected surge of needed medical care following an emergency. Medical surge involves rapidly expanding the capacity of
the existing healthcare system when an emergency overwhelms
day-to-day operations due to insufficient medical personnel,
equipment, supplies, and beds. Working with other state agencies,
the Pennsylvania DOH has the lead role in planning for the federally defined Emergency Support Function (ESF),[8] which includes
public health and medical services. The ESF is the mechanism for
coordinating federal assistance in response to a disaster or medical emergency that overwhelms local and state responders. Along
with community and state agency partners, the Pennsylvania DOH
developed the Pennsylvania Modular Emergency Medical System
(PA-MEMS) in order to structure medical-surge efforts in the commonwealth. Within PA-MEMS there is a model for alternate care

sites, including a subacute/chronic care unit that is appropriate for sheltering those with special medical needs.

THE STATE RESPONSE

All emergency response in the United States is local, and when local resources have been exhausted, localities can call on the state for assistance. The state can further engage federal resources by requesting a federal emergency declaration.

Pennsylvania has a system in place to request assistance in the event that the emergency response capacity of a local entity is exceeded. When the county needs additional assistance that a state agency, such as the DOH, can provide, they call upon these resources through the use of an unmet needs request sent to the Pennsylvania Emergency Management Agency (PEMA). This request includes a description of the incident and the goals of the individual mission so that the state can identify the appropriate resources needed. This request protocol was put into place so that counties, the Pennsylvania DOH, and PEMA can assess which assets are available and provide the most appropriate resources to meet the counties' identified needs. The protocol calls for the county to contact the local EMA, who then decides if they can fulfill the request through local resources. If they cannot fulfill the request, it is then passed to the Pennsylvania DOH and PEMA, who review it and, where merited, formally approve the request. PEMA then assigns a mission number and the Pennsylvania DOH identifies and mobilizes resources when they receive the confirmed request from PEMA with a mission assignment number.

In addition, Pennsylvania has teams in place to provide care for medical surge through an emergency resource called a Surge Medical Assistance Response Team (SMART). SMART is a 200-strong volunteer group that typically responds to local events, although it is considered both a state and local asset. SMART owns 3 large tents, with a total capacity of 48 patient beds. One tent is usually configured as an emergency room and the other two as semiprivate patient facilities. The team also has diesel generators to run a heating system, lights, and medical equipment for 60 to 80 hours. Volunteers include emergency medical technicians (EMTs), paramedics, nurses, physicians, and logisticians. The team is a southeastern Pennsylvania (5 counties) regional asset, but is also designated as a State Medical Assistance Team (SMAT), so it also supports an additional 7-county area in Pennsylvania. SMART activates in southeastern Pennsylvania

(SEPA) at the request of a county emergency management agency (EMA). For events outside of the SEPA region, activation is through the Pennsylvania DOH or PEMA. Unlike Disaster Medical Assistance Teams (DMATs)—which are operated under the National Disaster Medical System and under the U.S. Department of Health and Human Services and therefore can be federalized—SMART is supported by state agencies (Pennsylvania southeast regional task force and Pennsylvania DOH), a nonprofit corporation (Healthcare Improvement Foundation), and a local health institution advocacy organization (Delaware Valley Healthcare Council).

EMERGENCY PREPAREDNESS PLANS

Although all residential health facilities are required to have emergency preparedness plans, currently neither state nor federal officials have the resources to evaluate such plans for completeness. While some facilities have extensive emergency preparedness, response, and recovery plans, others plan to call 911 in the event of an emergency. Local community services that are normally available to these facilities, such as 911, may be under considerable strain in a community-wide emergency. Ambulance services will likely be unable to transport individuals unless they are in critical condition. Supplies that are normally delivered on an as-needed basis may be unavailable, and local supplies can be exhausted with residents waiting for replenishment after a disaster or a significant emergency that affects a large region.

Even though emergency plans are required by federal and state regulation, plans developed by long-term care facilities are often underdeveloped and not reinforced with training and resources. Previous disasters, such as Hurricane Katrina, which struck the Gulf Coast in 2005, illustrated how problematic a lack of preparedness can be. There are published reports of 139 Katrina-related deaths in nursing homes in New Orleans, Louisiana, alone.[8] Although Hurricane Katrina is an extreme example, emergencies can impact long-term care facilities at any time, as one facility located in a Philadelphia suburb experienced in May 2011.

IMPACT FROM THE STORM

On a warm spring night in 2011, a torrential downpour hit the Philadelphia area. A long-term care and rehabilitation facility with 112 residents in a suburb of Philadelphia had a dilapidated roof that had not yet been fixed. The downpour caused significant leakage and flooding into the building, so much so that water was coming out of the electrical sockets inside the facility. Alarmed, the facility managers called the fire department, who determined that 9 inches of water had accumulated behind the drop ceiling. The fire department was concerned about the integrity and habitability of the building and called for an evacuation. The storm continued with forecasts for more thunderstorms on the way.

The affected long-term care facility did not have a robust emergency plan. They did not have an independent transportation plan in the event that an evacuation was required, and this necessitated the involvement of local ambulances and a diversion of other local resources to fulfill this need. They also did not have a preexisting relationship with the local emergency management agency.

When the evacuation was announced, local EMS ambulances would be called to transport a small number of patients with significant medical issues to the hospital, including residents on ventilators. Protective shelter, outside of the damaged facility, was needed immediately for the remaining residents and staff. All of the residents were senior citizens, many of whom required medications, regular medical attention, and mobility devices such as wheelchairs. Five residents were bariatric patients, patients who had limitations due to their weight (averaging 500 pounds) and exceeded the working load limit and dimensions of support surfaces such as beds, chairs, wheelchairs, and toilets. Bariatric patients present significant challenges in evacuation emergencies, as special routes of exit may be required. Additionally, many of the residents were nicotine dependent, smoking every few hours. The municipal 911 responders contacted the county EMA to request resources.

EMERGENCY RESPONSE

The ambulance chief in the affected county who responded to the scene had been trained to call upon SMART and asked the county's emergency management agency to coordinate getting SMART to the long-term care facility. The county emergency manager was out of the state on family leave when the emergency call came through. The small staff of the county EMA left in charge was not sure how to coordinate and manage the SMART asset and suggested that the ambulance chief contact the neighboring county's EMA. In addition, there was some concern about the time required to send a request up through the state system, and the ambulance chief decided to activate the resource directly. The chief had an existing relationship with members of SMART, formed through professional interactions and joint exercises. An adjacent county had recently participated in a live exercise with SMART and they contacted SMART directly, rather than following the process for an unmet needs request.

The residents needed a safe and secure environment in which to wait until a more permanent evacuation solution could be determined. With the threat of additional storms and the medical fragility of many of the residents, SMART would be able to provide temporary shelter adequate for patients with special medical needs, as well as sufficient personnel to assist the staff at the long-term care facility. The SMART leaders believed they were assisting with a temporary step in the evacuation. However, SMART did not have the capacity for the number of residents that needed to be moved and cared for.

The neighboring county's EMA provided support for the incident, although command and control always remained with the EMS chief and township fire marshal of the county in which the incident occurred. This is standard incident management protocol.

The SMART team arrived at 3:00 AM, within 30 minutes of receiving the call, initially with 15 SMART volunteers. A total of 30 to 35 SMART volunteers responded to the event and stayed until the incident ended, a little more than 13 hours later. SMART initially focused on shelter and transportation for residents. They provided a safe space under a large tent in the parking lot of the facility where the residents could wait until they could be transferred to a more permanent shelter. SMART divided the tent into three different areas separated by curtains. One area held residents, one area was designated for toileting and was equipped with portable commodes, and one area was used as an administrative center. SMART remained concerned about the threat of high winds and lightening, which could prove dangerous in the tent structure provided.

The long-term care facility housed patients with varying degrees of medical needs. Some patients had physical disabilities, some had cognitive disabilities such as dementia, and some residents were relatively healthy, requiring minimal medical intervention. The facility's nursing staff cared for the patients, triaging those who should be transported to medical facilities, such as the resident who was due for a dialysis treatment. There were a few residents who had medical needs, including ventilator dependency, deemed critical enough to be transferred to the hospital. Those who were transferred to hospitals did not have their medication sent with them because of the need to get all residents out as quickly as possible. Medicare will only pay for a prescription to be filled once, so there were a variety of administrative hurdles that had to be overcome in order to ensure the residents received appropriate medications once they arrived at the hospital. The long-term care facility did not have duplicate patient medical records to send with patients. In order to address this issue, the administrative staff of the nursing home moved the photocopier into the tent and copied all of the patients' charts.

For those residents who did not need hospitalization, the nursing home staff identified appropriate placements. Once facility staff identified an alternate placement, they contacted family members to let them know where their loved one was being transported. Some family members took residents home. This created administrative challenges at the scene in order to avoid having family members wandering around the area, creating potential privacy violations as well as security and safety concerns. Staff had to identify family members as they arrived and arrange for a holding place for them to wait while the resident was brought to them. For residents who could not stay with family, facility staff called other local long-term care facilities to identify open beds. This task was made more difficult by the need to screen beds to match gender, smoking status, level of care needed, and whether the facilities accepted the residents' insurance.

The responding EMS chief worked to identify wheelchair-accessible transportation to move the evacuees from the temporary shelter to identified long-term care facilities. Ambulances could only transport individuals on a stretcher and could not accommodate wheelchairs. Many of the residents had custom-built wheelchairs that allowed for the greatest level of individual mobility, so it was important to transport the residents with their chairs. Only one county-owned, wheelchair-accessible van was available. The EMA called the local school district to ask for assistance, and they provided wheelchair-accessible buses. The school district shared their buses after students were dropped off at school, but requested that the buses be returned to the school district to transport the children home after school. Each bus could only hold two to three wheelchairs at one time.

The transport of the bariatric patients was another challenge. These five residents required special stretchers as well as ambulances with lift capability. Southeastern Pennsylvania only had two ambulances per county that could accommodate bariatric patients. Therefore, to move the five residents, the commander had to call upon all of the units from two counties.

The temporary care of the residents until a bed and transportation could be identified was a joint effort between the SMART team and the facility staff. Because the bed capacity of the tent set up by SMART was less than half of the number needed, all the patients had to remain sitting at some point and everyone was crowded together. The primary needs became toileting and feeding the displaced residents. Toileting activities for the evacuated residents were difficult because there was a lack of privacy for residents that used diapers and the portable toilet facilities were not wheelchair accessible. Eventually, screens were set up to facilitate a semiprivate space for changing diapers and using commodes. SMART members disposed of all waste after the response. It took approximately 10 hours to get all the residents placed and another 3 hours to pack up the tent and equipment the SMART team brought to the response. Although the incident response lasted 13 hours, crowding was gradually relieved as residents were transported to more permanent facilities.

SMART carried Meals Ready to Eat (MREs) as food provisions. This food was inappropriate for the majority of the facility residents, most of whom required specialized nutrition including low sodium diets or diets appropriate for diabetics. The facility had an established relationship with a local restaurant and arranged to have boxed food delivered for the patients while the volunteers ate the MREs. Many of the residents became agitated after being in the tent for so many hours, and staff and volunteers worked to take residents out of the tent for smoke breaks once it had stopped raining. Some residents slept in the tent facilities, while staff and volunteers stayed awake during the entire response.

AFTER ACTION ANALYSIS

The incident described was resolved in a relatively brief period of time—13 hours. The long-term care facility staff evacuated the building safely, and the residents had shelter, food, and medication for many hours after they were ordered to leave the building.

Because there was a safe temporary shelter available to the residents, the staff of the long-term care facility were able to stay with their patients. After the initial transfer of the medically critical patients was completed, staff were fully involved in meeting the needs of the remaining residents. They ensured that the copied medical charts and medications accompanied most of the remaining residents during transfer and that the final shelter destinations met the residents' needs. The preference was not to send residents to hospitals where they would have been exposed to infections and unnecessarily taxed available medical resources. The cost of admitting the residents to a hospital would have been much greater than the cost of setting up a temporary special medical needs shelter until a more permanent solution could be identified.

This was the second time that SMART had been asked to support a local nursing home, although it was the first time they had been asked to provide shelter for nursing home residents. This experience resulted in SMART enhancing their supplies by including wheelchair-accessible portable toilet facilities as part of their assets. Following this incident, they also provided additional outreach and training to local EMAs and hospitals.

Overall, the response to the flood in the long-term care facility went very well; however, this case highlights the need for better planning by long-term care facilities prior to an emergency. It is not enough that they are licensed, but rather such facilities should make sure they have an in-depth emergency response plan for the safety of their residents and staff. Local public health was not involved in the response because the SMART and facility staff did not feel their expertise or services were needed; however, local public health agencies could have supported volunteers and staff to ensure the health and safety of the residents. These issues are often forgotten until the need arises, and by then, it is usually too late.

We gratefully acknowledge the valuable information provided to us by the SMART team leaders and volunteers.

DISCUSSION QUESTIONS

1. Which competencies described in the Appendix does this case demonstrate?
2. What challenges will responders face in evacuating a building filled with residents who have functional needs? What are some of the functional needs that the responders might be likely to encounter?
3. What considerations might the staff have when evacuating the building to ensure the safety of the residents?
4. What might be the response from the residents when they are told they must leave the building?
5. In some disasters, the phone systems may not be operational. How might family members be made aware of where their loved ones have been moved? Often, families spend considerable time investigating appropriate residential facilities. What if a family is unhappy with the placement after the evacuation?

6. In this case there was no larger disaster; school buses, a wheelchair-accessible van, and EMS resources could be used to support the evacuation. What would happen if this was part of a larger, community-wide disaster, such as during a hurricane, that required the use of those resources elsewhere? What if all local residential facilities needed to be evacuated? What can long-term care facilities do to plan for that eventuality? How could county and state EMS contribute?
7. How could the long-term care facility have improved its emergency plans to address the challenges it faced?

REFERENCES

1. Code of federal regulations: disaster and emergency preparedness. 42 CFR §483.75(m). Available at: http://www.hpm.umn.edu/nhregsplus/NH%20Regs%20by%20Topic/Topic%20Administration%20-%20Disaster%20and%20Emergency%20Preparedness.html. Accessed March 13, 2013.
2. Brown LM, Hyer K, Polivka-West L. A comparative study of laws, rules, codes, and other influences on nursing homes' disaster preparedness in the Gulf Coast states. *Behav Sci Law.* 2007;25:655–675.
3. Medicare and Medicaid programs: requirements for long-term care (LTC) facilities: notice of facility closure. *Fed Regist.* 2011;76(34):9503–9512. Available at: http://edocket.access.gpo.gov/2011/pdf/2011-3806.pdf. Accessed March 8, 2013.
4. The Pennsylvania Code. (1975). Chapter 209. Fire protection and safety programs for long-term care nursing facilities. Retrieved from http://www.pacode.com/secure/data/028/chapter209/chap209toc.html on September 7, 2011.
5. Department of Justice. Emergency management under title II of the ADA. In: ADA Best Practices Tool Kit for State and Local Governments. October 26, 2009. Available at: http://www.ada.gov/pcatoolkit/chap7emergencymgmt.htm. Accessed March 8, 2013.
6. FEMA. Guidance on planning for integration of functional needs support services in general population shelters. Available at: http://www.fema.gov/pdf/about/odic/fnss_guidance.pdf. Published November 2010. Accessed March 8, 2013.
7. Centers for Disease Control and Prevention. Public health preparedness capabilities: national standards for state and local planning. March 15, 2012. Available at: http://www.cdc.gov/phpr/capabilities/. Accessed March 8, 2013.
8. Khanna R. Katrina's toll on the sick, elderly emerges. *Houston Chronicle.* November 27, 2005. Available at: http://www.chron.com/news/nation-world/article/Katrina-s-toll-on-the-sick-elderly-emerges-1939354.php. Accessed March 8, 2013.

5 Hurricane Irene: Evacuation of Coney Island Hospital

Joseph A. Marcellino

INTRODUCTION

In the past 3 decades there have been a number of disasters that have impacted healthcare systems. In recent years, however, serious consideration has also been given to other significant events, including terrorist incidents, hazardous material spills, fires, and utilities and systems failures. Hurricanes and floods have always been major threats for the United States. Natural disasters, such as hurricanes and floods, have significantly impacted the operations of healthcare organizations, particularly hospitals and nursing homes. Some of these events have led to evacuations of healthcare facilities. As the evacuation of a healthcare facility is a difficult and complex process, it has always been considered an action of last resort, with the focus on safeguarding the health and lives of patients and residents.

The evacuation of a healthcare facility requires a coordinated systematic approach. There are a number of issues that need to be addressed prior to and during the evacuation process. The complexity of moving patients, staff, visitors, equipment, supplies, medical records, and other essential materials is daunting and requires planning, preparedness, and response based upon the nature of the incident. The implications of facility evacuations are much wider and far reaching than the immediate functional loss of healthcare services. These events also create social and financial burdens spanning across all sectors of the community.

The purpose of this case study is to review a hurricane event that recently impacted the East Coast. This event was Hurricane Irene, and I will share lessons learned from the evacuation of a hospital in New York City, from the preplanning stage, to the operational phase, and finally to the recovery.

CONEY ISLAND HOSPITAL

The 2011 "visit" of Hurricane Irene to the East Coast brought with it the reality that hospital and nursing home evacuations are no longer relegated to our brethren in the states along the Gulf Coast. Several facilities located in the New York City metropolitan area were evacuated, including Coney Island Hospital located in Brooklyn, New York.

Those involved were able to successfully evacuate, shutter, and reopen a major teaching hospital in a timely, effective, and efficient manner. The hospital safely evacuated 280 patients in less than a 9-hour time frame, shuttered the hospital in less than 16 hours postevacuation, and was able to reopen and accept patients 24 hours after the storm passed.

BACKGROUND

The evacuation of multiple healthcare facilities is a large task with many moving pieces. As numerous agencies and organizations are involved, it is imperative that each unit fulfills its specific role and responsibility to ensure a successful city-wide evacuation. In order to do this, some agencies and organizations give up some control while other agencies take on additional responsibilities. With a task of this magnitude, it is essential that there is a unified evacuation where one entity has the majority of control.

In New York City, the roles and responsibilities of the Office of Emergency Management (OEM) are clearly specified and include planning and preparedness for critical emergencies that may happen in the city. There is a wide range of possible emergency events that can impact the city, encompassing those with public health implications to events involving transportation and Emergency Medical Services (EMS). The planning and preparedness division of the OEM reviews all potential emergencies and formulates a response. The OEM has developed a monitoring system known as "watch command," which is maintained 24 hours a day and interacts with all of the major city agencies and other public and private enterprises. The watch command system monitors all the emergency service frequencies in New York City, makes a situational assessment, and facilitates a possible escalation when they determine that a city-wide emergency exists. When an emergency occurs, one of the OEM's critical responsibilities is to coordinate the city-wide response involving multiple agencies, both public and private.

The OEM includes teams of professionals, such as emergency responders, interagency coordinators, logistics teams, incident command teams, information mapping teams, and many other highly specialized individuals, to help support emergency management operations and responses. The OEM reports directly to the mayor and has the critical responsibility of defining and activating emergency action plans, including the coordination of local and mass evacuations in the city of New York.

To ensure and facilitate an appropriate response to a possible evacuation, specific evacuation plans help guide the actions of the city and multiple agencies. These plans outline the responsibilities and actions that need to be performed by individual agencies, healthcare facilities, and other partner organizations so that there is careful coordination during an evacuation involving several healthcare facilities.

STORM TRACKING AND NOTIFICATION

The watch command division of New York City's OEM works jointly with the National Weather Service to monitor weather patterns and the potential of weather emergencies for the city and then OEM develops contingency plans to address the events. For instance, a hurricane event will be identified by its hazards, or potentially damaging events. These hazards include rip currents, high surf, high seas, and battering waves. In addition to these hazards, high winds will be anticipated with a potential for tornados and storm-surge situations, including significant rain and flooding. The definition of *storm surge* is the abnormal rise of water caused by the wind and pressure forces of a hurricane. It is interesting to note that throughout history this has been the greatest hazard and cause of fatalities from hurricanes, although this is changing. Additional hazards, including inland flooding caused by excessive rainfall, are likely when tropical storms make landfall, especially where there are preexisting complications. The forward speed of the storm also plays a significant role in the amount of rainfall in a given area.

The city also identifies and utilizes data from the National Oceanic and Atmospheric Administration, including forecast modeling. This computer modeling describes zones known as SLOSH—sea, lake, and overland surges from hurricanes—and calculates the potential levels that water may rise both at the coast and inland. These models guide governmental agencies in the development of regional evacuation plans.

The OEM for the city of New York has created hurricane evacuation zones. These zones coincide with the strength and category of a hurricane, following the national standards, which measure hurricane intensity (i.e., Category 1 to Category 5). New York City has the probability of experiencing a significant coastal storm event. This is due to its demographics, topography, and location in relation to the Atlantic Ocean. Due to the city's topography, its harbor and surrounding coastal areas in Long Island and New Jersey become a funnel through which severe weather events can impact New York City—commonly called the New York blight.

Hurricane evacuation zones for the city fall into three categories. Hurricane evacuation zone A, also classified as a Category 1 hurricane, requires 275,000 people to evacuate. In a Category 2 hurricane, also known as hurricane evacuation zone B, the estimated number of evacuees would be approximately 955,000. A Category 3 or Category 4 hurricane is classified as hurricane evacuation zone C. This impacted area would force approximately 2,400,000 individuals to be evacuated.

DECISION MAKING: EVACUATIONS

The authority for making decisions for New York City is rooted with the mayor. The office of the mayor has emergency powers that include recommending and ordering a cessation of nonessential services. The mayor has the authority to open shelters for a *voluntary* evacuation when indicated. If the conditions of the emergency change, the mayor may *recommend* an evacuation. If the conditions worsen, the mayor has the executive emergency powers to *order and mandate* an evacuation. Organizations, businesses, and individuals located in any of the SLOSH zones could be directed to evacuate. Hospitals are also required to follow the executive orders of the mayor. The New York City Department of Health (DOH) and New York State Department of Health (State DOH) support and abide by the mayor's executive order.

As the emergency intensifies, the OEM will activate the city's Emergency Operation Center (EOC). The EOC is composed of numerous local, city, state, and federal agencies that work together to support an emergency operation. In addition to these various agencies, federal guidelines require emergency management agencies to receive additional help through what is known as *emergency support functions*. These emergency support functions are composed of groups that provide specified services in response to an emergency. These functions consist of utilities (e.g., electrical, sewer, water), security (e.g., city and state police, FBI, homeland security), and health and medical emergency support (e.g., city and state DOH, health agencies, and hospital associations). The EOC also supports and receives aid from public and private agencies such as the banking industry, Red Cross, home-care agencies, schools, and transportation groups in an emergency.

During a major city-wide event such as an evacuation, the OEM will also activate an evacuation support center. The OEM, together with the DOH and state DOH, the Health and Hospital Corporation of New York City (HHC), and the Greater New York Hospital Association (GNYHA), evaluate the need for evacuation by health-care facilities in potentially affected areas. Key elements in the evaluation include the following:

- Time of expected onset of hazardous weather conditions
- Expected strength of the storm
- Number of facilities in the potential impact area

This evaluation will be included in the discussions of the New York City coastal storm steering committee, and the decision to evacuate will be made by the mayor of New York City as advised by the commissioner of the OEM.

COASTAL STORM IMPACT ON HEALTHCARE FACILITIES

The city's coastal storm plan is activated when the OEM declares that a pending storm will probably impact the coastal area. The OEM calls upon its coastal storm steering committee, composed of selected leadership from city agencies, including the GNYHA, the DOH, and the HHC. This committee will hold a conference call to update the agencies about the storm conditions. After the call, the coordinator of the health and medical emergency support function will reach out to the state's DOH and the fire department (FDNY) to ensure that they are aware of the situation.

There are 62 acute-care hospitals and 179 nursing homes licensed by the state DOH in New York City. Of these, 24 hospitals and 63 nursing homes are located in one of three evacuation zones and may need to be evacuated in the event of a coastal storm. The remaining 38 hospitals and 116 nursing homes are expected to receive evacuees. Healthcare facilities located in coastal storm evacuation zones represent more than 25,000 of the over 73,000 certified licensed beds in the city.

Table 5-1 represents the number of nursing homes and hospitals that could be evacuated based upon the category and severity of the coastal storm.

There are five hospitals in New York City that are located in SLOSH zone A, including Coney Island Hospital. If an evacuation order is given, Coney Island Hospital, along with the other four hospitals, will be required to evacuate all patients.

Table 5-1	Coastal Storm Impact on Healthcare Facilities, by Zone[1-3]				
	Total	Not in a Zone	Zone A	Zone B	Zone C
Bronx Facilities	54	43	0	0	11
Hospitals	9	7	0	0	2
Nursing homes	45	36	0	0	9
Brooklyn Facilities	56	29	7	8	12
Hospitals	12	6	1	0	5
Nursing homes	44	23	6	8	7
Queens Facilities	68	45	3	16	4
Hospitals	12	10	0	2	0
Nursing homes	56	35	3	14	4
Manhattan Facilities	45	22	2	7	14
Hospitals	22	10	2	3	7
Nursing homes	23	12	0	4	7
Staten Island Facilities	14	11	3	0	0
Hospitals	3	1	2	0	0
Nursing homes	11	10	1	0	0
New York City Totals	237	150	15	31	41
Hospitals	58	34	5	5	14
Nursing homes	179	116	10	26	27

Sources: Data from New York City Office of Emergency Management, "National Study on Carless and Special Needs Evacuation Planning: Case Studies," 2008; and State Office of Emergency Management and New York City Office of Emergency Management, "New York Standard Multi-Hazard Mitigation Plan," 2007; and New York State "Guidelines for Hospital Evacuation Protocols," 2006.

Table	
5-2	**Necessary Actions for Potentially Evacuating Facilities**
Collect current census information (including the number of patients that would be discharged) and enter information into New York State's Department of Health data system, known as HERDS (Health Emergency Response Data System)	
Consider implementing emergency patient/resident discharge plans	
Determine the method of communication with the New York City OEM Unified Healthcare Facility Coordination Center once activated	

Table	
5-3	**Necessary Actions for Potential Receiving Facilities**
Collect information on the ability to receive patients from evacuating facilities (e.g., beds, staff) and enter information in HERDS	
Consider implementing emergency patient/resident discharge plans	
Determine the method of communication with the Unified Healthcare Facility Coordination Center once activated	

NOTIFICATION AND ACTIVATION

The OEM, with the city DOH and the HHC, has developed a task list for healthcare organizations that need to evacuate facilities or to receive incoming patients. Efficiency requires that hospitals collect and report accurate census information about their patients, review and consider implementing their facility's emergency discharge plans, and determine the best way to maintain open communication with other healthcare facilities and city agencies (see **Tables 5-2** and **5-3**).

ASSESSMENT

Once a decision to evacuate has been made by the mayor, the New York City OEM will activate the assessment phase of their emergency plan. The goal is to collect information and to put into place

Table	
5-4	**Healthcare Facility Task List: Necessary Actions for Evacuating Facilities**
Implement emergency discharge plans	
Determine patient/resident transportation requirements (use New York State's DOH transportation assistance level [TAL] criteria)	
Communicate the TALs to the Unified Healthcare Facility Coordination Center and enter the information into HERDS	
Work with FDNY personnel deployed to facility	
Report issues to the Unified Healthcare Facility Coordination Center	

Table	
5-5	**Necessary Actions for Receiving Facilities**
Identify surge areas	
Implement emergency discharge plans	
Communicate ability to receive patients from evacuating facilities (e.g., beds, staff) to the Unified Healthcare Facility Coordination Center and enter information in HERDS	
Report issues to the Unified Healthcare Facility Coordination Center	

the needed resources to carry out and coordinate the evacuation (see **Tables 5-4 and 5-5**).

CONEY ISLAND HOSPITAL, DAY BY DAY

Coney Island Hospital is a division of the HHC, which includes 11 hospitals and 10 health-related facilities. HHC is the largest municipal public hospital system in the country. The facilities are organized into seven networks, three of which include hospitals in Brooklyn. Coney Island Hospital is located in south Brooklyn, a borough of New York City, and is a certified 375-bed acute-care teaching facility. The hospital is located in SLOSH zone A, approximately six blocks from the Atlantic Ocean and less than one-third of a mile from the shore. The facility is situated approximately three feet above sea level.

The hospital is located in a large, urban area of Brooklyn. The area is largely composed of one- and two-family homes east and west of the hospital, giving a suburban feel to part of the neighborhood. To the south and north are large apartment complexes housing over 150,000 people. The neighborhoods surrounding the hospital have a residential and commercial population base with a limited heavy industry base. The hospital's catchment area also includes two colleges, numerous parks, the Gateway National Recreation Area, a minor league sports stadium, the city aquarium, a number of marinas, Sheepshead Bay Fishing Village, New York City Transit Authority train and bus depots, a naval reserve station, and the Coney Island beaches. The borough of Brooklyn's residential population is close to four million people. The next closest hospital is over four miles away.

The hospital employs approximately 2,800 personnel, with an additional 300 clinical staff consisting of attending physicians, medical students, interns, and residents. The campus of Coney Island Hospital encompasses a square city block and houses eight buildings, including two 12-story towers, an 8-story tower, a 4-story inpatient behavioral health center, an administrative and support building, a power plant, and a NYFD-EMS division station and repair facilities. The hospital has over 85,000 Emergency Department visits and over 425,000 outpatient visits per year. The average daily census for the hospital is 99% of its certified beds.

Coney Island Hospital's scope in preparedness is to ensure effective mitigation, preparation, response, and recovery to disasters or emergencies affecting the environment of care or adversely impacting the hospital's ability to provide healthcare services to the community. During a coastal storm event, the hospital prepares to provide medical services to the community. Coastal storm planning and preparations require the hospital to protect against potential damage to the facility caused by hazardous water and wind conditions during a storm. The hospital is also required to ensure the continuity of patient care and safety (e.g., maintain generators, fuel, inventory levels of food and water, etc.) and maintain its supplies, whether the hospital shelters-in-place (stay inside the building that you are in at the time of an emergency) or evacuates.

The hospital has a robust emergency management system that includes a comprehensive disaster system specifying policies and procedures in 3 specific plans: emergency management, emergency operations, and response. The response plan encompasses actions for 36 emergency events or types. These response plans identify how to activate the emergency response system and how to respond in an emergency by utilizing specific detailed steps and protocols.

The hospital reviews and updates its emergency plans on an as-needed basis. The emergency management system is overseen by a committee of senior leadership consisting of the chief executive officer; chief operating officer; chief medical officer; chief financial officer; chief nursing officer; and chairpersons of medicine, surgery, primary care, emergency medicine, and nursing. The committee is chaired by the emergency management director of the hospital and meets eight times a year to review, develop, schedule, and test emergency preparedness activities for the hospital. The hospital actively exercises its emergency management program by having a minimum of six drills per year, both internally and externally. On average, Coney Island Hospital has executed 20 exercises and disaster drills per year for the past 5 years. The hospital and its leadership are consistently proactive in utilizing recognized emergency management practices and national, regional, and local standards.

The hospital's emergency management team instituted the pre-established plans to respond to Hurricane Irene. They activated their emergency response system, incident command, and EOC. They utilized specific components of the emergency response plans for the evacuation during Hurricane Irene, including the bed management plan, the hospital surge plan, the coastal storm plan, the 96-hour action plan, and the evacuation plan. In addition, both hospital-specific and corporate-wide vendors were notified about the possible impending evacuation, and stockpiles of water, food, medical supplies, and pharmaceuticals were topped off to ensure continued operations.

Tuesday, August 23, 2011

On August 23, 2011, the New York City OEM was internally monitoring the storm. A decision was made by the OEM to send weather updates and storm-tracking information to all city agencies. The hospital's emergency management team began tracking the storm and instituted internal discussions with senior leadership on preparedness activities and contingency planning for a severe storm.

Coney Island Hospital, because of its location and its proximity to the ocean, is poorly positioned to shelter-in-place during a large coastal storm. Once a significant coastal storm has been identified and is being tracked, the hospital must review contingency plans for ensuring the safety of patients and staff. The proposed action plans are also discussed with the corporate offices of the HHC. Because the coming hurricane could have a potentially significant impact on New York City, it was likely that the hospital's only choice would be to evacuate. If a decision was made to evacuate, the hospital would start the process and collaborate with HHC to initiate an evacuation ahead of a mayoral order, which typically is issued only 24 hours prior to the storm making landfall.

Wednesday, August 24, 2011

Like those at New York City's command center, the hospital actively tracked the progress of the hurricane. During the day's storm planning, senior leadership from the HHC corporate offices initiated three conference calls with the hospital's senior leadership to discuss operations and possible evacuation. The hospital implemented its severe storm contingency planning committee and reviewed the possibilities for the institution. The options included sheltering-in-place, or a partial or full evacuation of the entire hospital. Each of these actions had implications for patient care, for staffing and the transfer of staff to other facilities, and whether the facility was to be closed. Throughout the day, senior leadership met informally with department heads and clinical chairs to discuss the options and prepare for the storm.

While the team at the hospital was busy planning, HHC's corporate office was in constant communication with both the mayor's office and the city's OEM. Although they discussed possible outcomes and contingencies throughout the day, at midafternoon hospital leadership and HHC's corporate office conducted a formal joint planning teleconference in preparation for Hurricane Irene. The key areas of discussions were staffing, the possibility of full evacuation, communication, and the transfer of supplies in the event of an evacuation (see **Table 5-6**).

Table	
5-6	**Topics of Discussion in Preparation for Hurricane Irene**

Staffing of evacuating facilities and receiving facilities. Evacuation of Coney Island Hospital would impact the staffing schedules, transportation needs, and bed management of the other 21 facilities that were part of HHC.
Staffing of the Special Medical Needs Shelters (SMNS). HHC is also required to staff the SMNS in New York City during major events.
Possible evacuation of Coney Island Hospital.
Designation of key senior leadership who would serve as points of contact at all HHC facilities during and after the hurricane.
Transfer of a sufficient supply of food and water for patients, staff, and visitors to the HHC facilities receiving patients and transferred staff.
Ensuring that the generators at all HHC facilities and the fleet of motor vehicles owned by the corporation have been fully fueled.
Transfer of sufficient medical supplies (including pharmaceuticals) and gases to the HHC facilities receiving patients.

Thursday, August 25, 2011

On the morning of August 25, the emergency management team maintained discussions with the city's OEM. In addition, numerous telephone conference calls were conducted throughout the day with both HHC corporate offices and other HHC hospitals. After briefly updating HHC and OEM, senior leadership at the hospital activated their EOC. Leadership outlined the actions to be taken and followed the pre-established policies and procedures by instituting relevant components of the emergency management, emergency operations, and emergency response plans. The EOC utilized a national procedure known as the Hospital Incident Command System (HICS).

With the activation of the HICS, the management team (i.e., senior leadership, selected clinical chairpersons, and department heads) governed the operations center. Assignments to maintain round-the-clock hours of operation and the scheduling of shifts were needed. It was decided that teams would work in 12-hour shifts and all duties were delegated.

A situation room where key individuals from the senior management team could discuss organizational and operational objectives was established within the EOC. Two individuals were selected as the incident commanders—the emergency management director and an associate executive director of the hospital. The CEO maintained the role of liaison officer to the external groups.

Senior leadership activated the rapid patient discharge process. For the hospital, the rapid patient discharge process identifies inpatients that can be discharged home relatively quickly with clinical follow-up. A team composed of the chief medical officer, the medical director, and clinical chairs of departments would lead clinical staff in the rapid identification, assessment, and discharge of patients. All the teams work in conjunction with social work, patient representatives, and discharge planning staff. The hospital also contacted other HHC hospitals as potential receiving sites, as well as a number of the voluntary hospitals throughout New York City. In addition, they contacted the other numerous vendors involved: medical supplies companies, pharmaceutical suppliers, food delivery and fuel delivery companies, and transportation services (i.e., commercial ambulette companies, car services, and buses).

Senior leadership also decided to close all clinical operations by the end of the day. Elective inpatient procedures were canceled as well as all on-site and off-site outpatient services. In addition, engineering services conducted a facility-wide review of the campus to assess how to shutter the facility.

In essence, the hospital was preparing for evacuation prior to the formal declaration and announcement by the mayor. It was understood by the facility that they could be in the direct path of the storm, which underscored the possibility for significant damage to the facility. Due to this risk, hospital leadership and the corporate offices of HHC decided to evacuate the hospital once the formal declaration was announced by the mayor.

Numerous agencies received weather updates via conference calls convened by the New York City OEM and the National Weather Service. During the calls, they learned details regarding the weather, the potential path of Hurricane Irene, and its potential impact on the New York region. Projections were that the storm would have a direct impact on the New York City harbor, including Staten Island, Brooklyn, and parts of Rockaway and Long Island. Officials discussed the trajectories of the storm, predictions of landfall affecting the coast, potential flooding, storm surges and wind speeds, and the amount of rain expected. Being in the direct path of the storm could have devastating consequences on the hospital.

Throughout the day, the corporate office maintained contact with the mayor and the OEM. It was understood that the mayor would formally announce the evacuation of healthcare facilities and those located in coastal storm SLOSH zone A later that day.

At 5:00 PM, the hospital was formally notified by telephone via the HHC corporate office that the mayor would be making the evacuation announcement and that the hospital was preidentified for evacuation. The mayor would order a formal evacuation for 8:00 AM the next day.

The hospital prepared for evacuation. With an inpatient census of 341 patients, the hospital implemented its rapid patient discharge process action plan and was able to discharge 67 inpatients that evening. However, the Emergency Department and Obstetrics and Gynecology (Ob/GYN) Departments were still seeing patients who required hospitalization, resulting in an increase to the inpatient census overnight.

In preparation for the next morning, the hospital applied its evacuation checklist of processes, procedures, and steps for evacuating the remaining patients and shuttering the facility. Shuttering the facility required the transfer of hospital operations, clinical, and medical equipment and supplies to other facilities; closure of clinical and administrative floors; securing and weatherproofing the facility; and the complete lockdown of the campus. A critical step prior to the evacuation was to identify the remaining inpatients and determine how and where to evacuate them. The team also had to identify, based on each patient's acuity levels, how the remaining inpatients were going to be transported. They utilized the New York State DOH transportation assistance levels (TALs), which included 5 categories, to guide the decisions on the type of transportation necessary for the evacuation the next morning. The 5 categories are:

1. The patient can ambulate
2. The patient can ambulate with assistance
3. The patient is wheelchair-bound
4. The patient needs a stretcher and is unable to ambulate
5. The patient may need an advanced life support ambulance

Determining the appropriate TALs category for each patient requires considering if a non-ambulatory patient can be transported by ambulance, providing only basic life support (BLS); or if the patient needs advanced life support (ALS) during transit due to recovery from procedures while hospitalized; or if the patient needs skilled care such as cardiac monitoring, intravenous or other invasive therapies; or if the patient is ventilator dependent. In anticipation of the pending evacuation, patients were identified and their TALs category determined by their primary care attending physician and the nursing staff.

While the inpatients were being categorized based on their transportation needs, a team of physicians led by the chief medical officer and clinical chairpersons made arrangements with other hospitals to receive the patients. They reached out to both HHC hospitals and other hospitals in the borough of Brooklyn with whom Coney Island Hospital had pre-arranged mutual aid agreements to ask if they could accept some of the evacuated patients.

The hospital contacted the transportation vendors where there were preexisting agreements and also contacted the New York City Regional Emergency Medical Services Council (REMSCO) and New York City OEM for additional transportation resources beyond the existing contracts. FDNY-EMS advised Coney Island Hospital that they would not be involved in the transportation of patients during the evacuation process and that it would be the hospital's responsibility to set up transportation.

The hospital also identified and contacted other transportation resources, including commercial ambulance and ambulette companies, car services, and the ambulance services from voluntary hospitals to help support the transportation of patients.

By midnight, the hospital was able to identify and make arrangements with five receiving hospitals. Two of the five hospitals were other HHC facilities—Kings County Hospital (Kings) and Woodhull Hospital (Woodhull), both located in Brooklyn. The other hospitals, also located in Brooklyn, included Long Island College Hospital (LICH), Kings Brook Jewish Medical Center, and Maimonides Medical Center.

Friday, August 26, 2011

On Friday, August 26, the hospital began evacuating at 8:00 AM. The team reassessed the hospital's inpatient population to identify which patients could be rapidly discharged. Of the 280 people who were hospitalized that morning, 82 patients could be discharged utilizing the rapid patient discharge process, leaving 198 inpatients to be transferred to other facilities.

Table	
5-7	**Evacuation Methods**
32 patients transported by ALS ambulance (private vendor utilized for non-emergency transportation)	
98 patients transported by BLS ambulance (private vendor utilized for non-emergency transportation)	
28 patients transported by ambulette (private vendor utilized for nonemergency transportation)	
25 patients transported by city buses (provided to facility for patient transportation)	
15 patients transported by Coney Island Hospital buses	

Simultaneously, the incident command team met with the transportation vendors and identified personnel from both the hospital and the vendors who could assist. The movement of the 198 patients required 26 ambulances, 12 ambulettes, 2 New York City Transit Authority buses, and a number of HHC corporate minibuses and vans, as listed in **Table 5-7**.

During the evacuation, the FDNY and the FDNY-EMS provided support personnel to help in the transportation process. FDNY-EMS personnel did not provide transportation resources and ambulances to support the evacuation process, but were at the hospital to assess the timeliness of the movement of patients out of the facility. The New York City Police Department helped control the traffic and the crowds of people who gathered during the evacuation process.

To simplify the evacuation, no medical records were sent with the transferred patients other than the required transfer packets. The hospital's evacuation policy recommends that the hospital pharmacy prepare and dispense a 3-day supply of each evacuated patient's medication to travel with him or her to the receiving site. However, the pharmacy was advised that there was no need to provide the medication because receiving facilities had sufficient supply. Because of the pending storm and stoppage of all New York City transit, the hospital filled approximately 238 prescriptions for the patients who were discharged home, regardless of their insurance coverage.

All of the hospital's ventilator-dependent inpatients were sent either to Kings or Woodhull. Because the number of ventilator-dependent patients exceeded the equipment at the receiving facilities, 16 ventilators were sent to the 2 HHC facilities (i.e., Kings and Woodhull).

In addition, clinical providers and support staff (e.g., physicians, interns, residents, nurses, and social workers) were assigned to Kings, Woodhull, and LICH. Pharmacists and pharmacy technicians were also assigned to Kings.

The hospital's Incident Command Center coordinated all hospital operations and maintained constant communications with other agencies, including OEM, HHC Corporate, and the accepting and receiving facilities in which patients were transferred to. The status of the patients was tracked throughout the process. Patients and their families were notified by hospital staff about both the evacuation and where their loved ones were being sent. Questions were addressed by patient representatives and by clinical staff when needed. The receiving facilities notified Coney Island Hospital of the patients' arrival and their new bed location. Once patients arrived at the new facility, their families were notified of their new whereabouts.

Simultaneously, efforts focused on securing (safely closing, protecting, and ensuring that the campus was not vulnerable to additional damage, potential thefts, or further destruction) all hospital departments. The Information Technology (IT) Department and communications services were redirected to an off-site location to ensure seamless exchange of incoming and outgoing information. The pharmacy continued operations until the hospital officially closed. Surgical services were also available.

Communication was maintained both internally within the hospital and externally to the responding and administrative groups. Both clinical and support staff were advised of their roles and responsibilities and where to report for work if they were being reassigned. The entire hospital staff was kept abreast by regularly scheduled announcements, email updates, and meetings held in hospital units and departments. All formal press inquiries and agency reporting was conducted through the hospital's CEO and through the press offices at HHC. The myriad of activities and processes and numerous phone calls, operational meetings, and situation awareness updates helped to ensure and accomplish effective, safe, and seamless evacuation of inpatients by 6:00 PM.

Complicating the evacuation process, the Emergency Department was not initially put on FDNY-EMS ambulance diversion and was required to maintain operations until Saturday. Patients who came to the hospital with a medical emergency were stabilized and then transferred. The hospital's contracted ambulance provider, Midwood Ambulance Service, was stationed at the ambulance bay with ALS and BLS support, ensuring the rapid transport of patients.

Saturday, August 27, 2011

Between Friday night and Saturday morning, the hospital's engineering and environmental staffs and hospital police made preparations to safely secure and shutter the facility. The hospital conducted a floor-by-floor walk-through of every room in the facility to ensure that appropriate procedures were followed. These procedures included closing, taping, and securing boards over windows where necessary; checking ventilation systems; and tagging and securing each room, unit, and ward. IT worked with HHC's corporate IT to transfer all the electronic documents, back up files, and power down the computer system at the facility.

During the closing process, the Engineering Department developed a checklist of items that needed to be done prior to closure. **Table 5-8** contains a summary of the items on the checklist.

By noon, the hospital completed all the work necessary to shutter the facility and was formally closed by midafternoon. FDNY-EMS placed the Emergency Department on diversion so that no ambulances would bring patients to the hospital. Senior leadership contacted HHC corporate offices, the city's OEM, DOH and state DOH to notify them of the formal closure of the facility.

The hospital's incident command center maintained operations until 3:00 PM and most of the personnel was then transferred to an off-site location. The CEO, emergency manager, and some senior leadership conducted a final walk-through of the facility and then transferred operations to a "stay team" composed of staff from hospital police, environmental services, and engineering. Before they went home for much needed rest, it was agreed that the incident command team and senior leadership would all return as a soon as possible as the weather permitted. During the Saturday evening hours and overnight untill Sunday morning, the CEO, emergency manager, and some key senior leadership members maintained contact with the stay team for situational updates.

During the storm, the stay team assessed potential threats, ensured that the facility remained secure and that critical plant operations continued, and performed emergency repairs. The stay team's responsibilities are listed in **Table 5-9**.

Table	
5-8	**Hospital Closure Checklist**

Inspect and clear all roofs and roof drains. Remove any loose objects. Clean roof drains.
On grounds, clear all catch basins of debris.
Inspect and test operation of all sump pumps and alarms. Check that pits are clean of any debris.
Top off diesel generator tank. Test and start primary and secondary emergency generators.
Contact vendors for critical systems and secure agreements for emergency site service calls for Monday, August 28, 2011. Purpose was to inspect, repair, and ensure normal operation of critical controls systems.
Inspect boiler and burner controls.
Ensure emergency generator and switchgear systems are operational.
Install additional pumps in below-grade and first-floor electric distribution and machine rooms.
Secure all windows and roof doors. Visually check all areas. Close open windows. For larger glass, duct tape interior side.
Board up first-floor lobby single-pane large glass with plywood.
Position plastic, duct tape, plywood, and tools throughout buildings. Bring in ground dumpsters and barrels needed to contain leaks.
Install sidewalk scaffold in front of Hammett Main Entrance to protect it from the potential of falling debris.
Have contractors secure the construction site. Support construction fence. Remove and secure all loose objects. Install pumps in excavated portion. Increase protection around existing building (a new wing of the Emergency Department was under construction).
Place sand bags around all ground-floor entrances to main building, Tower Building, Hammett, and boiler/generator room.
Run temporary electrical feed for backup to sump pumps. In case of loss of one service, this would allow a quick switch to a separate line.

Table	
5-9	**Stay Team Responsibilities**

Hospital police radios were distributed to engineering staff and elevator mechanics.

Secured campus. Hospital police closed and locked all pedestrian entrances to the campus and secured the gate blocking the main car entrance on Ocean Parkway.

Avenue Z exit of campus was left open for EMS to access the EMS station.

Staff checked all roofs again. All rooftop mechanical equipment was checked. All access panels were resecured to ensure they were not subject to wind damage.

Off-site notification for the fire alarm was disabled. System was taken off-line. If an alarm should sound, in-house staff were to respond, determine cause, and notify FDNY if needed.

Elevator mechanic performed rounds of elevator machine rooms for all buildings during the storm. Protected and covered equipment as needed. The decision to keep the elevator mechanic on-site as part of the response team was to ensure that equipment was protected and could be repaired quickly, as well as to respond to anyone being trapped in an elevator car so FDNY would not have to be called.

Hospital police and engineering staff continued rounds of the main building, Hammett, Tower, and boiler room during the storm. Contained leaks, covered equipment, and checked below-grade pipe space for water.

Identified leaks around old windows and from some roofs. Water shorted out an electrical panel and smoke head in the Emergency Department machine room. During Sunday morning high tide, water from below, from construction site, and from Con Ed vault backed into crawl space.

Additional pumps were moved into place, sandbars were installed around transformers, and the outside manhole was pumped out.

Sunday, August 28, 2011

On Saturday evening and early Sunday morning, Hurricane Irene made landfall and wreaked havoc upon the city. The hospital sustained minor damage, which was minimized due to the prior actions and the monitoring by the stay team during the storm.

Members of the incident command team and senior leadership met at the facility at 7 AM Sunday morning. Separate teams conducted a facility-wide assessment of damage, examining building exteriors, roofs, and the hospital grounds. Once completed, many hospital personnel (i.e., engineering, environmental services, hospital police, pharmaceutical services, central supply, and other facility personnel) were recalled to the hospital to repair the damage, clean up, and prepare the facility to reopen.

Table 5-10 summarizes the damage noted and the steps taken to remediate damage caused by the storm. Table 5-11 reviews the actions taken to reopen the facility.

By 5:00 PM that evening, hospital leadership contacted the city and state DOHs and the HHC corporate office for authorization to reopen. Upon receiving approval from the state, the hospital CEO determined that the hospital could reopen at 7:00 AM the following Monday morning. Personnel from the EOC and the incident command center notified the hospital's department heads and they, in turn, notified the clinical staff that had been assigned to the other hospitals. All were advised to report to work at their regular reporting times once all of the patients were transferred back to the hospital. By Sunday night, hospital personnel were reporting to work. The incident command staff contacted the receiving hospitals and transportation arrangements were made to repopulate the facility.

By 10:00 AM the following morning, the hospital was ready to accept inpatients. A total of 117 inpatients were returned to Coney

Table	
5-10	**Recovery from the Storm**
Some broken windows noted in courtyard.	
Two damaged trees on campus. Small branches and leaves scattered around.	
Construction site excavation area flooded, threatening to leak into basement again at high tide.	
Engineering staff began to pump out water. Contractor responded set up on pumps. Water in main building pipe space. Continue to pump out.	
Removed sandbags from all the hospitals ground floor entrances and windows.	

Table	
5-11	**Reopening Coney Island Hospital**
Hospital grounds opened to employees at 7:00 AM. Pedestrian and vehicle entrance opened.	
Fire alarm vendor repaired damaged smoke head, inspected and tested all main panels, corrected system troubles, and put system back online.	
In-house staff inspected vacuum compressor, medical air compressor, oxygen tank, and medical gas panels.	
Emergency generator inspected, equipment tested.	
Tested nurse call program. Ensured the system was operational.	
Heating Ventilation and Air Conditioning/Controls checked chillers serving Emergency Department, Hammett, and Tower for damage and operation.	
Inspected and tested rooftop units. Put everything back in service.	
Engineering staff repaired damage to Pediatric Emergency Department. Replaced tiles, painted walls.	
During the rest of week, crews continued to clear main building pipe space of water. Repairs were made to outpatient clinics, damaged ceiling tiles were replaced, and so on.	

Island Hospital. By noon, the Emergency Department was formally removed from diversion and was able to receive ambulances from the city's 911 call system.

CONCLUSION

This case identifies evacuation processes and describes an evacuation of a healthcare facility based on an actual event in real time. Various preparations necessary to appropriately evacuate a healthcare facility included triage, determining transportation assistance levels, and command and logistical considerations. This event utilized and implemented specific policies and procedures to ensure that there was a seamless, timely, and effective evacuation. Preplanning and teamwork were essential, especially in the coordination among hospitals and transportation resources. The action of preplanning, training, coordination, and utilization of multiple resources made for an evacuation that was completed safely within 9 hours.

In conclusion, evacuations take time, need preparation, and utilize multiple resources. The basis for success is to always follow the four C's: communication, coordination, consideration, and common sense when you have to evacuate a healthcare facility.

DISCUSSION QUESTIONS

1. Which competencies described in the Appendix does this case demonstrate?
2. What prepared Coney Island Hospital to respond to this hurricane? Was their response effective?
3. Would you have made the same decisions as the administrators? Why or why not?
4. How important is it to know the "rules and regs" of preparedness?
5. Should hospitals be fully prepared for disasters at a time when they may not have enough money to operate? Should they stock supplies?
6. Should staff be expected to stay on the job?

REFERENCES

1. National Study on Carless and Special Needs Evacuation Planning: Case Studies. New York City Office of Emergency Management. New York, NY; 2008.
2. New York Standard Multi-Hazard Mitigation Plan. State Office of Emergency Management and New York City Office of Emergency Management. Albany, NY and New York, NY; 2007.
3. Guidelines for Hospital Evacuation Protocols. New York State. Albany, NY; 2006.

Section

II

Man-Made and Technological Events

Case

6 Rescue Following a Mine Collapse in Chile, 2010

Annette B. Ramírez de Arellano

BACKGROUND

The collapse of a mine in Copiapó, Chile, in 2010 was limited in time and place and produced no casualties. Nevertheless, the disaster trapped 33 men half a mile underground for 69 days and captured the imagination of people throughout the world. The incident has therefore been called both a "global drama" and a "massive experiment."[1(p. 2)]; and the protracted process of supporting and extricating the miners has been described as perhaps "the greatest rescue operation since Noah's ark."[2]

Throughout the ordeal, the miners and the rescuers faced public health decisions concerning an array of issues from sanitation and food distribution to morale and mental health. How these issues were handled sheds light on disaster management. The mine collapse and its complex resolution provide lessons in decision making and information flows. A clear chain of command and a delineation of responsibilities—both functionally and geographically—proved essential. An ability to partner with others, wherever these happened to be, was also evident. Moreover, the rescue team was able to manage the information flow so that the families of those at risk were kept updated and all received the same news at the same time. While this placed a particular burden on the authorities, it also fostered respect, built trust, and avoided confusion and miscommunication. The mine rescue, therefore, exemplifies leadership and communication. Both were essential under conditions of prolonged, extreme stress when the stakes were very high and the probability of success was low.

THE MINE RESCUE

On August 5, 2010, a group of miners entered the San José copper and gold mine in Copiapó, Chile, for their regular work day. Halfway through their shift, when many were on lunch break, they heard a massive explosion followed by the sucking sound of a drastic atmospheric change. The latter phenomenon, known as *el pistón*, produces a deafening noise and generates winds "so strong that they plaster a working man to the wall."[1(p. 21)] The men, accustomed to the moods and movements of the mine, knew that this was a major catastrophe. It did not take long for both those trapped inside the mine and those outside to take stock of the situation: A massive rock (later estimated to weigh 700,000 tons, the equivalent of two Empire State Buildings or 150 *Titanics*)[1](p. 34) had blocked off the entrance to the mine, which was wide enough to allow trucks to drive into the depths of the earth. Those on the surface realized that the only possible access to the miners was through the ventilation shafts. But when rescuers attempted to enter the mine by way of these shafts, the mine began to shift, the shafts collapsed, and the rescue workers had to be pulled out. The miners were now, in fact, entombed.

The mine, located in the Atacama Desert, presented a number of challenges and had been the site of previous accidents. It spiraled downward like an asymmetrical corkscrew, reaching a depth of approximately 2,300 feet into the rock. Over time, the mine had been honeycombed and gouged out, leaving certain sections perilously fragile. Some vertical surfaces had been reinforced with iron rods, but the horizontal roofs were thin and unprotected. There were no accurate maps of the mine, as the mining process altered its configuration on a daily basis. Not surprisingly, the miners considered the mine not as an inanimate environment, but as a living, breathing, temperamental beast that could exact a price for its metal wealth.

In addition to being an exceedingly intricate maze of tunnels, the mine was dark, dusty, and damp. Each of these characteristics presented special problems. The mine's depth made the miners difficult to reach; any communication, if feasible, would take a long time to achieve. The darkness meant that the miners could be easily lost and disoriented. Moreover, they would not be able to detect potential dangers such as falling rocks, slippery surfaces, and crevices, among others. Dust is an occupational hazard of most mining operations, and the destabilized San José mine was no exception. The collapse unleashed a cloud of dust and debris that covered everything it touched, enveloping the men in a thick layer of dust. At the same time, many surfaces were slimy. This damp surface combined with the high heat (95–100°F) and overall humidity (95%) to create a stifling environment in which the men were exposed not only to extreme discomfort, but also to a wide range of infections and sores. If the miners were to remain there a short time, these risks would be tolerable; during a long stay, these could become life threatening.

The rescuers, therefore, had a very clear mission with two objectives that they had to address simultaneously: locate the men and devise the means to extricate them—or, in the words of the chief mining engineer, André Sougarret, "get there and get them out."[3] In the absence of a natural entry into the mine, the rescue team knew they had to bore into the depths of the rock to establish communication with the miners and assess their status. They also had to begin planning the rescue strategy, called Operation San Lorenzo in honor of the patron saint of miners. These simple goals, in turn, involved hundreds of activities requiring an increasingly large and complex cast of characters from all over the world.

THE PLAYERS

The Miners

The miners were at the center of the rescue. Cut off from all communication and access to resources for an indefinite period of time, they had to muster and husband whatever resources were at hand. A group of 33 men between the ages of 19 and 63, they had different experiences, lifestyles, beliefs, and skills. Mining involves a variety of tasks, and the group reflected these in their functions. Some were drivers, and could therefore handle mechanical equipment. Some had some training as electricians, and could create some system of lighting. But others had just recently begun to wield a pickax, and had limited skills and scant understanding of their job. Importantly, the mine had a foreman, and he was in charge of keeping his men on task and enforcing discipline as needed. Over time, some of the miners assumed other roles that were in keeping with their personalities and beliefs. One, for example, acted as spokesperson; he also served as cheerleader and court jester. Another enjoyed writing and kept a log of their activities; a third wrote poetry. A fourth was a lay preacher and held prayer sessions on a regular basis, while a fifth who had received some training in nursing and first aid took charge of his colleagues' health needs. Although some of the miners were unionized, the union was less of a player than those directly affected, who quickly established their group identity by calling themselves "the 33."

The Rescuers

The second major group of stakeholders was the rescuers, who represented a diversity of authority and expertise. At the national level, the president of Chile, Sebastián Piñera, assumed a major role in the rescue, becoming very visible in the process and ensuring that all resources were available. At the outset, he stated that the country would "do everything humanly possible" and "spare no effort" to save the miners.[4](p. 31) Once he made this commitment, he cast a wide net to secure whatever was needed to further the rescue. As part of the national team, several members of his cabinet played a role in the operations. Shortly after the disaster happened, the minister of labor assumed the role of spokesperson. But as the rescue began, it was the minister of mines, Laurence Golborne, who had the responsibility for commandeering all needed expertise and materials and orchestrating the effort. He was also the key person informing the press and other media and communicating with the miners' families. Although an engineer and manager by training, Golborne had scant knowledge of the mines and believed in Lee Iacocca's dictum that it was important to "hire people brighter than himself and then get out of their way."[5](pp. 57–58) He selected André Sougarret, an experienced mine engineer from Codelco, the state copper mining company, to direct the all-important rescue operation. As those in command realized the complexity of their mission, they drew on expertise from around the world. U.S. know-how, Canadian technology, Israeli materials, and Australian equipment all played a part in the massive effort to save the Chilean miners.

Other members of the presidential cabinet who had key functions were the minister of health, who had oversight for the physical and psychological condition of the miners, and the leaders of the National Office for Emergencies, which oversaw the makeshift village that rose in the vicinity of the mine. The minister of foreign relations identified resources in other countries that could be brought to bear on the situation. He thus met with representatives of several mining countries, including Australia, Canada, Perú, South Africa, and the United States to see what expertise or technology they could offer.[4](p. 32) Other government players included the police, the militia, the Chilean navy, and the National Services of Geology and Mineralogy, whose responsibility was monitoring conditions in the mines.

The government authorities, in turn, identified needed staff and expertise; as a result, the rescuers grew to include more than 300 experts, each with special knowledge or skills—from drilling and cartography to nutrition and psychiatry—that could contribute to getting the miners out. Organizationally, there were two teams, one at the national level and one on site. In Santiago, the key ministries reached out to others and secured all needed resources; they also sifted through the many offers of manpower and technology that came from a variety of sources, separating well-intentioned philanthropy from opportunistic product placement. At the mine, a team of experts oversaw four areas critical to the rescue mission: mining engineering; medicine and health, including psychological support; services to families; and media and information.

The Miners' Families

The miners' families constituted the third major group of stakeholders. Being on the surface, they could serve as a voice for the miners when they were not accessible. The collectivity of parents, wives, children, and siblings were a constant reminder of the urgency of the rescue. They were not loath to hold the authorities accountable for everything that was done or not done. The families quickly became a powerful and vocal force, requesting information and being on site at all times. They moved to the vicinity of the mine, creating a makeshift settlement in the middle of the Atacama Desert. Born in shared grief but sustained by hope, *Campamento Esperanza* (Camp Hope) was a visible presence of the families' concerns and expectations for a successful outcome. The camp carried out an array of activities and enterprises, including convening periodic meetings among the dwellers as well as with the authorities and celebrating religious rituals. Over time, the camp had not only tents and trailers to house the families, but also multiple shrines; a canteen; and a variety of businesses, schools, and sports facilities. The jerry-built city eventually had a population of 2,000 persons in need of basic services, including power and water, food, health, and education. A Center for the Orientation and Support of Families (COAF, for its Spanish acronym) was instrumental in providing community and mental health services and information to the families in the new settlement. *Campamento Esperanza* soon evolved into a complex village with shuttle bus service, live entertainment, and even a resident clown for comic relief.

Other Players

Other players were only marginally involved, even when they were major stakeholders. Surprisingly absent from the rescue efforts were the mine's owners. As a private enterprise, the San José mine was ostensibly under the aegis of its owners. But because they faced possible liability issues and even criminal charges, they kept a low profile and did not assume a central role in the rescue. Moreover, the president of Chile recognized that the task required national attention and global resources, and was therefore beyond the scope of any private company. In Golborne's words, "We were not part of the problem. But we appeared as the responsible party, not only from the political perspective but also from a legal standpoint."[6(p. 6)] Despite the corporate distance kept by the mine's owners, the company's insurance company, the Chilean Insurance Association, covered the miners' health expenditures and provided vital medical and support personnel to care for the workers' physical and mental conditions.

TWO ANGLES OF VISION: FROM ABOVE AND FROM BELOW

Initially, the rescue team was not sure if the miners had survived the massive collapse; indeed, President Piñera and Minister Golborne had been told that the chance of finding any of the men alive was only 2%.[1(p. 84)] Nevertheless, the team was under extreme pressure to locate the men, and to do so as quickly as possible. With the existing entrances to the mine all closed, the only option was drilling holes to see if they could find any signs of life. In order to maximize the possibility of finding anyone within the maze of tunnels and crevices within the mine, Piñera had asked that multiple rigs begin boring into the mine.

On August 9, when Sougarret took charge of the search and rescue operation, machinery to perform the operations was already on site, but there was no strategy to guide the work. The head engineer's main task was therefore to coordinate the drilling and devise a systematic way to achieve the goal: inserting a 3.5-inch drill bit to find the miners, "a needle with a 2,300 foot journey, in search of a mine shaft."[1(p. 77)] Sougarret knew that speed and precision were trade-offs, but that both were necessary. In his words,

> Time was our enemy. We had to drill quickly because the veins that cut across the deposit are made of granite. But we had to drill slowly, because the bottom layer is rubbly. The mine seemed to be a jigsaw puzzle with pieces that did not fit together.[7]

He therefore decided to use different drilling techniques with varying degrees of precision and speed. The operation began with 10 rigs drilling at different points and different angles in order to maximize the chances of success. The drilling took place all day, every day, with three shifts of 8 hours each.[6(p. 12)] As expected, the speedier drills tended to veer off course, and any correction slowed down the process. Additionally, the rescue planners faced a number of unknowns, including how and where the miners were, and how accurate the drilling actually was. The head engineer estimated that, barring no major obstacles, the boreholes would advance at a rate of 325 feet per day. At best, it would take at least a week for the drill bit to reach its goal.

Following the collapse and the *pistón*, the miners had scrambled, either on foot or by truck, toward the mine's shelter, which was far enough from the landslide to remain intact. Once they got there, they saw that they were all right, and that all 33 in that shift were accounted for. Some had gotten bruised in the process of fleeing to safety, but there were no broken bones or other major injuries. Still, they were trapped, completely cut off from any source of help. They tried to make noise and even set a fire in the hope of sending signals to the surface, but received no response.

There was also still some concern that the collapse had caused casualties. The driver of the truck had passed another miner driving up the ramp. Had he made it through? The timing suggested that he might have been crushed as the mine caved in. However unfortunate their current fate, the 33 knew they had escaped death, and wondered if their coworker had also survived.

Although the mine had tunnels and other large areas in addition to the shelter, the latter now became the center of the men's lives. The designated 540-square-foot reinforced space with a metal door provided some respite, although it was "little more than a hole in the wall with a ceramic floor, reinforced ceiling, two oxygen tanks, a cabinet filled with long-expired medicine and a tiny stash of food."[1(p. 24)] The men were used to taking refuge there as soon as they heard a strange explosion or crack. The miners knew that this space would provide some degree of protection and would be the most likely target of the rescuers' efforts. They also realized that they were buried very deep, and that any breakthrough would take days. In the meantime, the only alternative to despair was making do with the resources at hand.

An inventory of the shelter's provisions was not encouraging. The two tanks of oxygen were put to immediate use, and the men took turns breathing from these as soon as they locked the door against the dust storm unleashed by the collapse and the *pistón*. Although the emergency cache of food had been restocked that very morning, it was designed to feed only 20 men over a span of 48 to 72 hours. Now, the need was of an altogether different magnitude, and the supply was so small that it was, in the words of one of the miners, Víctor

Zamora, "humiliating for a working man."[4](p. 203) The shift foreman took stock of what he had to feed his "troops": 10 liters of water, 1 can of peaches, 2 cans of peas, 1 can of salmon, 16 liters of milk (8 banana flavored, 8 strawberry flavored), 18 liters of juice, 20 cans of tuna fish, 96 packets of crackers, and 4 cans of beans.[1](p. 24) Severe rationing was therefore required, with "meals" being spaced out as the days of confinement stretched out. Their diet consisted of spoonfuls of tuna and crackers, with a few sips of milk. It was estimated that they were consuming only 100 to 150 calories per day.

Physical conditions were challenging at best. It was dark most of the time, as the few sources of light began to give out. Some of the men had watches, and the face of one watch could be backlit to change colors every 12 hours. This allowed the men to know when it was day and night. Nevertheless, the initial period was one of chaos and anxiety, a result of the men's understandable fears and frayed tempers. Factions and cliques formed, limiting cooperation. But within days, this gave way to greater order and an established routine. In an attempt to nurture a sense of normalcy and cohesion, the foreman took on the job that went with his title: he "guided, prodded and motivated the men under his command."[1](p. 51) At the same time, the men established a democratic system of decision making, everyone voting at key points, with a majority deciding on specific courses of action.

Two other leaders—one charismatic, the other religious—emerged from the ranks, and they helped raise morale and establish a regular routine. The men agreed that food had to be made to last, and that everyone should have the same portion. Initially they ate every 12 hours, but as food dwindled, the period between meals became commensurately longer. The men waited until everyone had his ration, then ate together. They also prayed together and had a daily meeting at 1:00 PM to make communal decisions. During the rest of the day, the men did chores and rested. One major task was digging wells, which ensured that they would have an ample supply of water. Those that had special talents were able to put them to use. The prayer group was led by the lay preacher. The miner who had had training in first aid became the de facto medic. The electrician used the batteries of two trucks to power light and charge the miners' helmet lights.[8] One miner made a set of dominoes from recycled materials. Another kept a log of all activities. In some cases, job titles were less important than personal attributes and talents. Over time, this division of labor helped to keep the men engaged and united during their extended period of relative helplessness.

STAGE 1: GETTING THERE

Sougarret's estimate that a drill would reach the miners within a week was only partly accurate. On August 16, one of the drills appeared to have reached a workshop located across from the refuge where the miners were expected to be. But the drill had reached an empty cavern that was not on any of the maps.[9] It had therefore bypassed the shelter. For the miners, who could hear the sound of the approaching drill, this was devastating. The realization that this hopeful attempt had missed them altogether raised new anxieties concerning whether they would be found. Still, they heard the buzz of multiple drills and were ready to take action if one of these were to break through into their space.

On the morning of August 22, when the rescue team's GPS system indicated that the drill was only some 150 feet from the target, the drilling slowed down to prevent rock shards from breaking off and injuring the miners below. The goal was to puncture a clean hole.[1(p. 118)] At 5:50 AM, when the drill finally broke through, the responses of the miners and those of the rescue team were immediate and joyous. Above ground, the rescue workers hugged and jumped up and down, awaiting further instructions. One member of the rescue team pounded the tube with a 16-pound hammer, to see if there was a response. Below, the miners were momentarily stunned at the sight of the drill. They had anticipated, prayed for, and rehearsed this moment. But now their excitement got in the way of the plan they had designed. Instead of first stabilizing the area to make sure that no loose rocks came down from the roof, which was a priority, they carried out other activities before the drill was pulled up. After allowing themselves a brief celebration, they took a can of spray paint to make sure that the returning drill head looked noticeably different from the one that had begun the journey into the rock. The men also began taking turns striking the protruding tube with a metal wrench, hoping to be heard above. Sougarret used a stethoscope to confirm that the pounding sound he heard was indeed coming from the depths of the mine. Finally, the miners used a piece of elastic ripped off one miner's underwear to tie a plastic bag to the drill. This contained a letter from one of the miners to his wife, providing the first communication in 17 days. But most important was a crumpled piece of paper, addressed to no one and everyone. Its message: "We are all well in the shelter, the 33." This succinct text conveyed much essential information: the men's location, their condition, and their survival as an intact group. Moreover, the message was hopeful and positive, rather than a cry for help.[10(p. 19)]

After the drill head was pulled up, it took approximately 6 hours for the rescue team to dismantle the entire apparatus. Once the rescuers discovered the painted head and found the plastic bag, the excitement quickly spread throughout the team. Minister Golborne would later describe the moment as "one of the happiest moments of [his] life," unleashing a "state of grace."[11] Although protocol called for one of the authorities to communicate the momentous news to the families, all lines of communication went awry. The fact that signs of life had been discovered in the mine spread rapidly throughout Camp Hope, which became "a delirious scene of tears, smiles, hugs, and waving flags."[1(p. 126)] The minister called President Piñera, who flew to Copiapó as quickly as possible.

After allowing themselves some time for celebration and thanksgiving, the authorities and the leaders of the rescue team knew that the flurry of excitement and shared relief was only the end of the beginning. As the head psychologist later said, "It was the best and the worst case scenario: the men were alive; now they had to be fed and maintained for an indefinite period of time."[12] The team then launched the next stage of the rescue: taking care of the men's physical and mental health and planning their ascent from the mine.

One of the first items to enter the mine was a remote control video camera that was manipulated from above. The idea was to give the rescue team some idea of the condition of the men. The video showed that the miners, most stripped down to their underwear to deal with the extreme heat, looked thin and scruffy. But the picture was grainy and the camera's audio did not function. Nevertheless, this was a harbinger of things to come: separated by 2,300 feet and many tons of rock, the miners and the rescuers would increasingly depend on an array of technology to bring them together.

STAGE 2: SURVIVAL AND RISK MANAGEMENT

The first priorities for the rescue team were hydrating and feeding the men and addressing their immediate medical needs. In order to send food down to the mine, the drilling team reinforced the borehole that had broken through to the refuge. Using a long hose made of PVC, they coated the walls of the hole with a metallic gel to ease the passage of a capsule that would be able to reach the men.[13] This system became their lifeline, serving as a conduit for sending the items they needed for both survival and comfort. Each capsule, a mere 5.5 inches in diameter but 5 feet long, was a hollow cylinder that operated like a pneumatic tube. This was stuffed with plastic containers full of supplies, and lowered by pulley to the refuge.[14] The capsules were soon known as *palomas*, or pigeons, because they flew from the surface to the shelter with scheduled regularity, connecting the survivors with their families and the rescuers. The system, which expanded to two other boreholes, was used not only to deliver food and pump oxygen, but also to send medications, toiletries, letters, clothes, boots, and even cots, among other items. Practically anything that could be compressed or rolled up into a diameter of 5 inches could be sent. The *palomas* were soon very busy, making some 40 trips per day. This, in turn, required a team of miners called *palomeros* to be on hand to receive and distribute the supplies and to return the capsule with letters and dirty clothes. This system functioned like a rudimentary post office. On the surface, each family had a cabinet where they would place the items and letters they were sending to their loved ones. And in the mine, an area was set aside for the men to leave the items they wanted sent up the shaft.

Having been entombed for 17 days with a mere spoonful of food as their main means of sustenance, the men dreamt of eating steaks and empanadas. Their diet, however, was carefully supervised by the medical staff, and closely followed the recommendations of physicians and nutritionists. After surviving on such few calories, the men could not shift to their pre-cave-in diet without hazarding, quite literally, a shock to their systems. After being severely malnourished and hungry for 17 days, the miners faced the danger of refeeding syndrome, a potentially fatal complication of starvation. Either too much food or the wrong kind of food could aggravate their altered metabolism, resulting in fluid and electrolyte disorders, with a variety of complications. Nutritional guidelines therefore called for avoiding a diet with an "inappropriately high protein-calorie intake."[15] The plan was to begin feeding the miners limited calories and a narrow repertoire of nutrients, and gradually increase both the caloric intake and the variety of foods.

At the outset, the men were told to double the amount of water they drank. The *palomas* sent them edible gels with protein and vitamins.[16] During the first day, their main food was 200 milligrams of Supportan, a milk-based, high-energy nutritional supplement enriched with omega-3 fatty acids, antioxidants, and fiber.[17] Over the next few days, the amount of supplement was increased fivefold. The physicians also sent down urine test strips so that the miners could measure the extent to which their bodies were affected by the lack of food. The tests showed that about half the miners were dehydrated and excreting ketones and myoglobin into their urine, a sign that their muscles were breaking down.[18] Information on the miners' health was then used to design their basic diet. The menus were adapted for those with special needs, including a diabetic and one who was on a special diet.[16]

Once the miners were nutritionally stabilized, they ate five times a day and were fed a greater variety of foods. The number of calories also increased, reaching 2,200 calories per day. Eventually they were even able to enjoy the traditional Chilean foods that they had so longingly craved. Nutritionists at the Chilean Ministry of Health prepared the daily menus, keeping tabs of calories and the different types of nutrients. These menus were then sent to a company that specialized in food preparation and delivery. Food portions were individually vacuum sealed and transported to the mine site, where they were rethermalized and packed into plastic tubes before they went via *paloma* on their journey to the center of the earth.[16]

In addition to basic sustenance, several of the men required medical attention. The minister of health, Dr. Jaime Mañalich, was in charge of health surveillance, collecting information and providing advice. He and his colleagues also established a close relationship with the miner who functioned as a medic. This miner oversaw the 33's ailments and ministered to their needs. Mañalich, who is both a physician and an epidemiologist, sent down a survey that each miner had to complete. This provided an inventory of their health problems and established a baseline for their care. The diabetic needed insulin, and this was sent in one of the first *palomas*. Another suffered from silicosis and required an inhaler.[18] Other immediate concerns were dental and dermatological. Without toothpaste or toothbrushes, dental hygiene was nonexistent. Two of the men had developed severe dental infections and had to be treated with antibiotics. And because the combination of cuts, heat, humidity, and dirt created the perfect environment for fungal and other infections, many of the men required topical treatment for these. In addition, the men were sent thermal socks made with a copper fiber that attacks bacteria, thereby eliminating odor and infection.[14]

The medic served as medical monitor, reporting to the physicians above. He took the miners' temperature and blood pressure and kept track of their weight with a scale that had been sent down. He also immunized the men against influenza, pneumonia, and tetanus.[19]

One health issue that had to be addressed was the men's request for cigarettes. Some were addicted smokers who were coping with withdrawal symptoms; one of the first items they had requested was cigarettes. This placed the medical authorities in a quandary. While they were reluctant to foster the smoking habit, they also realized that this was not the appropriate time to get the miners to quit. The medical team originally tried sending nicotine patches. When this did not satisfy the smokers, the physicians sent them two to four cigarettes per day. But this restriction was eventually lifted as the number of smokers increased and the demand for cigarettes rose. Dr. Jean Romagnoli, who was responsible for the men's physical conditioning and nutrition and was himself a smoker, supported the smokers' pleas, arguing that, in this particular case, common sense should prevail over orthodox medical advice.[1(p. 199)] When the men requested wine and beer, however, their petition was denied. Alcohol is not part of the miners' culture, because drinking in the mine is seen as a potential safety hazard.[20] Physicians felt that alcohol would affect their intellectual capacities at a time when they needed to be alert at every moment. Another concern was that nondrinkers would give their ration to others, who would then imbibe more than their share.[21]

The health team recognized that addressing the men's most obvious needs and physical conditions was only part of their job. The miners' emotional health posed equally important challenges. The men had faced a number of major psychological threats, any one of which could have triggered a breakdown. These included a lack of basic resources (food, water, air); an absence of craved substances, including nicotine and melatonin; sensory deprivation and lack of environmental clues; an upheaval in daily routines and circadian cycles; crowding and lack of privacy; lack of medical care; estrangement from loved ones; changes in roles; and uncertainty.[22(p. 62)] All of these had to be addressed. At the same time, the experts recognized that during the first 17 days the miners had faced these threats with organization, solidarity, determination, and resiliency, factors that boded well for their survival and recovery.

The mental health experts agreed that the key to the miners' well being was to keep them "busy and well-supported."[8] This, in turn, meant that leadership had to be established, with the men assigned different tasks and held accountable for these. Experts in psychiatry and psychology were consulted in order to devise strategies that would keep the men from descending into depression or showing signs of anxiety, irritability, listlessness, and hostility.

Because of the similarities in the physical and psychological conditions that astronauts and miners face, experts from the U.S. National Aeronautical and Space Administration (NASA) were brought in for their expertise in handling the effects of extreme confinement in potentially hostile environments.[23] On August 30, 2010, only 8 days after the miners had been found, two physicians, a psychologist, and an engineer from NASA arrived in Chile to advise on the miners' nutritional, medical, and psychological needs. Because there are approximately 20 different body functions that are linked to cycles of day and night, the NASA consultants recommended that these cycles be replicated artificially to restore the men's normal circadian cycles.[24(p. 69)] Using generators, light-emitting diode (LED) lamps, and other equipment, the topside team worked with the miners to restore lighting in the mine.[4(pp. 120–121)]

The psychologists, both local and imported, also underlined the importance of organization and keeping the miners occupied. The NASA team stressed the importance of routine daily activities such as playing cards, reading, and watching movies.[1(p. 157)] The organization that had already been created within the mine provided the structure for keeping the men engaged. But the division of labor that was already in place became more elaborate, as teams were formed to help with the upcoming rescue task. The medic was so busy monitoring the men's conditions and reporting to the minister of health and other physicians that he named an assistant to help with the task. And, given the many communications and deliveries that went to and from the mine, the *palomeros* were usefully employed sorting out and delivering the mail.

The behavioral experts also pointed out the benefits of maintaining a hierarchical system and clear command-and-control lines. In mining operations, the shift foreman is "sacred and holy"[25] and therefore a recognized leader. The foreman was thus given increased recognition and responsibility; he was the one who represented the 33, communicating with the president, the minister of mines, and Sougarret. Although other miners would emerge as spokesmen and assume other leadership roles, the occupational hierarchy was maintained even under altered circumstances. The 33 were divided into 3 working groups of 11 men each, with each one doing an 8-hour shift. Each group had a leader, or *capataz*, who reported to the foreman[1(p. 145)] Now that the men were fed and cared for, they had greater energy and could begin to perform a number of chores. These included reinforcing weak walls and clearing debris[1(p. 146)] Security patrols checked the mine to detect any signs of trouble and to clear loose rocks from the roof of the mine. The men also had to maintain their living areas to be as habitable as possible. Their living space expanded beyond the shelter, and areas within the mine were zoned for different uses. There were places for sleeping, for eating and recreation, for showering, and even for smoking.[26] There was also an area set aside as a restroom, but this varied over time: The mine had one chemical toilet that was moved periodically to dissipate the smells. When the toilet was full, the miners dug holes to bury their waste.[5(p. 125)]

A routine was established. Much of it revolved around meals, because it took more than an hour for all 33 rations to reach the mine. The routine began with breakfast, followed by a work shift that included not only tending to the mine, but also taking care of trash and emptying the makeshift area that became a latrine. The *palomas* also required constant attention, as the system operated around the clock. All the men had lunch together, after which they had another work shift and took care of their personal needs. They also held prayer sessions and sessions with the medical staff and the psychologists. Finally, the miners instituted a session called *mostrando las cartas*, or "showing your cards," in which they discussed any disagreements, plans, or concerns.[3]

Communication was a linchpin of much of the operation, and a broad array of technologies—from the rudimentary to the high tech—was used to connect the miners with their families and the rescue team. Shortly after the initial video was made, a telephone link was established with the mine. This was the creation of an ingenious inventor who had developed a telephone small enough to fit into a *paloma*. Although the rescuers had little faith in the modest contraption, the inventor was given two hours to install and test his $10 device. The phone was packed with instructions and a half mile of Japanese fiber-optic cable and sent to the mine; two of the miners wired the phone to the cable. One hour and 45 minutes after the telephone's arrival, it was tested and found to work.[1(pp. 133–134)] Shortly after that, Minister Golborne was speaking to the shift foreman, who said the men were waiting to be rescued. Golborne assured him that everyone was doing everything possible to bring them up as soon as possible.[4(p. 94)] The miner then asked about the fate of the coworker who was exiting the mine at the time of the collapse. Had he made it through? The minister reported that everyone was alive, and that their friend had made it to the surface unharmed.[1(pp. 134–135)]

After this initial conversation, the telephone's inventor talked to the miners on a daily basis, becoming, in his own words, their "psychologist, counselor, friend, courier, and love messenger."[4(p. 94)] The medical team also used the device to communicate with the medic. The link was used by the mental health experts, who held regular conference calls with the men. Through this means, the psychologists built a profile of the group and its individuals.[27]

Additional technology was put in place to provide the miners with news and carefully prescreened entertainment. Several electronics companies donated a number of tiny gadgets that could help the miners. These included three small projectors that allowed the miners to watch movies, videos of loved ones, and soccer games, and small speakers to listen to the *rancheras* (Chilean country music) and reggaeton of their preference.[28] Nevertheless, the rescue team controlled the technology sent to the mine; iPods were not allowed because they would isolate the miners and break the team spirit the rescuers were intent on nurturing.[14]

Almost a month after the cave-in, a fiber-optic communications link was installed. This allowed the men to communicate with their families through a live video feed and permitted those above ground to see the miners (although not vice versa, at least in the beginning). Each of the trapped men was given a 4-minute slot to talk to his family. When the miners complained that this was too short, they were given 5 and later 8 minutes apiece every other day.[4(p. 123)]

This system supplemented the written word, which remained the principal means of communication to and from the mine. With increased interaction between the miners and their families, a new issue arose. The chief psychologist in charge of the miners, concerned with mitigating their anxieties and keeping up their morale, was intent on sparing them from any demoralizing news conveyed by their relatives. Worried that the families would be communicating their anxiety and problems, including money woes, he had a team screening their communications, withholding letters that contained bad tidings. Any letters from the miners with information that could upset their families were also intercepted.

While this two-way censorship sought to protect the men and families from information that could concern or depress them, it also represented a violation of their privacy. The psychologist's paternalism therefore clashed with the miners' and families' basic autonomy and right to free expression. When the miners realized that the authorities were tampering with the letters they were sending and receiving, they were furious. They forcefully requested that the practice end because it was patronizing and infantilizing.[1(p. 156)] In response, the chief psychologist defended his actions by stating that controlling the content of all communications was "nonnegotiable" in order to avoid misunderstandings and potential hostilities.[21] The struggle escalated: The miners refused to speak to the psychologists, who, in turn, threatened to withdraw some of the treats on which the men depended.[27]

The conflict became even more acrimonious when some of the psychologists on the team objected to the censorship practice, siding with the miners. A psychiatrist who was consulting on the rescue also expressed his opposition to the control of information, thereby giving greater weight to the miners' position. Moreover, the families began exerting political pressure, and aimed their pleas and protests at Minister Golborne.[29] The miners wanted the government to fire the chief psychologist, but he had been hired by the private insurance company that covered the miners' health care and was therefore not directly accountable to the Ministries of Health or Mines. Instead, the psychologist took a week off to allow tempers to calm down.[1(p. 178–185)] During his leave, his temporary replacement ended the censorship, lifting all restrictions and allowing the mail to go through unchecked.

The psychologists rationalized the dispute and even saw it as a salutary sign that the men, having had their basic needs met, were now focused on other issues and were more forcefully asserting themselves.[30] Moreover, mental health experts, such as Dr. Jorge Díaz, thought that it was better for the miners to focus their anger and complaints on an external target rather than turning on each other.[27] After the chief psychologist returned from his brief leave, he gradually renewed and normalized his prior relationship with the men. The lack of restrictions, however, resulted in families sending "contraband" to their men. This included candy bars that could rot their teeth, and even pot, which had the potential of altering the men's behaviors and creating cliques.[1(p. 186)]

Throughout the process, the men were informed as to what was happening on the ground. But the rescue team was reluctant to give them a firm date for their rescue: there were just too many unknowns. Nevertheless, the men were told that they were likely to remain underground for a few months. In the meantime, the rescuers were working to design the means of extracting them as expeditiously as possible without jeopardizing their safety.

STAGE 3: GETTING THEM OUT

Planning for the rescue of the men had begun as soon as the cave-in occurred, but the task accelerated once the miners were found. At the same time, prudence and patience were all-important in making the right decisions. The technical team knew that they had to drill the smallest possible hole into which a capsule large enough to hold one man could fit. It was estimated that this hole had to be approximately 28 inches in diameter, or "the size of a bicycle tire, with no wasted space for luxury, no elbow room for comfort."[31]

As with the initial probe, there were multiple alternatives, called plans A to J, for drilling the all-important opening. These were winnowed down to three, which were then presented to President Piñera. Faced with the choice of three different methods, he opted for "all three of them because technologies may fail, but we cannot fail."[6(p. 19)] This built-in redundancy meant that each option had two backups, and that failure of one method would not jeopardize the overall rescue mission. Because the hardness of the rock and the depth of the mine posed unprecedented challenges, different strategies would maximize the chance of success.

The three plans differed in origin, approach, technology, speed, and precision. Moreover, they would enter the mine at different angles and target different points. Plan A used an Australian drill, the Strata 950, and relied on equipment that was already in Chile. Although the site supervisor had to come from Ontario, the technology was available and they could start quickly. This drill is able to drill a perfectly straight hole, and could therefore be aimed at the miners' shelter. The drill's precision is gauged constantly and the machine can self-correct.[32] But the technology has certain drawbacks. One is that the rig requires 4.5 gallons of water every second to lubricate the drilling process and to flush the ground rock back up to the surface.[33] Because the Atacama Desert is the driest in the world, enormous water tankers had to be brought in to operate the machine. Dependence on water also meant that the miners had to engineer drainage and holding pools to keep their living quarters dry.[25] Another disadvantage is that the Strata is known as a *raise borer*, which means that it must drill twice. Three drill bits create an initial pilot hole, and this hole is subsequently widened by reaming from the bottom up. Additionally, the pace is slow, so this was nicknamed the "tortoise plan."

Plan B relied on the Schramm T130, a drill developed in Pennsylvania that was then in use in a mine in northern Chile. Convinced that his machine could do the job quicker and more safely than other alternatives, the manufacturer of the drill bit used in this machine actively lobbied the Chilean Ministry of Mines to give this technology a chance. He developed a PowerPoint presentation to show how it worked, and made his case to the Chilean authorities.

The Schramm had succeeded in rescuing 9 miners who had been trapped for 77 hours in the Quecreek mine in Pennsylvania 8 years earlier, and thus had a credible track record.[32] Unlike the plan A drill, which relies on the rotation of the drill bit, the Schramm is a *downhole hammer*, or percussion drill that uses air-powered bits to pound the rock 20 times per second as the drill rotates. This dual action works particularly well in hard, brittle rocks and dry conditions, and therefore appeared to be particularly promising in the San José mine.[32] It was estimated that this technology could chew through 3 feet of rock in an hour.[33] In contrast to the slow-and-steady plan A, plan B was referred to as "the hare."

Once the authorities agreed to give this method a chance, the company recruited their most skilled operator to handle the drilling. The fact that he was drilling water wells for the U.S. Army in Afghanistan was no obstacle; Jeff Hart had the reputation for being "the best in the world at drilling large holes with the T130" and was therefore enlisted to help in Chile.[34] He knew the equipment well and had the experience and the endurance to do the job. He and another member of his team who was also in Afghanistan, flew to Dubai, Amsterdam, and Santiago, from where they were taken to Atacama. There, the drill was waiting for them. Nevertheless, additional equipment— some 26,500 pounds of it—had to be sent from the United States to the site.[35]

Although the T130 was fast, it needed a pilot hole to guide it and prevent it from veering off course. One of the original boreholes used in the *paloma* system was therefore sacrificed to the new objective. The 6-inch hole would guide the bit, which the drillers would enlarge twice: first to a width of 12 inches and then to one of 28 inches to accommodate the rescue pod that would bring the men up.[36] The use of the existing pilot hole allowed the drillers to send the rock cuttings down the existing hole, thereby reducing the complexity of the operation.[37] It was anticipated that this alternative could reduce the men's entrapment by half, getting them out in 60 days.

The ancillary equipment was transported from Bethlehem, Pennsylvania, to Copiapó by United Parcel Service (UPS). Once the Chilean embassy contacted the UPS office in Washington, DC, the company got in touch with LAN Airlines to fly the shipment. Because it was part of a humanitarian mission, the UPS Foundation funded it as an in-kind charitable gift.[35] Tractor-trailer teams loaded the machinery and drove it to Miami, from where it was flown to Chile. Only 3 days elapsed from loading in Pennsylvania to delivery in Copiapó, where plan B was about to get underway.

The third alternative, plan C, relied on an enormous Canadian rig—Rig 421—brought in from another Chilean mine. Used primarily for oil and gas exploration, the rig was an impressive piece of technology, requiring more than 40 trucks for its delivery. With a footprint the size of a football field and towering 147 feet in the bleak Atacama landscape, this rig represented the "heavy artillery," at least visually. It was reputed to be very fast, but it was designed for soft terrain, which this was certainly not. Moreover, it took 9 days to get it built and fully operational, thereby delaying its starting date. Nevertheless, the sight of plan C was reassuring to the rescue team and encouraging to the miners' families. Minister Golborne now urged everyone to "place their bets," leading many to choose their "favorite" in the race to reach the trapped miners. For his part, chief mine engineer André Sougarret calculated the potential speed of each drill and estimated that plan A would reach the refuge on December 1, plan B would reach its target (the mine's workshop) on October 10, and plan C would reach an intermediate shaft on October 30.[38]

The dates gave hope to the rescue team, and the fact that all drills were operating at all hours of the day and night suggested that the government's estimate of a rescue date—by Christmas—was unduly conservative. But because the technology was largely untested in the Chilean environment and circumstances, there was still much uncertainty and anxiety surrounding the enterprise. Minister Golborne was intent on providing hope at the same time that he guarded against unreasonable expectations.[39] Not surprisingly, all plans suffered setbacks, which increased doubts concerning not only when but also whether they would reach their goal.

Although the drilling for plan B began a week after the start of plan A, it made quick progress during its first 4 days and was faster than initially announced. Then, on the fifth day, the drill stalled. The air pressure collapsed; the machine spun, but no rock was being ground. The engineers stopped the drilling and pulled up the machine to inspect the hammer.

The evidence was obvious: the drill head was shredded. Football-sized chunks had been torn off the tungsten-steel shaft. A video camera . . . revealed the missing pieces had become entangled with iron. . . . Rods used to reinforce the mine . . . had sabotaged the rescue tunnel.[1(p. 169–170)]

The drill hole was clogged with metal, and there were no magnets strong enough to lift the pieces up the shaft. A Chilean engineer suggested using an open metal jaw that would enclose the fallen chunks and carry them up the shaft. This technique, called *la araña*, or the spider, was not taken seriously until the engineer met with Minister Golborne, who approved it immediately. The spider was sent down and reeled up. Once on the surface, the spider was cut with a blowtorch to release its "prey." The spider's catch was a tungsten hammerhead, which could be replaced. Plan B was saved, although several precious days were lost in the process.[1(p. 172–174)]

To complicate matters, while plan B was at a standstill, plan A also broke down temporarily. A leaky hydraulic hose forced the machinery to stop and had to be repaired. These setbacks occurred as plan C was about to start, so that there was at least one method to raise everyone's hopes that the rescue would eventually succeed. Plan C took off with such speed that officials thought it would overtake the other two methods and reach the miners first.[40]

Plan B suffered a second setback when the bit snapped and one of the drill heads detached from its base, landing on the floor of the mine. While no one was injured in the process, the head was picked up by the miners. One of them called the rescue team to report the find and ask the inevitable question, "What is it doing here?"[1(p. 193)] Despite these glitches, plan B continued to make faster progress than its "competitors." By the end of September, Minister Golborne could announce that the miners would be freed by the second half of October.[1(p. 209)]

On October 2, 2010, the minister reported on the status of the three strategies. Plan A would require an additional 30 days to create the first shaft, after which it would have to widen its entire length with another round of drilling. Although plan B was temporarily stalled in order to change its hammerhead, it was already two-thirds of the way drilling the full 28-inch wide tunnel. Plan C was also drilling the wider opening, but had reached only one-third of its length. Barring further mishaps, plan B seemed to be headed for success, and final plans for the rescue were put in place.[41]

While the drilling of the shaft received the most attention, the vehicle that would bring the miners to the surface was also of vital importance. The model was the *Dahlbusch Bomb*, a German system developed in 1955 when three miners were trapped in a German coal mine following an underground fire.[42] The system had been redeployed several times since then in different mining rescue operations. Its construction was entrusted to the Chilean navy, who, in turn, consulted Clinton Craig, the NASA engineer who had been sent to Chile. Other than the diameter and the overall height for the device, there were no specifications.[31] Craig returned to the United States and convened 20 NASA engineers to produce a design that would meet the needs of the "internauts." After listing the functions that the capsule had to perform, they developed a comprehensive list of 75 elements that needed to be incorporated into its design. No detail, however small, was overlooked. The capsule had to be operated by a single person; it also had to withstand the friction of traveling up and down the mine shaft, so it had to have lateral wheels. It needed a window or a mesh door to allow for ventilation and visual access to the surrounding shaft. The floor of the capsule had to be able to open up in case it got stuck and the passenger had to rappel down to the shelter. A consultation with medical experts yielded additional features: The capsule had to include an oxygen tank, a light, and a flat space in the bottom of the pod for the men to stretch their legs.[31] Other requirements were a camera, a biomedical monitor, and a means of two-way communication. With these and other specifications, the Chilean navy went to work. In the process, what NASA had called the "escape pod" and the Chileans called the "rescue capsule" was baptized the *Fénix*, or Phoenix, conjuring the image of the mythical bird that rose from the ashes. In keeping with the contingency planning that was the hallmark of the entire rescue, it was decided to have "a pair and a spare": Three Phoenixes with slight variations among them were built, each ready to raise the 33 from the depths of the mine.[43(p. 23)]

On September 25, the test capsule arrived at the mine, where it was greeted with applause from the inhabitants of Camp Hope. Phoenix 1 looked like a space capsule, although it was designed for an altogether different environment. It was not self-propelled, but rather relied on an Australian-made system of pulleys and a large crane to move it up and down the shaft.[44] It was, in effect, a highly customized elevator that would bring the men up the mine and into the sunlight. Sporting the colors of the Chilean flag, the Phoenix 1 weighed 924 pounds and had an interior height of 6 feet, 4 inches. Its interior diameter measured 21 inches, which meant that the more corpulent miners would face a tight squeeze. The vehicle had retractable side wheels to ease its passage as it traveled down the hole, and a bottom hatch that would allow the men to exit if necessary.[45] It was now poised to be tested; but first, the opening had to be completed.

On the morning of October 9, 33 days after it had begun and 1 day ahead of Sougarret's estimate, plan B broke through. The "cesarean section on Mother Earth" was done.[46] The last struggle with the rock was won inch by inch, with repeated stops to check that all was well.

With the drill jutting more than 2 feet into the miners' workshop, the job was completed. There was now a 28-inch opening descending more than 2,000 feet into the mine. Jeff Hart, who was at the controls when the Schramm T130 reached its target, thought that his heart had exploded before realizing that he had just completed "the most difficult hole [he] had ever drilled."[47] The celebration was commensurate with the previous ordeal. Inside the mine, the effect was almost as dramatic as the initial cave-in. The final burst caused a dust storm reminiscent of the *piston*, but this time the flying debris represented liberation rather than entrapment. As the men "hugged and hooted,"[1(p. 226)] the rescuers were enjoying their own celebration. Jeff Hart was showered with champagne and all of Camp Hope seemed to erupt in a frenzy of joy, relief, and pent-up feelings. The hundreds of journalists who had descended on the Atacama were now part of the celebratory party, although the final chapter of the evolving narrative was still pending.

The technical staff still had a lot of work to do. Plan A, which was the slowest, was aborted; plan C was continued in case a backup was needed. Now the authorities and their experts had to decide whether or not the shaft, once completed, should be sheathed with metal tubing. Installing a casing would reinforce the shaft and make it safer; moreover, the casing would provide a smoother surface for the wheels of the Phoenix. But it would delay the actual rescue by 3 to 7 days, which also had inherent risks. The tubing was estimated to weigh 400 tons, and would require a special crane to install it.[1(p. 202)] Moreover, it would have to be installed in sections, any one of which could buckle and jam. The risks and benefits of each alternative had to be carefully weighed. Minister Golborne urged caution, reminding everyone that no one had been rescued yet and that their task was not over until the last man had left the mine. The available evidence was presented to eight geologists, and each one gave a different answer.[6(p. 22)] Inspection videos of the opening shaft together with geological tests revealed that no casing was required other than in the section of the shaft closest to the surface. Minister Golborne announced it was not necessary to line the entire duct. Instead, only the first 315 feet, which were the most fractured, would be sheathed.[4(p. 153)] Even this careful assessment, however, was modified after being put to the test. During a probe, the metal sleeve providing the casing jammed. The hole was angled 11 degrees off vertical before plunging straight down, and the sheath had to be reduced in length by almost half: Only the first 180 feet of the shaft were encased.[48]

On October 11, Phoenix 1 was ready for its trial run. It went down into the shaft, suffering minor scratches, but basically without a hitch and even "without raising any dust,"[48] stopping some 40 feet above the miners' shelter before returning to the surface.[45] After three other trials, the vehicle was pronounced fit to do its work and the rescue was scheduled to begin the following day. Then, however, it was one of its siblings, the Phoenix 2, that was used to bring the men up.[42]

THE RESOLUTION: THE ASCENT OF "THE 33"

As the final hardware was put in place for the rescue, other aspects of the process were also underway. The men began undergoing preparations for their return home. The logistics of the process involved sending to the surface the souvenirs they had amassed during their stay in the mine. They had received sports jerseys signed by soccer star Pelé and other sports luminaries, rosaries blessed by the pope, bibles, flags, and mementos and photographs from their families. The ascending *paloma* traffic intensified as the men sent their belongings home in anticipation of their return.

A more important type of preparation required getting the men physically conditioned for the final stage of the rescue. Weeks before the Phoenix was ready to be launched, the miners had begun a regime to increase their physical fitness. They began with light calisthenics and progressed to more strenuous exercises. Although the capsule's ascent was expected to last less than half an hour, several measures were necessary to make sure the men could stand immobile for as long as an hour. In addition, the exercise regime sought to protect the men's lungs and cardiovascular health, prevent bodily fatigue, and assuage psychological stress. With few precedents to guide him, Dr. Jean Romagnoli designed an exercise regime based on a preventive model to meet the men's needs. He had been in close contact with the miners from the time they were found and had communicated with them by phone and video on an ongoing basis. Now, the men were encouraged to perform 20 minutes of aerobic exercise every day.[49] They wore biomedical monitoring equipment that allowed the medical staff above to manage each individual's routine and establish a profile for each individual based on key indicators such as heart rate, breathing rate, skin temperature, and blood pressure levels.[50] The workout was designed to raise the blood from the lower extremities to the trunk to avoid fainting, and to prevent lactic acid from building up and causing cramps. The regime also included cardiovascular exercises to burn fat. Elastic bands were sent down to help the men strengthen their arms and buttocks.[51] To illustrate the exercises, Romagnoli videotaped himself doing squats and lunges, hoping to encourage the men to get themselves in better shape for the most important trip of their lives.[52]

Additionally, the men had to be prepared to deal with what awaited them postrescue. The psychologists discussed some of the issues they could anticipate upon rejoining their families.[53] The miners also received training to face a new experience: Dealing with the news media. Because the story of the collapse, entombment, and rescue had created much interest in their shared and individual stories, the miners needed help in handling the attention that they were likely to command. An employee of the Chilean Insurance Association, the entity covering the men's medical care, began giving them media training and pointers on public speaking.[54] With the 33 men having become "among the most wired and media-savvy disaster victims in human history,"[1(p. 161)] they were aware of the general furor their story elicited. Their speech teacher, described as "practically evangelical in his effort to turn the shy and confused miners into media stars," stressed that there were financial dividends to successful use of the media; his daily lectures soon became quite popular.[1(p. 191)] The lecturer began with the basics: the differences between an interview and a press conference, the need to focus only on the questions asked, and how to tell their personal tale in the best way possible.[5(p. 140)] These pointers were supplemented with three memoranda prepared by one of the team psychologists working with several journalists and intellectual property lawyers. The titles of the memos indicate their scope and content: "Post-Rescue: Proposed Suggestions," "Possible Questions You May Be Facing," and "Suggestions for Dealing with the Press."[24(p. 82–83)]

Finally, the men were outfitted and prepared to deal with the ascent to the surface. The trip on the Phoenix 2 was meticulously planned to meet the needs of the men and their families. The rescue team was also attentive to how the event would unfold before the eyes of the world. By the time the capsule was ready to extricate the men from the mine, some 2,000 news reporters were camped out in the vicinity of the mine.[55] With the repeated ascents of Phoenix 2 being transmitted in real time in Chile and beyond, no detail of the disaster's final resolution would escape notice.[56]

Because the rescue capsule was likely to twist around several times during its 15- to 20-minute trip, the men faced the possibility of motion sickness. They were therefore switched to a diet of liquids, vitamins, and minerals, and told to abstain from food during the 6 hours prior to their ascent.[57] What was expected to be their last meal in the mine consisted of some salt, french fries, and an energy drink favored by athletes.[4(p. 157)]

Although the miners would emerge one by one, they would all be wearing similar clothes and follow the same protocol. Each miner received new socks and underwear, a sweater, and a green moisture-resistant, fireproof jumpsuit with his name embroidered on the chest.[57] The men also got helmets, gloves, and special sunglasses designed to protect them from the sun's ultraviolet rays when exiting the capsule. The helmet was equipped with communication gear so that the rescue team could keep constant contact with each man during his trip through the shaft. Each miner would also wear a bio-medical belt with vital signs sensors that would be monitored by the medical staff on the surface. In the event of a panic attack or any other problem, the staff would be able to talk to the miner and reassure him. Moreover, the speed of the winch could be increased to shorten travel time.[58]

With everything in place for the rescue to begin, the first of six rescue workers was winched down to the mine the night of October 12. Their role was to assess each miner's condition and prepare him for his ascent; they made sure each man wore the biomonitor belt, was harnessed inside the capsule, and carried sunglasses to wear as soon as he approached the glare of the sun and the many cameras that were waiting for him. The order of ascent had already been set, but the list was not publicized until shortly before the rescue. First to be extricated were "the most capable"; these tended to be not only the healthiest, but also the most skilled in handling the equipment. The minister of health described the requirements as follows: "They have to be psychologically mature, have a great deal of mining experience, and be able to handle quick training on how to use the harness and oxygen mask in the Phoenix capsule."[59] The rationale for this was that the initial group should be able to address any glitches, and let their fellow miners know what to expect. This initial group was followed by the weakest and ill, and included a diabetic, a hypertensive, and others who had dental infections or skin lesions. The rest would follow in a predetermined order, with the shift foreman the last to ascend.[60]

In the early morning of October 13, *Operación San Lorenzo* entered its final stage. Under the glare of the media, each miner made his trip on the Phoenix 2, emerging to the cheers of the rescue team, the emotional welcome of his family, the interest of the media, and the amazement of the one billion persons who watched from all points of the globe. Following the prescribed reentry protocol, each miner met with three family members of his choosing before being greeted by President Piñera, Minister Golborne, and key members of the rescue team. The miner then went through an inflatable tunnel and was taken by gurney to a medical triage station, where he underwent a 2-hour physical examination, received antibiotics, and had a special eye examination. From there, each miner was flown to Copiapó Regional Hospital, a 15-minute helicopter flight. Each was to remain in the hospital at least 2 days, for stabilization and observation. There, those with problems would be treated.[18]

The ascent of the 33 was as smooth as the prior wait and uncertainty had been difficult, and each miner emerged in his own way: raucous and cheering, quietly thankful, shy and bewildered, or praying and reverent. Beating the estimated time of arrival, all of the 33 were extricated in less than 23 hours. Then the 6 rescue workers were brought to the surface. Before embarking on the last trip of the Phoenix 2, however, they unfurled a banner saying "Mission Accomplished Chile." The first rescue worker to enter the mine was the last to leave. Once he was on the surface and Operation San Lorenzo had ended, President Piñera placed a metal lid over the rescue shaft, thereby sealing the mine.[6(p. 25)]

The rescue was indeed over, and all of Chile rejoiced in the outcome of what could have been a tragic disaster. With all the miners on the surface, the president requested that all place their helmets on their chest and sing the *canción nacional*, or national anthem, thus concluding the public act of celebration. The Chilean president described the rescue operation as "so marvelous, so clean, so emotional, that there was no reason not to allow the world to see it."[61] The media described the rescue as "flawless," and President Barack Obama pronounced it a "tribute not only to the determination of the rescue workers and the Chilean government but also the unity of the Chilean people who have inspired the world."[62]

AFTERMATH OF THE RESCUE

After acknowledging the end of the 33's long shift, President Piñera stated that neither Chile nor the miners would ever be the same again. In fact, what the miners experienced during the 69 days they were trapped was likely to mark them for life. Although the psychologists who treated the miners repeatedly extolled their resiliency, most of the 33 have suffered symptoms of posttraumatic stress disorder (PTSD). They had been counseled that their lives were likely to change, but many did not fully grasp the degree to which the experience in the mine would upend their work, their family relations, and their sense of self.

The Chilean Insurance Association, which covered the miners' health services, extended their coverage for 6 months following the rescue. For some, this was not long enough to resolve their health issues. Although the psychologists urged the men to give themselves "time and space,"[63(p. 65)] a year later most were still processing the experience and manifesting a variety of behaviors suggestive of PTSD. These include intrusive disturbances (nightmares, flashbacks), avoidance (establishing a distance from the experience), and hyperarousal (reacting to loud noises, bright lights, and sudden events).[64] Dr. Jean Romagnoli, who supervised their care while they were in the mine, believes that it is the men's present circumstances rather than their past ordeal that has traumatized them: "They are taking uppers, downers, stabilizers. It is not pills they need, but the tools to deal with fame and the tools to renovate themselves."[65] The physician's view is that the men have not had alternative employment, and that, rather than PTSD, is at the root of their problems. He sees the men as suffering from broken promises: "They were promised jobs with Codelco [the state mining company]. There were many promises that were seemingly gone with the wind or swallowed by the mine."[66] Although each man received approximately $10,000 and the gift of a motorcycle from a Chilean philanthropist, and benefited from trips to Disney World, England, and the Holy Land, these perquisites have not replaced the stability of a job.

The murky occupational picture has, in turn, led to financial uncertainty. Not long after the disaster, the owners of the San José mine filed for bankruptcy, putting the survivors out of work. Under Chilean law, the miners are first in line to receive the proceeds from the sale of the company's assets, a process that is subject to litigation.[6(p. 25)] In the meantime, the miners have found different means to support themselves. Four went back to mining, but two decided they could not handle the inevitable flashbacks and fears. Most of the men have sought other options. Fourteen of the 33 applied for retirement benefits, and after August 22, 2011, they began receiving monthly benefits.[67] Seven went on medical leave, largely because they suffer from sleep disturbances. Five of the men are small businessmen or have begun selling food and produce, and one is studying electronics.[66] The more mediagenic have been able to parlay their experience, fame, and talents into trips and motivational speeches, cobbling together new careers for themselves.

All 33 miners still hope for settlements from two lawsuits that have been filed. The first is against the government agency that oversees mine safety, holding it accountable for allowing the San José mine to continue operating despite repeated violations and sanctions. The miners seek $541,000 each in their suit.[65] In addition, the men are suing the mine owners for an undetermined amount. The government is also suing the owners of the mine, hoping to recover the $18 million they spent on the rescue.[6(p. 25)] All of these lawsuits are expected to take a long time to be resolved.

The men also expect to reap financial benefits from the sale of their story. Before they were rescued, the 33 made a pact not to sell literary or movie rights to their shared ordeal unless all benefited equally. Negotiations leading to a final deal took time; even more than a year later, when both movie and book deals have been signed, any payoff is well in the future.

While the increased visibility of the miners has made them celebrities, it has also made them targets. Some Chileans have criticized them for suing the government after the state did so much to rescue them.[67] Additionally, other miners have turned on them, stating that the 33 have benefited from the collapse and have not advocated for measures that could help all miners. The 33 have also been accused of becoming "too cozy" with the government and cashing in on their fame.[68]

The collapse of the mine at Copiapó has therefore come full circle, from disaster to survival and successful rescue to a kind of political tug-of-war and even reality show. The story continues to unfold as the miners remake the lives that took an unwanted and unexpected turn on August 5, 2010. At times, their individual stories have eclipsed their collective experience and the far-ranging and well-orchestrated activities that led to their rescue. While it is often said that the miners "rescued themselves" through their own organization and the careful husbanding of their limited resources, there is no doubt that others were also instrumental in the operation's final success. The rescue team's achievements cannot be overstated: Never had so many been rescued from so deep after so many days. There were setbacks and glitches, diverse opinions and moments of tension. But at each step of the way, good planning, scientific data, practical know-how, and global technology were brought to bear in the decision-making process. "What if . . . ?" was invariably asked, and there was always a hedge against any risk or gamble. With 33 lives at stake, Chile resolved to rescue the miners regardless of time and cost. In the process, the rescue team made history by developing a number of best practices that had never been tried before, and effectively rewrote the book on disaster management.

DISCUSSION QUESTIONS

1. Which competencies described in the Appendix does this case demonstrate?
2. There were several key decision points over the course of the 2 months during which the rescue took place. What were these, and how were they resolved?
3. Any major endeavor in disaster management health involves trade-offs. What were some of the trade-offs made during the Copiapó rescue? Indicate the rationale behind the decisions made.
4. What was the leadership role assumed by the various stakeholders?
5. Which specific national, cultural, and religious values did the rescue operation incorporate? What purposes did these serve?
6. Many disciplines and areas of expertise were brought to bear during the rescue operation. What were some of these, and how did they contribute to the final outcome?

REFERENCES

1. Franklin J. *33 Men*. New York, NY: G.P. Putnam's Sons; 2011.
2. Gavshon MH, Magratten D. Chilean miners rescued, but were they saved? *CBSNews*. August 22, 2011. Available at: http://www.cbsnews.com/8301-18560_162-20093598.html. Accessed March 19, 2013.
3. Sequera V. Straight-talking engineer was behind Chile rescue. *LubbockOnline.com*. October 16, 2010. Available at: http://lubbockonline.com/world/2010-10-16/straight-talking-engineer-was-behind-chilean-miners-rescue. Accessed March 17, 2013.
4. Pino Toro M. *Buried Alive*. New York, NY: Palgrave Macmillan; 2011.
5. Cherwin A. *Rescate: La Historia de los 33*. México: Grijalbo; 2011.
6. Useem M, Jordan R, Koljatic M. Leading the rescue of the miners in Chile. 2011. Available at: http://kw.wharton.upenn.edu/wdp/files/2011/07/Leading-the-Miners-Rescue.pdf. Accessed March 20, 2013.
7. Wurgaft R. El jefe del rescate, André Sougarret, se muestra cauteloso. *El Mundo*. October 12, 2010. Available at: http://www.elmundo.es/america/2010/10/12/noticias/1286838442.html. Accessed March 20, 2013.

8. Time, heat could take toll on trapped miners. *NBCNews.com*. Available at: http://msnbc.msn.com/id/38816833/ns/world_news-americas/t/t. Accessed March 17, 2013.

9. Fuentes F, Rodríguez M, Pizarro C. André Sougarret: "Yo dependo de lo que diga el presidente, pero hasta ahora me quedo." *La Tercera*. August 23, 2010. Available at: http://diario.latercera.com/2010/08/23/01/contenido/pais/31-36352-9-andre-sougarret-yo-dependo-de-lo-que-diga-el-presidente-pero-hasta-ahora-me.shtml. Accessed March 19, 2013.

10. Ibáñez C. *Los 33 de Atacama y Su Rescate*. Santiago, Chile: Origo Ediciones; 2010.

11. Useem M. *The Leader's Checklist, Expanded Edition: 15 Mission-Critical Principles*. Philadelphia, PA: Wharton Digital Press; 2011.

12. Iturra A. Rescate minero: un referente mundial [video]. January 25, 2011. Available at: www.youtube.com/watch=AOcAPNfhvig. Accessed July 11, 2011.

13. Franklin J, Tran M. Trapped Chilean miners start receiving food and water. *The Guardian*. August 24, 2010. Available at: http://www.guardian.co.uk/world/2010/aug/24/trapped-chilean-miners-food-water. Accessed March 19, 2013.

14. Moffett M. Inventions ease the plight of trapped miners. *The Wall Street Journal*. September 30, 2010. Available at: http://online.wsj.com/article/SB10001424052748704116004575522343755639692.html. Accessed March 20, 2013.

15. National Institute for Health and Clinical Excellence (NICE). *Drug Therapy Guideline No. 46.00: Guidelines for the Prevention and Treatment of Adult Patients at Risk of Developing Refeeding Syndromes*. London, England: Author; 2007.

16. Bonnefoy P, Mackey R. Miners no longer forced to order in. *The New York Times*. October 15, 2010. Available at: http://thelede.blogs.nytimes.com/2010/10/10/15/miners-no-longer-forced-to-order-in/. Accessed July 14, 2011.

17. Fresenius Kabi. Supportan drink product features. Available at: http://www2.fresenius-kabi.com/internet/kabi/gb/fkintpub.nsf/Content/Product+Features+Supportan+Drink. Accessed March 20, 2013.

18. McNeil DG Jr. Defying predictions, miners kept healthy. *The New York Times*. October 13, 2010. Available at: http://www.nytimes.com/2010/10/14/world/americas/14medical.html?pagewanted=all&_r=0. Accessed March 20, 2013.

19. Barrionuevo A. Trapped Chilean miners forge refuge. *New York Times*. August 31, 2010. Available at: http://www.nytimes.com/2010/09/01/world/americas/01chile.html?pagewanted=all&_r=0. Accessed March 19, 2013.

20. Mosteiro JP, Sukni F. La angustia de la mina se combate con liderazgo, disciplina, y objetivos. *La Gaceta*. September 25, 2010. Available at: http://www.intereconomia.com/noticias-gaceta/internacional/%E2%80%9C-angustia-mina-se-combate-liderazgo-disciplina-y-objetivos%E2%80%9D. Accessed March 20, 2013.

21. Peregil F. La NASA se posa en la mina San José. *El País*. September 4, 2010. Available at: http://elpais.com/diario/2010/09/04/internacional/1283551208_850215.html. Accessed March 20, 2013.

22. Salud mental y catástrofes: el caso del rescate de los 33 mineros sepultados en Chile. *Norte de Salud Mental*. 2011;9(39):56–70.

23. Entwistle J. NASA provides assistance to the Chilean miners. Nasa Blogs website. October 29, 2010. Available at: http://blogs.nasa.gov/cm/blog/NES _Teachers_Corner/posts/post_1286984937675.html. Accessed March 20, 2013.

24. Ibáñez C. Psicología positiva y catástrofes: el caso del rescate de los 33 mineros de Chile. *Norte de Salud Mental.* 2011; 9(39):68–70.

25. Franklin J. Luis Urzúa, the foreman keeping hope alive for Chile's trapped miners. *The Observer.* September 4, 2010. Available at: http://www.guardian .co.uk/world/2010/sep/05/luis-urzua-chile-trapped-miners. Accessed March 19, 2013.

26. NASA psychologist assists trapped Chilean miners [Morning Edition transcript]. National Public Radio. October 5, 2010. Available at: http://www .npr.org/templates/story/story.php?storyId=130342897. Accessed March 20, 2013.

27. Franklin J. We know best: doctors tussle with miners. *The Sydney Morning Herald.* September 18, 2010. Available at: http://www.smh.com.au/action /printArticle?id=1933967. Accessed July 15, 2011.

28. Mineros chilenos piden 'reggaeton' y rancheras. *El Siglo de Torreón.* August 31, 2010. Available at: http://www.elsiglodetorreon.com.mx/noticia/553773 .mineros-chilenos. Accessed July 22, 2011.

29. Álvarez R. Golborne decidió levantar la censura a las cartas que envían familiares a los 33 mineros. *AreaMinera.* September 8, 2010. Available at: http://www .aminera.com/noticias-2010-mineria/27166.html. Accessed July 22, 2011.

30. Mineros de Chile cumplieron un mes atrapados: están "cansados." 26Noticias website. Available at: http://www.26noticias.com.ar/mineros-de-chile -cumplieron-un-mes-atrapados-estan-cansados-117246.html. Accessed March 20, 2013.

31. Parker L. To design miners' escape pod, NASA thought small. AOL Original. October 9, 2010. Available at: http://www.aolnews.com/2010/10/09/to -design-miners-escape-pod-nasa-thought-small/. Accessed March 20, 2013.

32. Yang J. From collapse to rescue: inside the Chile mine disaster. *TheStar. com* October 10, 2010. Available at: http://www.thestar.com/news /world/2010/10/10/from_collapse_to_rescue_inside_the_chile_mine _disaster.html. Accessed March 20, 2013.

33. Emergency mine rescue [NOVA video]. PBS. October 26, 2010. Available at: http://www.pbs.org/wgbh/nova/tech/emergency-mine-rescue.html. Accessed March 20, 2013.

34. Walsh E. Why American drilling hero Jeff Hart will not be at Chile mine for miners rescue. *San Francisco Examiner.* October 12, 2010. Available at: http:// www.examiner.com/article/why-american-drilling-hero-jeff-hart-will-not -be-at-chile-mine-for-miners-rescue. Accessed March 20, 2013.

35. Butler S. UPS moves a mountain of machinery for trapped Chilean miners. UPS website. September 17, 2010. Available at: http://blog.ups.com/2010/09 /17/ups-moves-a-mountain-of-machinery-f. Accessed July 28, 2011.

36. Fountain H. Plan B turns out to be fastest path for rescue. *The New York Times.* October 12, 2010. Available at: http://nytimes.com/2010/10/13 /world/americas/13rock.html?pa. Accessed July 27, 2011.

37. Chilean miners' families file $27 million lawsuit. *Latin American Herald Tribune.* Available at: http://www.laht.com/article.asp?ArticleId=368954&C ategoryId=14094. Accessed August 18, 2011.
38. Chile mine rescue chief: how we dug out the miners. *BreakingNews.* October 16, 2010. Available at: http://www.breakingnews.ie/world/chile-mine-rescue -chief-how-we-dug-out-the-miners-477900.html. Accessed March 19, 2013.
39. Golborne L. Management in times of crisis: the miners' rescue. Lecture given at: National Museum of Natural History, Smithsonian Institution; October 11, 2011; Washington, DC.
40. U.S. State Department. Timeline of Chilean mine rescue, IIP/WHA. Bureau of International Information Programs, Western Hemisphere Affairs; 2011.
41. Detienen 2 de 3 perforaciones para rescate de mineros en Chile. *Milenio.* October 2, 2010. Available at: http://www.milenio.com/cdb/doc/noticias2011 /d9cff78f9e4c88e6e0efd703f4f077e8. Accessed March 20, 2013.
42. NASA-designed capsule helps free Chilean miners. *The Engineer.* October 13, 2010. Available at: http://www.theengineer.co.uk/channels/design -engineering/news/nasa-designed-capsule-helps-free-chilean-miners /1005467.article. Accessed March 20, 2013.
43. Stromberg J. Deep thinking: the rescue team devised—and tested—new technology to save the miners. *Smithsonian.* January 2012:23.
44. 'Phoenix' sparks hope for trapped miners. *France 24.* September 26, 2010. Available at: http://www.france24.com/en/print/5098133?print=now. Accessed August 3, 2011.
45. How the Phoenix capsule works. *FoxNews.* October 12, 2010. Available at: http://www.foxnews.com/scitech/2010/10/12/phoenix-rescue-capsule-save -chilean-miners/. Accessed March 19, 2013.
46. Kraul C. Chile rejoices as all miners are rescued. *Los Angeles Times.* October 14, 2010. Available at: http://articles.latimes.com/2010/Oct/14/world/la -fg-chile-miner-rescue. Accessed June 22, 2011.
47. Warren M. Jeff Hart, Chile mine driller from Denver, becomes rescue hero. *HuffPost Denver.* October 9, 2010. Available at: http://www.huffingtonpost .com/2010/10/09/jeff-hart-chile-mine-dril_n_757060.html. Accessed March 20, 2013.
48. Trapped Chilean miners prepare for ride to freedom. *NBCNews.com.* October 11, 2010. Available at: Available at: http://www.nbcnews.com/id/39612897 /ns/world_news-americas/. Accessed March 20, 2013.
49. Sherwell P. Trapped Chilean miners emerge to fame, movie contracts— and angry wives. *The Telegraph.* October 9, 2010. Available at: http://www .telegraph.co.uk/news/worldnews/southamerica/chile/8052941/Trapped -Chile-miners-emerge-to-fame-movie-contracts-and-angry-wives.html. Accessed March 20, 2013.
50. Zephyr Company. Case study: Zephyr provides physiological monitoring of Chilean miners during San José Mine rescue operation. Available at: http://www.zephyr-technology.com/media/CaseStudies/ZCS -007-CaseStudy-HC_ChileanMinerRescueOperation.pdf. Accessed March 20, 2013.

51. Moffett M. Chile miners work out before rescue. *The Wall Street Journal.* October 7, 2010. Available at: http://online.wsj.com/article/SB1000142405 2748704689804575536490309185222.html. Accessed March 20, 2013.

52. Special exercises for trapped Chilean miners [video]. *Wall Street Journal.* October 6, 2010. Available at: http://online.wsj.com/article/CC432ACF-2A07-4467 -83E9-3D62C8A6C354.html#!CC432ACF-2A07-4467-83E9-3D62C8A6C354. Accessed March 20, 2013.

53. Ibarra A. La última carta del sicólogo a los mineros: "Hay una vida nueva a tu disposición." *El Mercurio.* October 23, 2010. Available at: http://www.emol. com/noticias/nacional/2010/10/23/443094/la-ultima-carta-del-sicologo-a -los-mineros-hay-una-vida-nueva-a-tu-disposicion.html. Accessed March 19, 2013.

54. Scholfield P. Chile's trapped miners: monitored and media-trained. *BBC News.* September 22, 2010. Available at: http://www.bbc.co.uk/news/mobile /world-latin-america-11388894. Accessed August 5, 2011.

55. Kraul C. Health experts monitoring trapped miners in Chile brace for unexpected ailments. *Los Angeles Times.* October 11, 2010. Available at: http:// articles.latimes.com/2010/oct/11/world/la-fg-chile-miners-medical-20101011. Accessed March 19, 2013.

56. Torrens M. Bienvenidos al circo minero. *LaInformacion.com.* October 13, 2010. Available at: http://noticias.lainformacion.com/mundo/bienvenidos-al -circo-minero_nsJPUwi7a4ZZAFLPZC8Pm1/. Accessed March 20, 2013.

57. Rescue crews test "Phoenix 1" capsule in Chile. *NECN/CNN.* October 11, 2011. Available at: http://www.necn.com/pages/print_landing?blockID=329 591&feedID. Accessed August 3, 2011.

58. Padgett T. Chile celebrates as miners emerge from underground. *Time.* October 13, 2010. Available at: http://www.time.com/time/printout/0,8816, 2025106,00.html. Accessed July 22, 2011.

59. Cunningham B. Drilling rig reaches trapped Chilean miners leading to rescue. *SMN.* October 11, 2010. Available at: http://www.realestateradiousa .com/2010/10/11/drilling-rig-reaches-trapped-chilean-miners-leading-to -rescue-video/. Accessed March 19, 2013.

60. Chilean miners prepare for rescue operation. *BreakingNews.* October 12, 2010. Available at: http://www.breakingnews.ie/world/chilean-miners-prepare -for-rescue-operation-477406.html. Accessed March 19, 2013.

61. All 33 Chilean miners rescued in flawless operation. *FoxNews.* October 13, 2010. Available at: http://www.foxnews.com/world/2010/10/12/rescued -chilean-miner-returns-surface/. Accessed March 19, 2013.

62. Jackson D. Obama: Chile mine rescue has "inspired the world." *USA Today.* October 13, 2010. Available at: http://content.usatoday.com/communities /theoval/post/2010/10/obama-chile-mine-rescue-has-inspired-the-world/1. Accessed March 20, 2013.

63. Iturra A. Una experiencia de intervención psicológica en catástrofes: el caso de los 33 mineros chilenos. *Norte de salud mental.* 2011; IX(39): 63–67.

64. Zimmerman R. Buried alive: how will mental health of Chilean miners fare? MedScape website. Available at: http://www.medscape.com/viewarticle /730393. Accessed May 18, 2011.

65. Franklin J. Chilean miners live in poverty a year after saga. *The Washington Post*. August 4, 2011. Available at: http://articles.washingtonpost.com/2011 -08-04/world/35268981_1_chilean-miners-jean-romagnoli-epic-rescue. Accessed March 19, 2013.

66. Rausell F. No tenemos donde caernos muertos. *El Nuevo Día*. August 5, 2011. Available at: http://www.elnuevodia.com/notenemosdondecaernos-muertos-1032002.html. Accessed March 19, 2013.

67. Los 33 mineros de Chile: un año después de su famoso rescate de las entrañas de la tierra. *Progreso Hoy*. August 3, 2011. Available at: http://www .progresohoy.com/noticias/n-455/. Accessed March 20, 2013.

68. Vergara E. Protesters throw fruit at Chile's rescued miners. *The Washington Post*. August 6, 2011: A13.

7

The Lessons of Tragedy: The 2004 Madrid Train Bombings

Pietro D. Marghella and Isaac Ashkenazi

INTRODUCTION

Just 1 year after the Al Qaeda attacks on 9/11, David Campbell, the former CEO of St. Vincent's Medical Center in New York City, was invited to address the plenary session of the annual American College of Healthcare Executives' Congress in Chicago, Illinois. Shortly after the attacks, Campbell wrote an important article about the experience he and his staff encountered as the level I trauma center closest to the World Trade Center.[1] In that article, Campbell detailed eight lessons learned (which will be discussed later in this case) that were intended to help healthcare organizations become better prepared for dealing with the aftermath of mass casualty events.

In addition to discussing the important lessons for hospital organizations learned as a result of the historically unprecedented attack, Campbell issued a clear warning to the assembled healthcare executives:

> 9/11 should be considered a *catastrophic casualty anomaly*, in that there were more fatalities than there were survivors requiring critical care support. Had the reverse been true, it is arguable whether the healthcare infrastructure of New York City and its surrounding environs could have absorbed the casualty load and provided adequate resources to support the victims.[2]

He called for enhanced disaster planning at the organizational level and emphasized the importance of coordinating it into a community-wide plan.

In the United States, the issue is, in part, one of surge capacity. In a system dominated by managed care, hospital beds are profit centers. As such, hospitals must maintain maximum bed capacity in order to remain profitable. The net result is that the vast majority of our hospitals—especially those in urban areas, which are also the highest threat venues for terrorist attacks and large-scale disasters—are forced to operate with little to no excess capacity for sudden spikes in patient loads. In the event of an attack or disaster where the 9/11 paradigm is reversed, there will be "no room at the inn," and healthcare infrastructure in the area closest to the locus of the event will run the risk of imploding.[3]

A second issue is one of *siloization*. Siloization is used to describe disparate organizational entities with a common mission focus—such as hospitals and the mission of healthcare delivery (*and* disaster response).[4] Under normal (albeit, dysfunctional) conditions, the "silos" exercise vertical leadership within their own organizational continuums. This prevents them from seeking collaboration and sup-port from one another for the purpose of bolstering or improving their overall efficacy to maintain their mission when environmental duress (i.e., a disaster) descends. Under these conditions, the silos should be considered at-risk of collapse when that duress descends.

Whether a function of an overall lack of surge capacity or the inability to break out of their silos and work together for the common mission of pre-event coordinated response, this is exactly what happened to the healthcare infrastructure of Madrid, Spain, in the wake of the terrorist attack on the *Cercanias* (commuter train system) on the morning of March 11, 2004 (called 11-M). According to the U.S. Defense Intelligence Agency's *Defense Executive Intelligence Review*, published just one day after the attacks, "The 11 March train bombings in Madrid resulted in a mass casualty incident that over-whelmed the disaster response system. Local ambulance services and hospital emergency department resources were woefully inadequate to handle the estimated 1,500 casualties, many with serious trauma and burn injuries."[5]

It is important to note that Madrid is a highly westernized metrop-olis with a well-developed and modern medical and public health infrastructure sector. It therefore seems somewhat incongruous that its infrastructure should so quickly collapse under the weight of a disaster event that produced a casualty load of 2,062 victims (the official Spanish government casualty toll of the attack). In an era where it is entirely reasonable to expect that there will be future ter-rorist attacks generating catastrophic levels of casualties, this event stands as an important marker to help preclude similar collapses from occurring. The purpose of this case is to examine the conditions of the Madrid train bombing disaster and the attendant inability of the healthcare infrastructure to adequately absorb the casualty load.

THE ANATOMY OF THE ATTACK RESPONSE

The attack consisted of a total of 10 explosions aboard 4 commuter trains during the peak of the Madrid rush hour on a Thursday morn-ing (see **Figure 7-1**). All of the affected trains were traveling on the same line and in the same direction between *Alcalá de Henares* and the *Atocha* station in Madrid. It was later reported that, in all, 13 improvised explosive devices (IEDs) had been placed on the trains. The explosions took place between 7:39 AM and 7:42 AM, and all emer-gency services were immediately alerted.

Figure 7-1

10 bombs in 4 commuter trains.

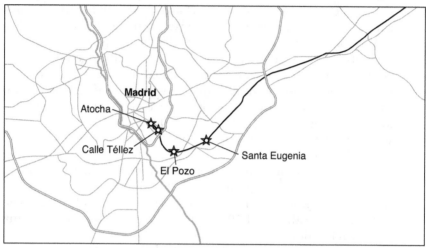

Station	Time of attack	Number dead	Number injured
Atocha	07:38	29	115
Calle Téllez	07:39	64	165
El Pozo	07:41	67	56
Santa Eugenia	07:42	27	52

Source: Adapted from interactive infographic 'Madrid train bombings: March 11, 2004' guardian.co.uk © Guardian News and Media Limited 2011.

Initial emergency treatment and triage was carried out by emergency medical services (EMS) near the scenes of the blasts, and the victims were subsequently transferred to Gregorio Marañón University General Hospital (GMUGH) and Doce de Octubre University General Hospital, among other hospitals, including Clínico San Carlos, Hospital de la Princesa, Hospital de la Paz, Hospital Fundación de Alcorcón, the El Niño Jesús Hospital, and the Hospital Central de la Defensa. A small field hospital was also set up by the Servicio de Asistencia Municipal de Urgencia y Rescate (SAMUR)—Madrid's emergency medical system—in a sports facility in an area near the *Atocha* station attack zone. The vast majority of survivors were evacuated by ambulance, and many others were taken to hospitals and temporary treatment locations by private vehicles. Most casualties arrived at treatment facilities between 8:00 AM and 11:00 AM. According to official information, by 9:00 PM that evening, 1,430 casualties had been treated, 966 of whom were taken to 15 public community hospitals. The 2 largest public hospitals in Madrid, GMUGH and Doce de Octubre University General Hospital (with 1,800 and 1,300 beds, respectively), received around 53% of those casualties. The other victims were treated in primary care facilities and near the scenes of the blasts. Many other casualties with mild injuries were received at different facilities on the days following the blasts. Very few patients were taken to private hospitals. As noted, the explosions resulted in 2,062 casualties, 177 (8.6%) of which were immediate deaths at the scene. There were 14 subsequent deaths (in-hospital deaths) that occurred either on the same day or later on among the 82 victims who were reported to be in critical condition at 9:00 PM that day, bringing the total death toll to 191. According to official information from the Spanish government, the resources mobilized to care for the wounded and their families were unprecedented, with over 70,000 health personnel involved, 291 ambulances for transport, 200 firefighters, 13 groups of psychologists, 500 volunteers, thousands of donations of blood at hospitals and in 10 mobile units, and 1,725 blood donors from other regions of the country. The 112 emergency communication centers that were set up to handle calls from concerned citizens received more than 20,000 phone calls during the morning of the blasts.[6]

DISCUSSION

While an enormous amount of credit is due to all of the individuals involved with the response to the bombings, the events were nonetheless systemically overwhelming to the medical infrastructure of the city and merit careful analysis in order to extrapolate lessons learned.

Lopez-Carresi[7] breaks down the response failures into two categories: those that could be attributable the overall disaster response system of Madrid (and, by extension, Spain, as the event easily qualifies as an incident of national significance) and those that could be attributable directly to the medical system (although it should be noted that the two are clearly related to each other).

The disaster system response failures included the following:

- No existing interagency emergency planning to accommodate a response to a major incident.
- Disorganized treatment and lack of appropriate prioritization in the transportation of victims, leading to high numbers of uncontrolled evacuations.

- Contradictory orders from different response managers (i.e., lack of unified command and a designated incident commander).
- Each EMS response agency had its own radio frequency, they were incompatible with one another, and there were no tactical channels for responders in the field.
- No use of a standardized triage system or triage tags, leading to confusion between the triage system acuity ratings and the triage tag acuity designators.
- Multiple advanced life support (ALS) teams concentrating their efforts on one patient while leaving many others unattended (i.e., unwillingness of medical providers to accept a degradation in the standard of care and adopt a "for the greater good" paradigm of triage and treatment).
- The Military Central Hospital received only 5% of the casualty load, even though it permanently maintained the largest surge capacity assets for disasters and has served as the primary casualty-receiving center for most of the region's disaster drills since the early 1990s.[7]

The medical system response failures included the following:

- Hospitals in the Madrid response network had never been exposedto a disaster and mass casualty incident of that magnitude.
- None of the hospitals—with the exception of the Military Central Hospital—had conducted drills with the local EMS to determine patient spread loading and response requirements.
- There was no proper trauma system established in Madrid, and none of the hospitals in the response network had been specifically designated and accredited as a trauma center.
- There was uncertainty of the ability of any single hospital to deal with a sudden, significant surge of critical casualties; the result was initial chaos and an uneven distribution of those casualties to the available medical facilities.
- There was difficulty in the hospitals' ability to communicate with first responders at the scenes of the blasts.
- There were deficiencies in security at the hospitals (e.g., an excess of outside voluntary personnel), identification of the casualties, and adequate record keeping.
- Most hospital staffs were not acquainted with patterns of blast injuries (i.e., lack of sensitization and clinical training on asymmetrical event threats).

THE NEW NORMAL

In the "Era of Asymmetrical Threats,"[8] it is an unfortunate reality that war, terrorism, violence, natural and man-made disasters, and pandemic disease outbreaks have made threat omnipresent in our international environments. Like both the mornings of 9/11 and 11-M, we have virtually no way of knowing when the next event will occur. However, we do know that most catastrophic casualty events that have a reasonable opportunity for occurrence (like those encapsulated in the U.S. Department of Homeland Security's *National Planning Scenarios*) have the capacity to produce casualty loads that in some cases could quite dramatically exceed those realized in the Madrid train bombings.[9]

In all cases, one could legitimately argue that the medical infrastructure of the affected region (or, in some scenarios, nation) will invariably bear the preponderant weight in supporting the affected population. Logic would argue, therefore, that if we believe that there is a reasonable chance for a future occurrence, the medical infrastructure of our nations should be taking the necessary steps to enhance our ability to deal with catastrophic casualty streams. However, just as Spain failed to absorb the lessons of 9/11 and David Campbell's warning of future risk to the medical community as a key critical infrastructure and resource sector, we've still not accomplished any substantial means of enhancing the national posture of preparedness and healthcare readiness. Consider the litany of issues that remain endemic to the vast majority of the world's healthcare infrastructure:

- Our current, virtually universal triage protocols are highly subjective and are not focused on the true value of triage in the pure public health paradigm of disasters—protecting constrained and static resources.
- We neither engage in a cyclic, constantly repetitive deliberate planning process nor have any sort of commonality of approach in how we prepare for the healthcare and public health incident management mission.
- By failing to engage in deliberate planning, we miss the most important by-product of the planning process: identifying and resourcing the requirements needed to execute the surge mission.
- We continue to rely on absurd surge concepts that will prove to be impossible or at least futile to implement when disasters

occur (e.g., freeing up minimal care beds, cancelling elective surgeries, or parking cots in halls).

- We still continue to demonstrate a willingness to accept a reliance on shelters of last resort as a surge capacity resource (e.g., the Superdome during Hurricane Katrina); it's almost impossible to imagine a worse mistake.
- National systems like the U.S. National Disaster Medical System (NDMS) are still viewed as viable surge resources and considered assets of choice by less-than-well-informed (and politically appointed) leaders.
- The issue of who is in charge often leads to a stalled death match, weakening every effort across the operational continuum to advance surge capacity and capabilities.
- No one at the local, state, or national level of response claims responsibility for or has been apportioned direct surge capacity resources to meet the mission requirements of any large-scale disaster.
- For assets at the national level that are capable of responding as surge capacity resources (e.g., military assets), there is always the issue of the "tyranny of time and distance" and the fact that much of an affected population will already be dead, dispersed, or recovered (DDR) by the time major platforms can be put in place.

So the question that begs to be asked is this: Are these issues endemic to the mission of meeting surge capacity requirements in large-scale catastrophic casualty events capable of being overcome? The authors would argue that the answer is "yes," if we take on the following measures.

We have to recognize that meeting surge capacity requirements in our healthcare and public health sectors is a common interest across the operational spectrum (i.e., local/tactical, state/operational, and national/strategic). Gerencser, Napolitano, and Van Lee[10] describe this as a "mega-community" issue, the mega-community being a public sphere in which organizations and people deliberately join together around a compelling issue of mutual importance, all following a set of practices and principles that will make it easier to achieve the desired result. Commonality of purpose helps to build resilience, which may be described as the ability to function as normally as possible in an abnormal environment.

We should consider borrowing from proven constructs from other areas of national defense. Cebrowski and Gartska[11] coined the term *network-centric warfare* to describe a method of enhancing operational effectiveness and increasing dominance in the battle space by treating warfare platforms as part of an information management and information technology (IM/IT) networked architecture. This same concept, applied to the healthcare space to create a network-centric health emergency response (NCHER), focuses on using computers, data links, networking resources, and agile processes to link emergency preparedness and response resources to a highly integrated network that shares large amounts of critical information and coordinates and manages the resources, operations, and intelligence necessary for a multifaceted response to a community threat. NCHER can reduce siloization and dramatically improve healthcare and public health delivery response capability and efficiency.

We should "dump the three-ring binders" and move away (rapidly) from a reliance on static, written planning documents.[12] The voluminous tomes we produce to demonstrate the intensity of our planning efforts are useless; they do not maintain pace with the fluidity of threats that exist in our environment, and they are outdated the minute they are placed on a shelf. We need to leverage IM/IT systems that make planning and response a constant, "rheostatable" function within our healthcare organizations. Utilizing proper planning tools can contribute markedly to enhancing surge capacity, which is largely dominated by logistical management.

There is a pressing need to adopt national policy on an effective triage protocol. As previously noted, our current triage protocols are highly subjective, as they rely on the visual stimuli and emotional resonance perceived by the individual conducting the assessment. There is a pressing need to replace these protocols with an evidence-based, quantitative approach to assessing treatment prioritization. In the disaster environment, protecting limited surge capacity resources to facilitate the "for the greater good" paradigm is paramount.

Identifying alternate treatment locations of opportunity is far different than relying on shelters of last resort. The difference in the two is only deliberate planning. If you don't prepare in advance of a disaster, your chance of an adequate response and recovery diminish in equal (but inverse) proportion to the magnitude and impact of the event. There are traditional surge capacity initiatives (e.g., siting alternate care facilities in areas geographically proximal to medical treatment facilities) that have the capacity to work in a disaster if they're done with planning, foresight, and resources in advance of the event.

There needs to be a national disaster preparedness education campaign that targets the common denominator to every community: the family unit (consider what the U.S. "Stop, Drop, and Roll" campaign did for fire safety in the 1960s). Educating people on preparedness, mitigation, and response strategies can have a direct impact on the preservation of healthcare resources and the protection of limited surge capacity assets.

At the height of the Cold War, most nations had some sort of national civil defense program to accommodate a response to a large-scale disaster. In addition to providing healthcare and public health surge capacity assets for a response, the programs helped to sensitize populations to threat. One could argue that while we have dramatically decreased the threat of nuclear Armageddon, the panoply of asymmetrical threats and increasing levels of natural disasters has increased our level of risk.

We have to retool, or create wholesale, a new and improved NDMS. In concept, the construct of the NDMS remains valuable to the United States and should be considered for replication in foreign nations at risk of any large-scale natural or man-made disasters. However, in its present state, each portion of the tripartite system has significant shortfalls that must be addressed before the NDMS can conduct operations in its expected capacity. Examples of the NDMS's shortfalls include lack of dedicated or immediately available lift for the transportation mission; significant reductions in the number of participating civilian hospitals and the closure of Veterans' Affairs and Department of Defense facilities, resulting in reductions in hospital-based surge capacity; and the persistent conundrum of pulling response assets from extant medical infrastructure when an assumption of the *National Planning Scenarios* describes the risk of near-simultaneous disasters such as opportunistic terrorist attacks.

Finally, in the same vein that military organizations resource assets for traditional national security missions, disasters must be viewed as a persistent national security and safety threat. Organizations that exist primarily as response-contracting organizations (e.g., the Federal Emergency Management Agency [FEMA]) without standing apportioned response resources will never defeat the tyranny of time and distance when disasters occur, no more than a draft plan will defeat an enemy with a delayed counterattack.

The eight lessons that Campbell[1] learned from the 9/11 experience in New York are very useful for enhancing readiness in the healthcare sector and, subsequently, enhancing surge capacity:

1. Mass casualty events, especially those involving chemical, biological, radiological, nuclear, and high-explosive (CBRNE) agents,

require regional planning for regional response. This point supports the reduction of hospital-based organizational silos and the use of a network-centric architecture for improved healthcare response to disasters.

2. The increased risk of terrorist attacks requires adding comprehensive CBRNE protocols to hospital disaster plans. This point supports the migration of plans away from static tomes and the need to enhance training to breed familiarity with events that may very well produce unusual and uncommon clinical presentations.

3. The ability to share emergency information between and among healthcare providers and government agencies must be improved. This point supports the enhanced use of IM/IT resources to help open the information, intelligence, and communications apertures among and between both disparate agencies and organizations and those that were not traditionally part of the homeland security/defense institutions (i.e., the medical and public health communities).

4. That a regionalized system for collecting and sharing key information—before, during, and following a disaster—must be implemented. This supports the previous point about leveraging IM/IT capacity and engaging pre-event deliberate planning if there is to be any hope of successfully prosecuting the medically centric incident management mission. It follows that we must embrace a culture of preparedness instead of relying on repetitive, knee-jerk reactivity to drive our response activities.

5. The important role of behavioral health services in disaster planning and response must be recognized and addressed during and after mass casualty events. Post traumatic stress disorder (PTSD) and related illnesses will dominate the long term health sequelae of large-scale disasters, especially in certain special needs populations. It is vital that this is recognized and that behavioral health professionals are engaged throughout the disaster life cycle. This point also supports the need for pre-event education and sensitization to threat to help vulnerable populations understand and prepare for threats that now exist in their environment.

6. Disaster response must include a focus on both the immediate and longer-term effects on patients and staff. Those who may not have been directly impacted by a disaster are still potential witnesses to a dramatically traumatic event; they cannot be treated as those who gray into the background when the more pressing and urgent victims of the disaster begin to present.

7. Healthcare providers must develop plans that provide interaction with the public, especially in the areas of media relations,

volunteer management, community health and preparedness education, and the management of donations. The common denominator to all disasters is casualties; in as much, hospitals will be immediately placed at the forefront of public interest and have the greatest need for information management. Healthcare providers must be prepared beyond their normal, limited scope of clinical interest and professional demands.

8. The critical role of hospitals in local and regional disaster response creates a major financial challenge for hospitals that must be recognized and addressed. This point supports the function of deliberate planning as the means to identify and capitalize the resources necessary for response and surge capacity requirements.

CONCLUSION

The 2004 Madrid train bombings had all the elements of a "predictable surprise."[13] Terrorists attacked a transportation platform where there was a densely contained, highly vulnerable population at risk, virtually guaranteeing a high-impact, high-visibility mass casualty event. Because trains are closed environments, the explosions guaranteed blast overpressure, exacerbating the impact of the attack (i.e., the degree of injury intensity) on the affected population. The attacks followed the pattern of multiple, near simultaneous events that are the hallmark of terrorists, severely complicating response to the point of disruption or collapse. The disaster overwhelmed both the local and regional disaster response and medical infrastructure capacities, which were not experienced, trained, equipped, or resourced to support an affected casualty load of this magnitude. In a single day's attack, nearly all of the purposeful cascades that terrorists plan for were achieved. It is clear that railway systems will continue to represent one of the more singularly attractive targets for future terrorist attacks.

This, then, is the reality of why surge capacity planning is so important for anything related to a national mass casualty incident. The fact is, even for developed nations, in the event of a terrorist attack or a natural disaster with thousands needing medical attention, there will be insufficient resources to support the affected population if pre-event deliberate planning has not been done to address surge. The ability of our public health and healthcare system to respond to catastrophic events and save as many lives as possible will remain the single most important measure of national preparedness.

DISCUSSION QUESTIONS

1. Which of the competencies described in the Appendix does this case demonstrate?
2. Describe what is meant by the term *catastrophic casualty anomaly*, and what would an event in reverse of this phenomenon portend for a major metropolitan health system?
3. In the standard model of healthcare organizations functioning primarily as businesses in developed countries, what is the net effect of maintaining hospital beds as profit centers on the ability to maintain medical surge capacity within healthcare systems?
4. Provide a brief description of the theory of "siloization" and its impact on disaster response capacity in the medical and public health infrastructure.
5. Deliberate planning prior to a sudden-onset disaster is known to contribute markedly in enhancing incident response outcomes. Describe some of the major failures associated with a lack of pre-event deliberate planning in the Madrid train bombings.
6. What is the potential impact of not using standardized triage protocols for the first responder and first receiver communities tasked with responding to large-scale mass casualty events?
7. How might a "network-centric health emergency response" (NCHER) construct enhance a healthcare system's ability to respond to a catastrophic disaster?

REFERENCES

1. Campbell D. 9-11: a healthcare provider's response. *Front Health Serv Manag.* 2002;19(1):3–14.
2. Campbell D. 9-11: a healthcare provider's response. Plenary Session Presentation at the Annual Congress of the American College of Healthcare Executives, Chicago, IL; 2002.
3. Marghella P, Lehman C. Saving the many. *Homeland Defense J.* 2008;6(5):22.
4. Marcus L, Ashkenazi I, Dorn B, Henderson J. Meta-leadership: expanding the scope and scale of public health. *Leadersh Public Health.* 2008;8:1–2.
5. U.S. Defense Intelligence Agency. 11 March 2004 Madrid train bombings report. *Defense Executive Intelligence Review* (Unclassified). Washington, DC: Author; 2004.
6. Peral Gutierrez De Ceballos J, Turegano-Fuentes F, Perez-Diaz D, Sanz-Sanchez M, Martin-Llorente C, Guerrero-Sanz J. 11 March 2004: the terrorist bomb explosions in Madrid, Spain—an analysis of the logistics,

injuries sustained and clinical management of casualties at the closest hospital. *Crit Care.* 2005;9(1):104–111.

7. Lopez-Carresi A. The 2004 Madrid train bombings: an analysis of pre-hospital management. *Disasters.* 2008;32(1):41–65.

8. Hammes T. *Welcome to the era of asymmetrical threats.* Presentation made at: The 202 Medical Management of Chemical, Biological, Radiological, Nuclear, and High Explosive (CBRNE) Weapons of Mass Destruction course at the Uniformed Services University of the Health Sciences; 2002; Bethesda, MD.

9. U.S. Department of Homeland Security. The national planning scenarios. *National Response Framework.* Washington, DC; 2010.

10. Gerencser M, Napolitano F, Van Lee R. The mega-community manifesto. *Strategy + Business.* 2006;43. Available at: http://www.strategy-business.com /article/06208. Accessed March 13, 2013.

11. Cebrowski A, Gartska J. Network-centric warfare: its origin and future. *Proceedings.* 1998;124(139):32.

12. Marghella P, Josko W, Montella A. Dump the 3-ring binders. *Inside Homeland Secur.* 2010;8(1):57–61.

13. Bazerman M, Watkins M. *Predictable Surprises: The Disasters You Should Have Seen Coming.* Cambridge, MA: Harvard University Press; 2004.

Case

8

The *Deepwater Horizon* Gulf Oil Spill Disaster

James H. Diaz

BACKGROUND

In April 2010, the *Deepwater Horizon* oil platform exploded, burned, and sank in the Gulf of Mexico off the Louisiana coast, triggering a massive oil spill. From April until July 2010, Louisiana light crude oil gushed into the deepwater sea column at an unprecedented rate, making this the largest oil spill in the history of the offshore oil exploration industry. The *Deepwater Horizon* oil spill dwarfed all prior oil tanker spills in magnitude, impacted ecosystems, and caused extensive environmental damage to the Gulf Coast and its commercial fisheries and wildlife sanctuaries. A massive cleanup effort was launched and manned by over 55,000 oil field workers and untrained volunteers, mostly commercial and recreational fishermen, and the cleanup was coordinated by BP, the responsible party, and the U.S. government.

This case study will describe the chronology of the disaster, its key players, and several major public health issues, including the chemical toxicities of crude oil and dispersants as well as the acute health effects of chemical exposures in both oil spill cleanup workers and Louisiana's general population as compared to the acute health effects in cleanup workers and others following prior oil spills worldwide. In addition, this case study will describe the resolution strategies and outcomes of the oil spill and predict potential future chronic health effects in Louisiana cleanup workers compared to chronic health effects in first responders and cleanup workers following prior oil spills. Lastly, this case study will predict potential adverse ecosystem outcomes based on prior studies in the oil-rich North and Baltic Seas. It will assess the potential for adverse chronic health outcomes in exposed, vulnerable populations with high seroprevalences for genetic polymorphisms regulating the hepatic detoxification of chemicals in crude oil and dispersants.

On April 20, 2010, the 126 workers on the BP *Deepwater Horizon* were going about the routines of completing an exploratory oil well—unaware of the impending disaster. What unfolded would have unknown impacts shaped by the Gulf region's distinctive cultures, institutions, and geography—and by economic forces resulting from the unique coexistence of energy resources, bountiful fisheries and wildlife, and coastal tourism. The oil and gas industry, long lured by the Gulf reserves and public incentives, progressively developed and deployed new technologies, at even larger scales, in pursuit of valuable energy supplies in increasingly deeper waters farther from the coastline. Regulators, however, failed to keep pace with the industrial expansion and new technology—often because of the industry's resistance to more effective oversight. The result was a serious, and ultimately inexcusable, shortfall in supervision of offshore drilling that played out in the Macondo well blowout and the catastrophic oil spill that followed.[1]

OVERVIEW

At 9:45 PM central daylight time (CDT) on April 20, 2010, the *Deepwater Horizon*, a 9-year-old floating deep-sea oil-drilling platform, exploded and burned for 36 hours before sinking and triggering a massive oil spill in the northern Gulf of Mexico, 41 miles off of the Mississippi River delta in Louisiana (see Figure 8-1 and Table 8-1). The explosion killed 11 platform workers; 115 survivors were rescued at sea by responding civilian and U.S. Coast Guard (USCG) vessels and helicopters. From April 22, 2010, until the seafloor wellhead was capped on July 15, 2010, Louisiana light crude oil was released into the deepwater column at a rate ranging from 53,000 barrels per day (8,400 m^3/day) to 62,000 barrels per day (9,900 m^3/day) for a total crude oil spill of 185 million gallons, or 4.9 million barrels, over an area up to 6,800 square miles (180,000 km^2). **Table 8-1** identifies the failures in managing the drilling site, in the procedural and mechanical processes and in regulating the industry.

Table	
8-1	**Systematic Failures in the *Deepwater Horizon* Oil Spill Disaster**

Managerial Failures	Technical Failures	Regulatory Failures
1. Poor safety culture at BP exemplified by the Texas City, Texas explosion in March 2005 and the Alaska pipeline spill in Prudhoe Bay, Alaska in March 2006.	1. Improper selection of a liner well design rather than a long-string well design with a continuous steel casing between the seafloor wellhead and the oil and gas zone. The liner casing was selected because it was cheaper, faster to install, and could be cemented quicker than a long-string casing.	1. Like the initial federal response to the flooding and loss of life (over 1,000 persons dead in New Orleans following Hurricane Katrina), the initial federal response to the oil spill was also delayed and inadequate. Weeks elapsed before President Obama visited the Gulf Coast oil spill impact zones.

(continued)

Table	
8-1	**Systematic Failures in the *Deepwater Horizon* Oil Spill Disaster (*continued*)**

Managerial Failures	Technical Failures	Regulatory Failures
2. Priority on profits over safety. As a PhD-level petroleum geologist and seasoned BP executive, BP CEO Tony Hayward knew how to increase company profits by cutting production costs using faster drilling techniques and fewer safety test runs.	2. Inadequate stabilization of the liner production casing with the right number of centralizers ($n = 21$) to eliminate gas channeling as recommended by computer scenarios and by Halliburton engineers—only 6 centralizers were used because ordering more would have been costly and taken days to deliver to the rig by helicopters.	2. No clear lines of authority and effective communication among federal, state, and local officials and BP.
3. Decisions made on an ad hoc basis by middle management to save time and money, as exemplified by selecting a cheaper well-bore design with limited subsequent integrity testing.	3. Critical delay in diverting the drilling mud gushing over the rig from the unsealed well overboard before the channeled methane gas reached the rig deck and ignited an inferno.	3. Repeated underestimates of gushing oil flow rates by government scientists, making the federal government appear incapable of handling the oil spill. Later, this was admitted by Homeland Security Secretary Napolitano and Interior Secretary Salazar.
4. The use of generic offshore drilling plans and not specific plans designed for the *Deepwater Horizon*. There was a "walrus protection plan" designed for Arctic drilling, but no blowout preventer–failure backup plan.	4. Failure to engage the blowout preventer early in the crisis when it may have worked.	4. Ineffective enforcement of the offshore drilling moratorium that prevented new drilling, but allowed the MMS to issue permits and waivers for projects already underway.

Managerial Failures	Technical Failures	Regulatory Failures
5. No risk assessment and management plans in place with frequent disaster response training and mock disaster exercises.	5. Inadequate cement integrity and quality testing by Halliburton, the cement contractors.	5. No enforceable MMS regulations to require testing/retesting of blowout preventers, cement jobs, and pressure tests prior to abandoning a newly drilled well in order to install a production rig.
6. Poor communication among BP top management, onshore and offshore middle management, and onshore and offshore contractors, including Transocean (the rig operators) and Halliburton (the cement contractors).	6. Inadequate positive and negative pressure tests by BP and Transocean engineers in order to detect problems that could lead to a possible blowout, including gas channeling effects and ineffective cement seals (both of which contributed to the rig explosion and fire).	6. Insufficient numbers of properly trained MMS offshore inspectors. In April 2010, there were 5 inspectors for 23 offshore facilities (1 inspector per 5 rigs) in the MMS Pacific region and 55 inspectors for 3,000 offshore facilities (1 inspector per 54 rigs) in the MMS Gulf region.
7. Poor communication among the contractors as to their specific roles and responsibilities.	7. No clear abandonment procedures to ensure a sealed wellhead before the *Deepwater Horizon* drilling rig could cast off and turn the newly drilled well over to a production rig.	7. Cozy relationships between the MMS regulators and inspectors and the offshore oil and gas industry that MMS was charged with regulating.
8. A fragmentation of responsibilities among contractors when these responsibilities should have been carefully linked and choreographed.	8. Summoning an inadequate number of giant oil-skimming ships and storage vessels to receive skimmed oil.	8. "Boom war" outbreaks: The USCG distributed containment booms to local responders primarily based on political pressures from Gulf state governors, local officials, and congressmen rather than on scientific recommendations from NOAA and the EPA using satellite monitoring of oil slicks and their movements toward sensitive ecosystems, such as national parks and wildlife sanctuaries.

(continued)

Table	
8-1	Systematic Failures in the *Deepwater Horizon* Oil Spill Disaster (*continued*)

Managerial Failures	Technical Failures	Regulatory Failures
9. Insensitive and ineffective leadership exercised by top management, especially Tony Hayward, who took a vacation in the middle of the disaster to attend a sailboat race in England.		9. On-site bureaucratic behavior and government-speak exhibited by federal officials rather than timely and clear communications and behaviors expressing sensitivity and heartfelt sympathy for a population suffering yet another major disaster within 5 years of Hurricanes Katrina and Rita.
		10. A 6-month delay by the NIEHS in announcing requests for proposals (RFPs) for a necessary longitudinal cohort study (the Gulf Oil Workers' Study of 55,000 cleanup workers) that was open-ended and underfunded. This delay in starting the cohort investigation caused recall and response bias by study subjects, interfered with recruitment of exposed cases and unexposed controls, caused misclassification of exposed cases and controls, and limited the reliability of short-term biomarkers for subsequent chronic illnesses.

Abbreviations: EPA, U.S. Environmental Protection Agency; MMS, Minerals Management Service; NIEHS, National Institute of Environmental Health Sciences; NOAA, U.S. National Oceanic and Atmospheric Administration; USCG, United States Coast Guard.

This oil spill was the largest oil spill in the history of the petroleum industry. Its magnitude and impact on ecosystems caused extensive damage to marine and wildlife habitats. It impacted over 1,600 miles of shoreline, significantly spoiled over 800 miles of beach and marsh shoreline from Texas to Florida, and threatened the viability of the northern Gulf's commercial fishing and tourism industries (see **Figure 8-1**).[1]

A massive cleanup effort was launched as dispersed and weathered crude oil approached the U.S. coastline. In addition to the use of oil

Figure 8-1

The *Deepwater Horizon* Gulf of Mexico oil spill slick, as viewed from space on May 24, 2010, by the moderate-resolution imaging spectroradiometer (MODIS) on the United States National Aeronautics and Space Administration (NASA) Terra satellite. The oil spill stemmed from a methane gas explosion on the *Deepwater Horizon* oil rig 48 miles off of the Mississippi River Delta in Louisiana on the evening of April 20, 2010, which killed 13 platform workers. As much as 4.9 million barrels (200 million U.S. gallons) were released into the northern Gulf of Mexico between April 22, 2010, and July 15, 2010, when the leak was capped.

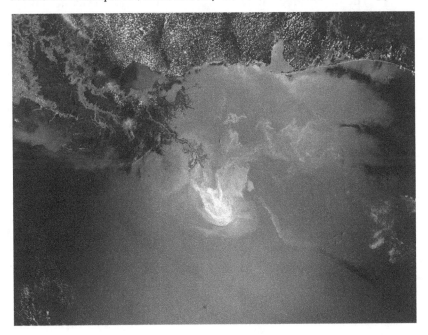

Source: United States National Aeronautics and Space Administration (NASA), NASA/ GSFC MODIS Rapid Response.

dispersants injected at the subsea wellhead site and sprayed on the sea surface by aircraft and surface vessels, several other remediation strategies were used in an attempt to protect coastal beaches, estuaries, and wetlands from oil slicks. These attempts included skimmer ships, floating containment booms, intentional burning of surface, and placing sand-filled berms and rock barriers around barrier islands and shorelines. The predominant dispersant used in the first month of the oil spill was the Nalco COREXIT 9527, later replaced by COREXIT 9500.[1] The volume of the COREXIT oil dispersants used in the cleanup effort was reported to have been 1.8 million gallons.[2]

HISTORY REPEATS ITSELF: THE *IXTOC I* GULF OIL SPILL, 1979

Juan Antonio Dzul was a teenager when the *Ixtoc I* oil rig exploded and sank in June 1979 in the Gulf of Mexico, 70 miles from the fishing town of Champotón where he grew up and still lives.[3] In a 2010 interview, he recalled:

> The oil covered the reefs and washed up on the shore. Fish died and the octopuses were buried under the oil that filled the gaps between the rocks where they live. Even today you can find stains on rocks a few centimeters deep, and if you stick something metal in them the smell of oil still escapes.[3]

The *Ixtoc I* oil rig exploded and sank in 160 feet of shallow water on June 3, 1979.[4,5] Approximately 10,000 to 30,000 barrels of crude oil per day were spilled into the southern Gulf of Mexico until two relief base wells stopped the flow 10 months later on March 25, 1980.[4,5] The only dispersant used in the *Ixtoc* spill was COREXIT 9527, and it was only applied to surface Mexican waters because the U.S. Environmental Protection Agency (EPA) considered COREXIT 9527 too toxic for U.S. waters.[4,5] Today, more than 30 years after the *Ixtoc I* spill, the Yucatan commercial fishery is 50% to 75% less productive annually than prior to the spill. The Kemp's ridley sea turtles did not return to Yucatan's beaches to lay their eggs for 10 years. However, there were few long-term adverse human health effects due to sparsely populated coastal areas and limited human exposures during cleanup efforts.[4,5] **Table 8-2** compares the magnitudes and outcomes of the *Ixtoc I* and the *Deepwater Horizon* Gulf oil spills.

THE KEY PLAYERS

Anthony B. "Tony" Hayward, PhD, CEO of BP plc

Tony Hayward is a PhD-trained geologist and British businessman who replaced Lord John Browne as the chief executive officer (CEO) of the oil and energy giant BP plc (public limited company) in 2007. Hayward had risen through the ranks at BP, starting as an offshore rig geologist in 1982, later assuming technical and commercial leadership roles with BP throughout the world. On December 18, 2006, during run-up elections to replace Lord Brown as CEO, Hayward was publically critical of BP management's handling of a major explosion at the BP Texas City

Table 8-2	A Comparison of the Magnitudes and Outcomes of the *Ixtoc I* and the *Deepwater Horizon* Gulf of Mexico Oil Spills[1-4]	
	Ixtoc I Oil Spill	*Deepwater Horizon* Oil Spill
Location: Gulf of Mexico	Bay of Campeche (62 miles northwest of Cuidad del Carmen, Yucatan, Mexico)	Macondo Canyon (41 miles off of the mouth of the Mississippi River)
Water Depth (Gulf water depth record = 10,011 ft)	160 ft	5,067 ft
Drill Depth (Gulf drill depth record = > 30,000 ft)	11,800 ft	18,360 ft (13,293 ft below the seafloor)
Date of Spill	June 3, 1979	April 20, 2010
Ultimate Causes of Spill	1. Flawed well design plan 2. Failed blowout preventer (BOP)	1. Drilling mud circulatory failure 2. Failed blowout preventer (BOP)
Operator	Pemex/Sedco (Sedco later became Transocean)	BP/Transocean
Crew	63	146
Deaths	0	11
Injuries	0	Unknown
Maximum Spill Flow Rate (1 barrel of crude oil = 42 U.S. gallons)	30,000 barrels = 1.26 million gallons	62,000 barrels = 2.6 million gallons
Total Volume of Spill (1 barrel of crude oil = 42 U.S. gallons)	3 million barrels = 126 million gallons	4.28 million barrels = 180 million gallons
Dispersants Used	COREXIT 9527 (only in Mexican waters)	COREXIT 9527, later COREXIT 9500
Area of Gulf Impacted	1,100 mi^2	6,800 mi^2
Shorelines Impacted	162 mi (Texas, Mexico)	1,600 mi (Texas to Florida)
Plugging Strategies	"Sombrero" containment cap, drilling mud plug, "junk shot" plug	Containment dome, "top hat" containment cap, drilling mud plug, "junk shot" plug
Spill Stopped	March 28, 1980, by relief wells permitting cementing	September 19, 2010, by relief wells permitting cementing
Cleanup Costs	$100 million	$40.9 billion to date

Source: The National Commission on the BP Deepwater Horizon oil spill and offshore drilling. Deep water: the Gulf oil disaster and the future of offshore drilling. Report to the President, January 20111; Biello D. One year after BP oil spill, at least 1.1 million barrels still missing—where in the Gulf of Mexico is the oil from the Macondo well blowout? Scientific American. April 25, 2011. http://www.scientificamerican.com/article.cfm?idone-year-after-bp-oil-spill-millions-of-barrels-oil-missing-barrels-still-missing2; Tuckman Jo. Gulf oil spill: parallels with Ixtoc raise fears of impending ecological tipping point. The Guardian. June 1, 2010. http://www.guardian.co.uk/environment/2010/jun/01/gulf-oil-spill-ixtoc-ecological-tippingpoint? INTCMPSRCH;[3] Schrope M. The lost legacy of the last great oil spill. Scientific American. July 14, 2010. Available at http:/www.scientificamerican.com/article.cfm?idthe-lost-legacy-Ixtoc-oil.[4]

Oil Refinery on the Louisiana–Texas border on March 23, 2005, that killed 15 workers and injured 170.[6] At a town hall meeting in Houston, Hayward said, "We have a leadership style that is too directive [sic] and doesn't listen sufficiently well. The top of the organization doesn't listen sufficiently to what the bottom is saying."[6] Later, on May 12, 2009, in a lecture on his role as BP CEO at Stanford Business School, he stated: "[O]ur primary purpose in life is to create value for our shareholders."[7]

As BP CEO, Hayward always pursued more value for BP shareholders by cutting the costs of increased production, and for himself, by collecting millions of dollars annually in bonuses and stock options. By early 2010, however, Hayward, a petrochemical geologist with years of industry experience, must have begun to suspect that his cost-cutting and risk-taking strategies, especially in the critical areas of safety and cross-training, could threaten his own BP stock value. In March 2010, a month before the *Deepwater Horizon* explosion and sinking, Hayward sold up to half of his BP shares and took over $20 million in profits.[8] BP shares later fell in value by over 30% and dividend payments ceased for months, cash-strapping large numbers of BP retirees and British pensioners.

Following the *Deepwater Horizon* oil spill, Hayward downplayed the spill and stated on May 17, 2010, that the spill would likely be "very very modest" and "relatively tiny" in comparison to the size of the ocean.[9] On May 30, 2010, Hayward was widely condemned for telling a reporter, "We're sorry for the massive disruption it's caused to their lives. There's no one who wants this thing over more than I do, I'd like my life back."[10] Hayward disputed claims of massive underwater plumes of oil suspended in the Gulf, which had been reported by marine scientists on three research vessels.

On June 17, 2010, in testimony before a congressional investigatory committee, Hayward launched his new damage-control strategy—diffusion of responsibility—by stating: "this is a complex accident, caused by an unprecedented combination of failures. A number of companies are involved, including BP . . ."[11] Later in June 2010, BP placed Bob Dudley in charge of handling the *Deepwater Horizon* Gulf oil spill, reporting to Hayward. On October 1, 2010, Bob Dudley, a Mississippi native, replaced Hayward as BP CEO.

President Barack H. Obama

In a television interview on June 8, 2010, President Barack Obama simply said that Hayward "wouldn't be working for me after any of those statements" following the oil spill.[12]

Although President George W. Bush was severely criticized for not personally visiting New Orleans and the Mississippi Gulf Coast immediately following the devastation of Hurricane Katrina in 2005, President Obama repeated the same public relations failure by not visiting coastal Louisiana after the oil spill in 2010 and by simply relying on his incident commander and agency heads to report secondhand for weeks on the environmental impact.

Admiral Thad W. Allen, U.S. Coast Guard

Admiral Thad Allen, a USCG Academy graduate and the son of a career USCG chief, was widely praised for his performance as the national incident commander during the aftermath of Hurricanes Katrina and Rita on the Gulf Coast from September 2005 until January 2006[13] (see **Figure 8-2**). Admiral Allen was appointed to a 4-year term as the

Figure 8-2

Admiral Thad W. Allen, Commandant, United States Coast Guard, 2006–2010, National Incident Commander, *Deepwater Horizon* Gulf oil spill, 2010.

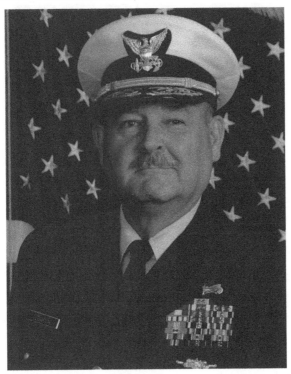

Source: Reproduced from Commandant's Corner, Official Portraits from the United States Coast Guard, U.S. Department of Homeland Security.

23rd Commandant of the USCG, ended his service as Commandant on May 25, 2010, and continued to serve the nation on active duty as the National Incident Commander of the *Deepwater Horizon* Gulf oil spill disaster. Admiral Allen retired from the USCG on June 30, 2010, but continued his service as the oil spill incident commander until October 1, 2010—the very same day that Bob Dudley replaced Tony Hayward as BP CEO.

Janet Napolitano, U.S. Secretary of Homeland Security

Secretary Janet Napolitano was confirmed as the third Secretary of Homeland Security by the Senate on January 20, 2009, after having served as attorney general of Arizona from 1999 to 2002 and governor of Arizona from 2003 to 2009 (see **Figure 8-3**). Because the

Figure 8-3

Janet Napolitano, Secretary, Department of Homeland Security.

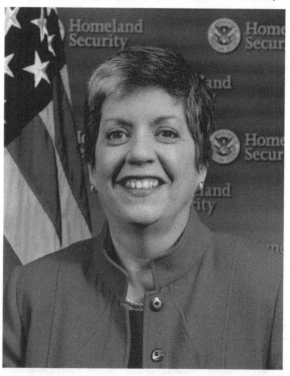

Source: Reproduced from the Department of Homeland Security. Available at: http://www.dhs.gov/secretary-janet-napolitano. Accessed April 22, 2013.

USCG operates under the Department of Homeland Security during peacetime, Admiral Allen was deployed by Secretary Napolitano as national incident commander during the oil spill disaster response, and he reported to Secretary Napolitano and the president. During early congressional investigations of the Gulf oil spill, Napolitano testified that the federal government had "limited capacity and expertise" in dealing with major offshore oil spills in very deep water.[14] In addition, Napolitano testified that "before the blowout, it is clear that there was an assumption that a [blowout preventer] would never fail."[14] Throughout the disaster, Napolitano must be credited with the following actions: (1) deploying and supporting Admiral Thad Allen as national incident commander, a proven leader with the expertise and regional credibility to oversee a major oil spill cleanup in the Gulf; (2) immediately and truthfully admitting that the federal government response was overwhelmed by the magnitude and technical complexities of the oil spill disaster and that only the offshore oil industry had the necessary technological response capacity; (3) pursuing the best estimates of daily oil spill flow rates and timelines to reducing flow rates and ending the oil spill; and (4) ultimately admitting, along with Secretary Salazar, that the government's early estimates of daily oil spill flow rates were inaccurate compared to the flow rates calculated by independent scientists.

Susan Elizabeth "Liz" Birnbaum, Director of the U.S. Minerals Management Service

Liz Birnbaum served as the general counsel to the U.S. House Committee on Natural Resources from 1991 to 1999, where she handled legislative and oversight activities for the Department of the Interior and its divisions, including the Minerals Management Service (MMS). In July 2009, she was appointed director of the MMS. The MMS was created in the 1980s and was directly charged with administering programs that ensured the effective management of renewable energy, traditional energy, and mineral resources on the nation's Outer Continental Shelf, including the safe exploration and production of oil and natural gas and the collection and distribution of revenues from mineral development on federal lands. The MMS had a long history of granting blanket exemptions from submitting comprehensive environmental impact statements to offshore drilling companies prior to undersea explorations on their offshore leases. A perennial problem at MMS Gulf Coast installations was a lack of fully trained technical inspectors for the large numbers of oil and gas exploration and drilling operations in the northern Gulf of Mexico. In recent years, the MMS had been plagued by scandals, including one in the Denver office in which eight employees were disciplined for partying with, having sex with, and receiving expensive gifts from their energy industry counterparts.[15] With a history of comfortable relationships with the oil and gas industry, the MMS could be considered a prime example of regulatory failures leading to the *Deepwater Horizon* oil spill disaster.

An example of the oil and gas industry's relationship with the MMS was the manner in which the MMS always deferred to the industry for developing and implementing safety protocols for monitoring and testing/retesting many of the critical aspects of offshore drilling practices, including mandatory cement stability tests and follow-up for negative pressure tests before wellheads on the seafloor could be plugged and temporarily abandoned.[1]

> Government also failed to provide the oversight necessary to prevent these lapses in judgment and management by private industry. MMS regulations were inadequate to address the risks of deepwater drilling. Many critical aspects of drilling operations were left to industry to decide without agency review. For instance, there was no requirement, let alone protocol, for a negative-pressure test, the misreading of which was a major contributor to the Macondo blowout. Nor were there detailed requirements related to the testing of the cement essential for well stability.[1]

In fact, these two insufficiencies in MMS regulatory oversight contributed to the final fatal string of five human errors that doomed the *Deepwater Horizon* and 13 members of its crew. This final fatal string of human errors included (1) no backup barriers to gas flow at the bottom of the well, (2) fewer centralizers (BP used only 6 centralizers to cut costs when Halliburton engineers recommended 21 centralizers) to keep the cement job evenly poured around the drill casing, (3) no cement integrity testing, (4) misinterpretation of a negative pressure test for potentially explosive upward pressure in the well, and (5) early removal of the drilling mud barrier to keep any excessive upward or "blowout" pressure under control. In retrospect, there was only one engineering failure in the *Deepwater Horizon* oil spill disaster, the failure of the blowout preventer—a failure assured by the five human failures.

In her letter of resignation as MMS director to President Obama and Secretary Salazar on May 27, 2010, Liz Birnbaum wrote:

> It's been a great privilege to serve as Director of the MMS [for less than 10 months]. I have enormous admiration for the men and

women of the MMS who do a difficult job under challenging circumstances. I'm hopeful that the reforms that the Secretary and the Administration are undertaking will resolve the flaws in the current system that I inherited.[16]

Kenneth Lee "Ken" Salazar, U.S. Secretary of the Interior

Secretary Ken Salazar is a native of Colorado who served as attorney general of Colorado from 1999 to 2005 and as a U.S. senator from Colorado from 2005 to 2009 (see **Figure 8-4**). On December 17, 2008, President-Elect Obama announced that he would nominate Salazar as his Secretary of the Interior, despite a mixed reaction from the national environmentalist movement, which accused him of being more oil

Figure 8-4

Kenneth L. Salazar, Secretary, Department of the Interior.

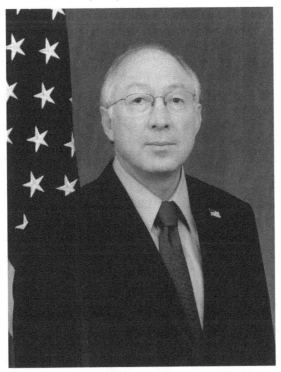

Source: Reproduced from the Department of the Interior.

shale industry oriented than environmentally oriented in Colorado.[17] Salazar was confirmed as Secretary of the Interior unanimously by the Senate on January 20, 2009. The Department of the Interior remains directly responsible for the activities of the former Minerals Management Service (MMS), now temporarily renamed the Bureau of Ocean Energy Management, Regulation, and Enforcement (BOEMRE).

Salazar can be credited with (1) enforcing the offshore oil-drilling moratorium imposed by President Obama after the oil spill; (2) establishing the Outer Continental Shelf Oversight Board; (3) directing the MMS to play a key role in investigating the oil spill, despite the service's oversight history; and (4) recognizing the deficiencies in the MMS division and giving the division a new director, Michael Bromwich, and name, the BOEMRE. Nevertheless, some could argue that Salazar should have resigned along with Liz Birnbaum after the oil spill disaster. As a former attorney general and U.S. senator from a mineral-rich state (Colorado), Salazar would have been very familiar with MMS responsibilities and was appointed by the president to oversee them.

In 2011, the BOEMRE was divided into two separate federal agencies: (1) the Bureau of Safety and Environmental Enforcement (BSEE), now responsible for safety, inspection, and enforcement of regulations of all offshore oil and gas operations; and (2) the Bureau of Ocean Energy Management (BOEM), now responsible for all energy exploration leasing and planning on the U.S. Outer Continental Shelf. Former BOEMRE interim director Michael Bromwich, an attorney and former inspector general for the Justice Department with no technical or oil and gas industry experience, was named by Salazar to head the BSEE and was criticized for halting all mineral exploration in the Gulf for almost a year. During this time, nearly 100 operating offshore oil rigs and all of their support vessels left the Gulf for lucrative, long-term (4 or more years) drilling contracts with the nationalized oil companies of Brazil (*Petrobras*) and Mexico (*Pemex*). Unlike the tourism industries of coastal Mississippi, Alabama, and the Florida panhandle, the coastal tourism, offshore and commercial fishing, and oil and gas support industries of Louisiana have never fully rebounded to a pre-oil-spill activity and economy.[18]

Jane Lubchenko, PhD, Administrator, National Oceanic and Atmospheric Administration

Dr. Jane Lubchenko, a renowned academic marine biologist, was nominated by President Barack Obama to serve as the administrator of NOAA, a division of the U.S. Department of Commerce

Figure 8-5

Jane Lubchenko, PhD, Administrator, National Oceanic and Atmospheric Administration of the U.S. Department of Commerce.

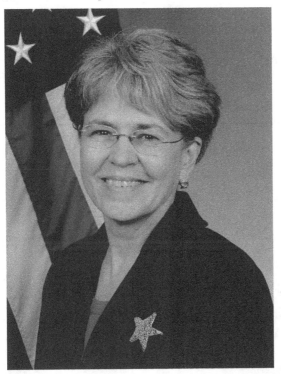

Source: Reproduced from the National Oceanic and Atmospheric Administration of the U.S. Department of Commerce. Available at: http://www.noaa.gov/lubchenco.html. Accessed April 22, 2013.

(see **Figure 8-5**). Following her confirmation by the Senate on March 19, 2009, she promised the nation that science would always guide the agency.[19] NOAA has remained the lead federal agency in monitoring the conditions in the Gulf and its coastlines following the oil spill, in directing the National Resource Damage Assessment (NRDA) process following the oil spill, in assessing the short- and long-term impacts of the oil spill on the marine ecosystem, and in ensuring that the fish and shellfish harvested from the Gulf of Mexico remain safe to eat. To date, Dr. Lubchenko has delivered on her promise to the nation.

Lisa P. Jackson, Administrator, U.S. Environmental Protection Agency

Lisa P. Jackson, a native of New Orleans, Louisiana, and a chemical engineer, was appointed by President Obama to serve as the 12th administrator of the U.S. EPA in 2009, after having served for 6 years as assistant commissioner, and later commissioner, of the New Jersey Department of Environmental Protection and as chief of staff for former New Jersey governor Jon Corzine (see **Figure 8-6**). Prior to that, she was employed by the EPA for 16 years. The EPA is not a cabinet department, but its administrator is normally given a cabinet rank. The EPA has approximately 18,000 full-time employees and an annual budget of over $10 billion. The EPA has a significant

Figure 8-6

Lisa P. Jackson, Administrator, U.S. Environmental Protection Agency.

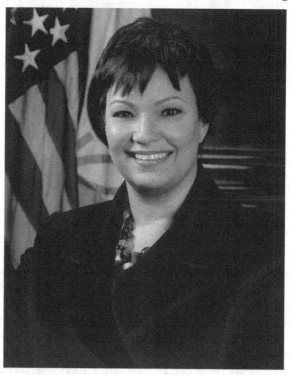

Source: Reproduced from the U.S. Environmental Protection Agency.

presence in southern Louisiana, where it monitors air quality at several stationary sites, many near petrochemical refineries, and reports its results to the Louisiana Department of Environmental Quality (DEQ), the Louisiana Office of Public Health (OPH) Section of Environmental Epidemiology and Toxicology, and to the public on its website. In response to the BP oil spill, the EPA monitored air, water, sediment, and waste generated by the cleanup operations. In addition, the EPA conducted toxicological testing on eight different dispersants on sensitive aquatic organisms (shrimp and fish) found in the Gulf of Mexico; and later confirmed that the dispersant COREXIT 9500 was no more or less toxic than the other seven dispersants tested.[20] Unfortunately, the EPA did not test the toxicity of the other COREXIT dispersant used by BP in the oil spill cleanup, COREXIT 9527, which contained the highly toxic industrial solvent, 2-butoxyethanol.[20] Administrator Jackson was frequently on site in New Orleans and coastal Louisiana after the oil spill and should be credited with directing the EPA to intensify its environmental monitoring operations and frequently reporting results to the responsible state agencies and to the public at large. However, the EPA was unsuccessful in getting BP to use any of the tested dispersants in the cleanup operations other than the two COREXITs produced by the its subsidiary, Nalco, and the EPA should have included COREXIT 9527 in its toxicological testing of dispersants on aquatic organisms for potential bioconcentration in the marine food chain.[20]

Following the *Ixtoc I* Gulf oil spill in June 1979, the EPA considered the dispersant, COREXIT 9527, too toxic for surface applications in U.S. waters.[4,5] However, later, following the *Deepwater Horizon* Gulf oil spill in April through September 2010, the EPA permitted an unprecedented amount of COREXIT 9527 to be applied to surface and, for the first time, to deep subsurface Gulf waters.

Local incident commanders and health department officials often accused the EPA of not rapidly releasing its test results to the public until confirmed by retesting. The EPA responded to this criticism by posting an article on its website entitled "Science to Support EPA's Response to the BP Oil Spill"—an excerpt from which is as follows:

> EPA's cadre of scientists is uniquely positioned to provide immediate and ongoing technical advice and expertise, as well as work to facilitate the gathering of data from air, water, waste and sediment samples from the affected area. In coordination with the Joint Incident Command, Agency scientists are communicating results and information to emergency responders,

citizens, and others in need of the latest scientific information. . . . Environmental data, including air quality and water samples, is updated daily on EPA's BP Oil Spill Response Web site as it is collected and validated by EPA's response teams along the impacted coastlines. This data is meant to determine potential risks to public health and the environment.[21]

RESIDENTS OF THE GULF COAST REPRESENTING THE MOST IMPACTED BUSINESSES AND INDUSTRIES

The impacts to those living along the Gulf Coast were dramatic and potentially life-changing.

Clarence R. Duplessis, Commercial Fisherman, Davant, Louisiana

Now, five years later [after Hurricane Katrina] we are facing the *Deepwater Horizon* oil spill. This is the worst of our problems because we have no answers, no solutions, only questions. As we watch our livelihood and even an entire culture being washed away by crude oil and chemicals that no one knows the long-term effects of, we ask: Will we have the mortgage payment next month? How long will this last? Will I be able to go oystering next year or ever again? How long will it take the fisheries to recover?[1]

Dean Blanchard, Owner, Dean Blanchard Seafood, Inc., Grande Isle, Louisiana

By mid-May 2010, tar balls and oil had started washing up on Grande Isle's beaches and wetlands. During his 30 years in business, Dean Blanchard had become one of the nation's major suppliers of Gulf shrimp and a millionaire. By mid-June 2010, Blanchard figured:

I've lost $15 million in sales in the last 50 days. That would have been $1 million in my pocket. We've got 1,400 vessels that go and catch shrimp and come to our facility. [Now,] basically we've lost all our customers because we can't supply them.[1]

Sheryl Lindsay, President, Orange Beach Weddings, Orange Beach, Alabama

In the wake of the oil spill, Sheryl commented:

> Every time the phone rang, all we got was another cancellation—
> or someone asking how bad it was down here. . . . Orange Beach
> is a popular spot for destination weddings and many of my brides
> come from out of state. . . . A lot of girls asked me what should they
> do—they were worried about the smell, about whether the guests
> could swim and the quality of the seafood.[1]

In 2009, Lindsay had taken out a small business loan for $55,000
to expand her business, but now she feared that she could not meet
the payments as her business diminished.

CHRONOLOGY OF THE DISASTER

March 2008. BP purchased offshore oil-drilling rights on the
Macondo Prospect located in Mississippi Canyon Block 252 (MC 252)
from the MMS at a federal oil lease sale in New Orleans.

February 2008. BP filed a 52-page environmental impact statement
for the Macondo well with the MMS indicating that "it was unlikely
that an accidental surface or subsurface oil spill would occur from
the proposed drilling activities."[1]

February 15, 2010. The *Deepwater Horizon* offshore drilling rig,
owned by Transocean and leased to BP, began drilling a subsurface oil well on the Macondo Prospect. The well was to be drilled at
18,000 feet (5,500 m) below sea level and then plugged and temporarily suspended for subsequent completion by a more permanent
rig structure for prolonged subsea oil production. Like Transocean,
owner of the rig, Halliburton was also a key subcontractor responsible for critical technical jobs, including the drilling mud and
well-cementing activities.

April 1, 2010. A Halliburton contract employee, Marvin Volek,
warns that the BP use of cement was "against our [Halliburton's] best
practices"[1]

April 17, 2010. *Deepwater Horizon* completes its drilling operations
and the well is prepared for cementing so that a production well can
subsequently retrieve the oil. The blowout preventer (BOP) is tested
and declared functional. A Halliburton engineer, Jesse Gagliano,
reports that using only 6 centralizers on the cement casing string

instead of the 21 centralizers that he has recommended "would likely produce channeling and a poor cement job."[1] Gagliano had earlier been informed that only 6 and not 21 centralizers could be helicopter-delivered to the rig in time for scheduled completion.

April 20, 2010. BP cancelled a recommended cement integrity test because it would have taken 9 to 12 hours and cost $128,000. The planned relocation of the *Deepwater Horizon* to another drill site was now 43 days overdue and had cost BP $21 million.

April 20, 2010, 9:45 PM CDT. Gas, oil, and concrete exploded up the well bore and ignited on the decks of the *Deepwater Horizon,* incinerating 11 platform workers whose bodies were never recovered and injuring 17 others, 2 of whom later died. Earlier that same day, BP officials had gathered on the platform to celebrate 7 years without an injury on the *Deepwater Horizon,* a 9-year-old, $560 million floating drill rig and the pride of the Transocean offshore oil exploration fleet.

April 21, 2010. USCG Rear Admiral Mary Landry named federal on-scene coordinator and estimated potential spill at 8,000 barrels per day. Two attempts to shut the BOP using remotely operated subsea vehicles (ROVs) failed.

April 22, 2010, 10:21 AM CDT. The *Deepwater Horizon* sinks—on Earth Day!

April 22, 2010. BP reported leak rate to be 1,000 barrels per day.

April 28, 2010. NOAA estimated the leak rate to be 5,000 barrels per day.

April 29, 2010. Louisiana governor Bobby Jindal declared a state of emergency and ordered the coastal deployment of oil containment booms.

April 30, 2010. Oil washed ashore at Venice, Louisiana, and President Barack Obama halted all new offshore oil drilling.

May 2, 2010. NOAA closed all commercial and recreational fishing in oil-spill-affected federal waters from the mouth of the Mississippi River to Pensacola Bay—an area of 6,814 square miles.

May 7–10, 2010. BP attempted to cap the spewing seafloor wellhead first with a 125-ton container dome and then a smaller and more maneuverable 5-foot "top hat" containment vessel both designed to receive drilling mud and debris to clog the well bore in a process known as a *junk shot,* industry slang for plugging the spewing wellhead with debris or junk, including bowling balls. Both strategies failed.

May 12, 2010. BP released undersea video of the leak and independent consultants estimated oil flow at 20,000 to 100,000 barrels a day—significantly greater than the BP estimate of 5,000 barrels a day and the USCG estimate of 8,000 barrels a day.

May 15, 2010. The USCG and the EPA authorize the use of underwater dispersants for the first time in U.S. waters.

May 22, 2010. President Barack Obama signed an executive order that established the Bipartisan National Commission on the BP *Deepwater Horizon* Oil Spill and Offshore Drilling.

May 23, 2010. BP rebuffed a direct order from the EPA to discontinue the use of COREXIT dispersants and select alternative dispersants.

May 25, 2010. Former USCG commandant Admiral Thad W. Allen was appointed the national incident commander of the Unified Command for the BP *Deepwater Horizon* oil spill.

May 27–29, 2010. BP initiated a process of forcing heavy drilling mud stored on barges into the well bore from the sea surface in a new type of plug strategy called *top kill*; it was later reported as a failure.

June 4, 2010. Tar balls washed ashore in Pensacola Beach, Florida.

June 16, 2010. BP agreed to fund a $20 billion escrow account administered by Kenneth Fineberg to compensate victims of the oil spill.

June 21, 2010. NOAA increased the commercial and recreational fishing ban from Atchafalaya Bay, Louisiana, to Panama City, Florida—an area of 86,985 square miles or about 36% of all federal waters in the Gulf of Mexico.

July 5, 2010. Weathered crude oil is spotted at the Rigolets Pass leading into Lake Pontchartrain surrounding New Orleans.

July 10–15, 2010. BP removed an ineffective containment cap and installed a new 40-ton, 3-ram capping stack on the gushing wellhead, designed for subsurface forcing of drilling mud into the well bore.

July 15, 2010. BP reports that crude oil is no longer flowing uncontrollably into the Gulf of Mexico.

August 2, 2010. The Independent Flow Rate Technical Group calculated that the well was initially dumping 62,000 barrels of oil per day into the Gulf; that was reduced to 53,000 barrels per day as capping procedures improved and crude oil reserves were depleted.

September 19, 2010. The double relief well drilling process was completed by BP and the federal government declared the Macondo well "effectively dead."[1]

October 1, 2010. Admiral Thad Allen stepped down as the national incident commander and Bob Dudley replaced Tony Hayward as BP CEO.

THE MAJOR PUBLIC HEALTH ISSUES

The *Deepwater Horizon* oil spill disaster presented multiple sources of toxic chemicals to vulnerable receptor populations on the Gulf Coast via several exposure pathways, including air, water, soil, sand, and seafood. The sources and mechanisms of chemical releases included the following: (1) oil booming, skimming, and burning activities, all of which exposed surface weathered crude oil and dispersant mixtures to photochemical and combustion effects with evaporative and solid particulate releases into the atmosphere; (2) the chemical, physical, and circulatory effects of oil and dispersant mixtures in the seawater column, which resulted in subsequent pooling of chemicals on the seafloor, in subsurface plumes, in estuaries and tidal marshes, and on beaches and tidal flats; and (3) the bioaccumulation effects of the more persistent constituents of crude oil, such as polycyclic aromatic hydrocarbons (PAHs), and dispersants that entered the marine food chain from the benthos to aquatic mammals. Oiled and dying pelicans and beached bottlenose dolphins and sea turtles often served as the earliest sentinels of offshore oil slicks approaching sandy beaches along the northern Gulf Coast.

The Chemical Constituents of Light Crude Oil

The chemical constituents of crude oil are often referred to as total petrochemical hydrocarbons and are divided into (1) the volatile organic compounds (VOCs), which will burn or evaporate quickly in surface spills and minimally bioaccumulate in seafood; and (2) the PAHs, which are more stable, can be activated by sunlight, and bioaccumulate to a greater extent in the seafood chain. The major monitored PAHs and VOCs and their levels of concern (LOCs) in air and in seafood during the *Deepwater Horizon* oil spill are depicted in **Tables 8-3** and **8-4**. On April 30, 2010, and again on June 15, 2010, trace levels of PAHs were detected in four seafood samples, but remained below LOCs.[22] VOCs remained below LOCs in air and seafood throughout the *Deepwater Horizon* oil spill.[22]

The acute health effects of liquid volatile crude may be divided into the shared effects of exposures to total petrochemical hydrocarbons and the specific effects of exposures to VOCs and PAHs, which may be compounded by sunlight (phototoxicity) and by heat. The shared acute health effects of crude exposures to VOCs and PAHs include dermal erythema, conjunctival irritation, lacrimation, mucosal

Table	
8-3	**Air and Seafood Surveillance for Polycyclic Aromatic Hydrocarbons (PAHs) during the *Deepwater Horizon* Gulf Oil Spill, 2010**

PAHs	Air Surveillance	Seafood Surveillance
Sampling and Analyzing Agencies	EPA, LADEQ*	LADHH, LADWF, NOAA[†]
Established Levels of Concern (LOCs)	24-hour screening LOCs	Screening LOCs in specific seafood by weight
Units for LOCs	ng/m^3	mg/kg
Benzo(a)anthracene	8.7	490–2,000
Benzo(a)pyrene	0.87	0.35–1.43
Benzo(b)fluoranthene	8.7	0.035–0.143
Benzo(k)fluoranththene	8.7	3.5–14.3
Chrysene	87	35–143
Dibenzo(a,h)anthracene	0.8	0.035–0.143
Indeno(1,2,3-cd)pyrene	8.7	0.35–1.43
Fluoranthene	NR	65–267
Fluorene	NR	65–267
Phenanthrene	NR	490–2,000
Pyrene	NR	490–2,000

*These [LOC] screening values are not indicators of potential health risks. They function as triggers for further evaluation when containment concentration values exceed the screening values.

[†]These [LOC] screening values are not indicators of potential health risks. They function as triggers for further evaluation when containment concentration values exceed the screening values [or highest level of screening LOCs in specific seafood by weight].

Abbreviations: EPA, U.S. Environmental Protection Agency; LADEQ, Louisiana Department of Environmental Quality; LADHH, Louisiana Department of Health and Hospitals; LADWF, Louisiana Department of Wildlife and Fisheries; NOAA, U.S. National Oceanographic and Atmospheric Administration; NR, not reported.

irritation, sneezing, coughing, bronchospasm, nausea and vomiting if ingested, and chemical pneumonitis if aspirated. Both PAHs and VOCs can cause myocardial depression with sensitization to endogenous catecholamines and precipitate angina or myocardial infarction during inhalation exposure, especially in enclosed and underventilated spaces. PAHs are phototoxic and can cause skin bronzing and

Table	
8-4	**Air and Seafood Surveillance for Volatile Organic Compounds (VOCs) during the *Deepwater Horizon* Gulf Oil Spill, 2010**

VOCs	Air Surveillance	Seafood Surveillance
Sampling and Analyzing Agencies	EPA, LADEQ	LADHH, LADWF, NOAA
Established Levels of Concern (LOCs)	24-hour screening LOCs "These [LOC] screening values are not indicators of potential health risks. They function as triggers for further evaluation when containment concentration values exceed the screening values."	Screening LOCs in specific seafood by weight "These [LOC] screening values are not indicators of potential health risks. They function as triggers for further evaluation when containment concentration values exceed the screening values."
Units for LOCs	$\mu g/m^3$	mg/kg
Total C12-C13 Aliphatics	NR	233
Ethylbenzene	43,000	NR
Isopropylbenzene	4,000	NR
Naphthalene	30	33–133
Toluene	3,800	NR
m-, p-, or o-xylene	8,700	NR

Abbreviations: EPA: United States Environmental Protection Agency; LADEQ: Louisiana Department of Environmental Quality; LADHH: Louisiana Department of Health and Hospitals; LADWF: Louisiana Department of Wildlife and Fisheries; NOAA: United States National Oceanographic and Atmospheric Administration; NR, not reported.

hyperpigmentation with solar keratosis formation and, later, skin cancers. In addition, viscous hydrocarbons can plug hair follicles if not washed off, causing oil acne ("oil boils") or oil folliculitis. The solvents in dispersants and VOCs can cause defatting dermatitis with lichenification and secondary infection, chemical contact dermatitis, and allergic, eczematous contact dermatitis in sensitive individuals.

VOCs are highly lipophilic and neurotoxic compounds that can cause biphasic central nervous system (CNS) effects with initial headache, dizziness, intoxication, vertigo, and ataxia, followed by obtundation, stupor, and coma with respiratory depression. Temporary glove-and-stocking peripheral neuropathies with allodynia, anesthesia, and paresthesias may occur after short-term VOC exposures to unprotected skin with painful, permanent peripheral sensory neuropathies not uncommon after long-term exposures, especially to hexanes and xylenes.

When crude oil is burned on the sea surface, the VOCs are mostly consumed or vaporized; PAHs are pyrolized into anthracenes and pyrenes, and particulates of the burned hydrocarbons are released into the atmosphere. The major contaminants of burned crude oil that were monitored in the atmosphere and their levels of concern (LOCs) are depicted in **Table 8-5**.

Table	
8-5	**Pollutants, Particulates, and Dispersants Monitored in the Air during the *Deepwater Horizon* Gulf Oil Spill, 2010**
Air Pollutants, Particulates, Dispersants	**Air Surveillance**
Sampling and Analyzing Agencies	EPA, LADEQ
Established Levels of Concern (LOCs)	LOCs in air: 24-hour screening levels (or longer), 1-time screening reference toxic concentration
Units for LOCs	$\mu g/m^3$, ppb
Pollutant: H_2S	0.07 $\mu g/m^3$ over ≤ 14 days
Pollutant: SO_2	10.0 $\mu g/m^3$ over ≤ 14 days
Particulate: PM10	150 $\mu g/m^3$ over 24 hours
Particulate: PM2.5	35 $\mu g/m^3$ over 24 hours
Dispersant: 2-butoxyethanol	330 ppb (1-time screening reference toxic concentration)
Dispersant metabolite: 1-(2-butoxy-1)-methylethoxy-2-propanol	7 ppb (1-time screening reference toxic concentration)
Abbreviations: EPA: United States Environmental Protection Agency; LADEQ: Louisiana Department of Environmental Quality.	

In addition to PAHs and VOCs, burning weathered and dispersed crude oil will release toxic gases (carbon monoxide, hydrogen sulfide, ozone, sulfur dioxide, and nitrogen oxides), traces of heavy metals ranging from arsenic to zinc, and particulate matter (PM) ranging from visible ash to respirable, ultrafine particulate matter 2.5 microns in diameter (PM 2.5), which have been associated with immediate cardiorespiratory symptoms and premature death. Although the 24-hour averages for PM 2.5 levels on June 12 and June 14, 2010, at Grande Isle, Jefferson Parish, Louisiana, exceeded the EPA's LOCs, atmospheric particulates remained generally present at normal levels for the Louisiana Gulf Coastline from April through July 2010.[21] Lastly, burning crude oil on the sea surface, rather than burning crude oil on shore or on barges, provides all of the ingredients for the formation of bioaccumulating polychlorinated dibenzodioxins, including seawater chloride sources, petrochemical hydrocarbons, and heavy metal catalysts both in crude oil and seawater.

The Chemical Constituents of Dispersants

Crude oil dispersants were developed for water surface application to break up oil slicks, to increase the rate of oil biodegradation by marine microorganisms, and to protect fragile coastlines supporting commercial fisheries and wildlife breeding habitats. Once the process of chemical oil dispersion begins, the physical turbulence created by winds, waves, and tides further disperses droplets or micelles of crude oil in the water column. To be effective, dispersants are composed of two types of chemicals: surfactants and solvents. The surfactants are the least toxic ingredients of dispersants and are designed to make the dispersants bind to spilled crude oil. Common surfactants in dispersants include petroleum distillates and dioctyl sodium sulfosuccinate (DOSS), derivatives of which continue to be used in laxatives and stool softeners (e.g., Colace, Dulcolax).

The solvents in surfactants are more toxic and are used to disperse and dissolve spilled crude oil. Commonly used solvents in dispersants include propylene glycol, a solvent used in many intravenous drug preparations, and 2-butoxyethanol, an industrial solvent used in paint thinners and strippers and in industrial and household cleaning compounds. Both propylene glycol and 2-butoxyethanol are glycol ethers that are hepatically metabolized to lactic and pyruvic acids by the alcohol dehydrogenase (ADH) enzyme system that also metabolizes ethanol (ethyl alcohol). Butoxyethanol can also be metabolized to ethylene glycol (antifreeze), a highly nephrotoxic glycol ether, by an alternate route in rodent models; it is unclear if this toxic route of metabolism occurs in humans when the ADH detoxification system becomes saturated by overdoses. The chemical constituents and the acute health effects of the two COREXIT dispersants used in the 2010 *Deepwater Horizon* oil spill cleanup are summarized in **Table 8-6**, and their chronic health effects are summarized in **Table 8-7**.

On June 30, 2010, the EPA reported its results of toxicity testing on eight oil dispersants, only one of which, COREXIT 9500, was

Table		
8-6	**A Comparison of the Acute Health Effects of the Two COREXIT Dispersants Used during the *Deepwater Horizon* Oil Spill Cleanup, 2010**	
Dispersants Used	**COREXIT 9527**	**COREXIT 9500**
MSDS-Listed Hazardous Ingredients	2-butoxyethanol (ethylene glycol monobutyl ether), Propylene glycol (1,2-propanediol), Dioctyl sodium sulfosuccinate (DOSS)	Hydrotreated light petroleum distillates, Propylene glycol (1,2-propanediol), Dioctyl sodium sulfosuccinate (DOSS)
MSDS-Listed Other Ingredients	Butanedioic acid, Sorbitan, 2-propanol	Butanedioic acid, Sorbitan, 2-propanol
Mucosal (EENT)	Lacrimation; acute irritation of eyes, nose, throat; metallic taste	Same
Dermal	Acute irritation, erythema	Same
Pulmonary	Cough, bronchospasm, aspiration pneumonitis if ingested	Same
Cardiovascular	Blood pressure instability, hypo-/hypertension, bradycardia	Same
Gastrointestinal	Acute nausea, then vomiting	Same
Neurological	Acute headache, inebriation, intoxication, depressed mental status, tremor	Same
Hematological	Oxidizing stress on red blood cells with hemolysis and hemolytic anemia, especially in patients with glucose-6-phosphate dehydrogenase (G-6-PD) deficiency	Same
Renal	Hemoglobinuria following acute hemolysis	Same

Table	
8-7	**A Comparison of the Chronic Health Effects of the Two COREXIT Dispersants Used during the *Deepwater Horizon* Oil Spill Cleanup, 2010**

Dispersants Used	COREXIT 9527	COREXIT 9500
MSDS-Listed Hazardous Ingredients	2-butoxyethanol (ethylene glycol monobutyl ether), Propylene glycol (1,2-propanediol), Dioctyl sodium sulfosuccinate (DOSS)	Hydrotreated light petroleum distillates, Propylene glycol (1,2-propanediol), Dioctyl sodium sulfosuccinate (DOSS)
MSDS-Listed Other Ingredients	Butanedioic acid, Sorbitan, 2-propanol	Butanedioic acid, Sorbitan, 2-propanol
Mucosal (EENT)	"Gas eye"—chronic blepharitis and conjunctivitis	Same
Dermal	Dry skin, lichenification, fissuring, secondary infection	Same
Pulmonary	Exacerbation of preexisting obstructive airways disease, occupational asthma	Same
Cardiovascular	NR	Same
Gastrointestinal	Elevated hepatic transaminases	NR
Neurological	Chronic tremor	NR
Hematological	Anemia, initially hemolytic, then renal	Same
Renal	Acute tubular necrosis followed by chronic renal failure possible in patients predisposed by genetic polymorphisms	Same

Abbreviation: NR, not reported.

used in the *Deepwater Horizon* oil spill cleanup.[20] The toxicity tests included a variety of cytotoxicity tests and tests of both androgenic and estrogenic receptor disruption.[20] The EPA concluded that all of the dispersants tested manifested some degree of cytotoxicity at concentrations between 10 and 100 parts per million (ppm), but none of the eight dispersants tested demonstrated any significant endocrine-disrupting activity via the androgen or estrogen signaling pathways.[20]

Prior Health Effects following Oil Tanker Spills

The acute health effects of prior oil tanker spills are compared in Table 8-8.[23–33]

Table 8-8	Acute Health Effects of Prior Oil Tanker Spills	
Tanker Spills (location, year)	**Study Designs**	**Acute Health Effects**
Exxon Valdez (Alaska, 1989)	Closed claims study.	1,811 claims: 506 sprains/strains, 264 respiratory symptoms, 150 cuts, 144 contusions.[23]
MV Braer (Scotland, 1993)	Case-control study.	Significant increase in headache, throat, and eye symptoms by day 1 of exposures; health quality remained significantly reduced in exposed cases at 6 months postexposure.[24, 25]
Sea Empress (Wales, 1996)	Case-control study.	Significant increase in medical and mental health complaints in exposed cases.[26]
Nakhodka (Sea of Japan, 1997)	Home interviews of 282 cleanup workers; 97 submitted urine samples.	Low back and leg pain, headache, eye and throat irritation related to duration of exposures; no increase in urine benzene indicator; 3 workers had slight increases in urine toluene indicator.[27]
Erika (Bay of Biscay, France, 1999)	Cross-sectional study in 1,465 professional and volunteer cleanup workers.	Skin exposures from decontaminating oiled birds associated with increased risks of dermatitis and eye irritation.[28]
Prestige (NW Spain, 2002)	Before-and-after cross-sectional study.	Significantly increased DNA damage and immunosuppression as measured by comet assays, CD_4 counts, interleukins (ILs)-2, -4, -10, and interferon gamma in preexposed versus postexposed patient blood samples.[29]
Tasman Spirit (Pakistan, 2003)	Case-control study.	Significant abnormalities in pulmonary function in exposed cases.[30, 31]
Heibei Spirit (South Korea, 2007)	Exposed cleanup workers versus exposed coastal residents study.	Significant increases in urine volatile organic chemicals and in mental health complaints in exposed cases; both cases and controls reported cough, sore eyes and throats, and skin rashes.[32, 33]

Prior Chronic Health Effects Following Oil Tanker Spills

The chronic health effects of prior oil tanker spills are compared in Table 8-9.[34–38]

Table		
8-9	**Chronic Health Effects of Prior Oil Tanker Spills**	
Tanker Spills (location, year)	**Study Designs**	**Chronic Health Effects**
Exxon Valdez (Alaska, 1989)	Follow-up study of closed claims participants 14 years later.	Increased prevalence of reactive airway diseases, neurological impairments, and multiple chemical sensitivities.[34]
Exxon Valdez (Alaska, 1989)	Mental health survey study 1 year postspill and again at 6 years postspill.	$n = 599$; increased odds ratios for anxiety = 3.6; posttraumatic stress disorder = 2.9; depression = 2.1. These adverse mental health effects were observed at similar levels up to 6 years postspill.[35]
Erika (Bay of Biscay, France, 1999)	Cancer-risk analysis based on water column and beach PAH measurements 4 months after spill and on modeling of atmospheric PAH levels.	PAH residues were greatest on rocky soil; the highest estimated cancer risk approximated 10^{-5} per lifetime.[36]
Prestige (NW Spain, 2002)	Survey study sent to 38 commercial fishermen's cooperatives, $n = 6,780$ (76% response rate) 1 to 2 years postspill.	Significantly increased prevalence of lower respiratory tract symptoms in fishermen participating in cleanup with a significant dose–response effect for exposures by hours, days, and activities.[37, 38]
Prestige (NW Spain, 2002)	Cross-sectional case-control study among exposed case fishermen ($n = 501$) and unexposed control fishermen ($n = 177$) 2 years postspill.	Significantly increased prevalence of persistent lower respiratory tract symptoms, elevated markers of airway injury (8-isoprostane, vascular endothelial growth factor, basic fibroblast growth factor) in breath condensates, and chromosomal lesions and structural alterations in circulating lymphocytes 2 years postspill.[37, 38]

LOUISIANA'S IMMEDIATE PUBLIC HEALTH EXPERIENCE

The Section of Environmental Epidemiology and Toxicology of the Office of Public Health (OPH) of the Louisiana Department of Health and Hospitals (DHH) closely tracked and evaluated over 300 cases of individual reports of acute health effects related to the BP oil spill using a sentinel, syndromic surveillance system that transmitted data directly to the OPH from physicians' offices, outpatient urgent care clinics, hospital emergency departments, Emergency Medical Services (EMS), and the Louisiana Poison Control Center. Ranked descriptions of the Louisiana state experience with the reported acute health effects related to the BP oil spill are summarized in **Tables 8-10** through **8-13**, and mirror similar acute health effects reported by oil spill cleanup workers and the general population following prior oil tanker spills worldwide (see Table **8-9**).

Table	
8-10	Active Surveillance for Acute Human Health Effects of the *Deepwater Horizon* Oil Spill in Louisiana: Ranking of Reporting Sources, Routes of Exposures, Agent Exposures, Locations of Exposures, Activities during Exposures, and Acute Healthcare Utilization

Rankings	Reporting Sources	Routes of Exposures (excludes other)	Chemical/ Physical Agent Exposures	Exposure Locations (excludes unknown)	Activities During Exposures	Healthcare Utilization Sites (by workers)
1	ED	Inhalation	Heat	Offshore	Offshore worker	ED or urgent care
2	PCC	Dermal	Odors and fumes	Shoreline	Onshore worker	Clinic or office
3	Urgent care	Ocular	Emulsified oil and dispersant	Coastal Terrebonne Parish	Boom deploy worker	Hospital inpatient (mostly one day)
4	EMS	Ingestion	Liquid crude oil	Coastal Jefferson Parish	Cleanup worker	Call, no care

Abbreviations: ED, Emergency Department; EMS, Emergency Medical Services; PCC, Patient Care Clinic.

Source: MS Canyon 252 Oil Spill Surveillance Report, Week 38, From 09/19/2010 to 09/25/2010, pp 1–7. Oil Spill Health Effect Summary. Louisiana Department of Health and Hospitals, Office of Public Health. Section of Environmental Epidemiology and Toxicology. Baton Rouge, LA.

Table	
8-11	Active Surveillance for Acute Human Health Effects of the *Deepwater Horizon* Oil Spill in Louisiana: Age Rankings of Those Reporting Symptoms

Ranked Age Distributions for All Reporting Symptoms	Oil-Related Workers Reporting Acute Health Effects (mostly male)	General Population Reporting Acute Health Effects (mostly female)
1	18–44 years	45–64 years
2	45–64 years	18–44 years
3	65+ years	0–17 years
4	0–17 years	65+ years

Source: MS Canyon 252 Oil Spill Surveillance Report, Week 38, From 09/19/2010 to 09/25/2010, pp 1–7. Oil Spill Health Effect Summary. Louisiana Department of Health and Hospitals, Office of Public Health. Section of Environmental Epidemiology and Toxicology. Baton Rouge, LA.

Table	
8-12	Active Surveillance for Acute Human Health Effects of the *Deepwater Horizon* Oil Spill in Louisiana: Syndromic Surveillance of Oil-Related Workers: Ranking of Symptoms

Organ Systems	Neurologic	Respiratory	GI	Cardiac	Skin	Eye
Ranking of Systems Reporting Symptoms	1	2	3	4	5	6
The Most Commonly Reported Symptoms by Organ System						
1	Headache	Sore throat	Nausea	Chest pain	Rash	Irritated eyes
2	Dizziness	Cough	Vomiting	Palpitations	Redness, itching	Blurred vision
3	Syncope	Dyspnea (SOB)	Diarrhea	NR	Dryness, chaffing	NR
4	Altered taste	Nasal stuffiness/ irritation	Anorexia	NR	NR	NR
5	Tremor	Wheezing	NR	NR	NR	NR

Abbreviations: GI, gastrointestinal; NR, not reported; SOB, shortness of breath.

Source: MS Canyon 252 Oil Spill Surveillance Report, Week 38, From 09/19/2010 to 09/25/2010, pp 1–7. Oil Spill Health Effect Summary. Louisiana Department of Health and Hospitals, Office of Public Health. Section of Environmental Epidemiology and Toxicology. Baton Rouge, LA.

Table						
8-13	**Active Surveillance for Acute Human Health Effects of the *Deepwater Horizon* Oil Spill in Louisiana: Syndromic Surveillance of the General Population: Ranking of Symptoms**					
Organ Systems	**Respiratory**	**Neurologic**	**GI**	**Eye**	**Skin**	**General**
Ranking of Systems Reporting Symptoms	1	2	3	4	5	6
The Most Commonly Reported Symptoms by Organ System						
1	Sore throat	Headache	Nausea	Irritated eyes	Rash	Weakness, fatigue
2	Cough	Dizziness	Vomiting	Blurred vision	Redness, itching	Sweats
3	Dyspnea (SOB)	Altered taste	Diarrhea	NR	Dryness, chaffing	Fever
4	Nasal stuffiness/ irritation	NR	NR	Anorexia	NR	NR
5	Wheezing	NR	NR	NR	NR	NR

Abbreviations: COPD, chronic obstructive pulmonary diseases, including asthma; GI, gastrointestinal; NR, not reported; SOB, shortness of breath.

Source: MS Canyon 252 Oil Spill Surveillance Report, Week 38, From 09/19/2010 to 09/25/2010, pp 1–7. Oil Spill Health Effect Summary. Louisiana Department of Health and Hospitals, Office of Public Health. Section of Environmental Epidemiology and Toxicology. Baton Rouge, LA.

MAKING FUTURE CHRONIC HEALTH PREDICTIONS BASED ON PRIOR EXPERIENCES

To determine future health effects, we could look at symptoms following previous oil spills. Only two prior oil tanker spills have provided any significant peer-reviewed and evidence-based results on the longer-term health effects of human exposures to coastal oil spills: the tanker *Exxon Valdez* oil spill in Alaska in 1989 and the tanker *Prestige* oil spill in Spain in 2002. In a master's thesis, O'Neill[34] studied the health status of oil spill workers 14 years after the *Exxon Valdez* oil spill and found a significantly greater prevalence of the symptoms of chronic airway disease among workers with higher exposures to weathered crude oil and dispersants, as well as a greater prevalence of self-reported neurological disorders and multiple chemical sensitivities. In 1993, Palinkas and colleagues[35] reported their results of a validated mental health instrument survey study 1 year after the *Exxon Valdez* oil spill and again 6 years postspill in 599 exposed subjects. There was a statistically increased odds ratio of anxiety, posttraumatic stress disorder, and depression following the oil spill, which remained significantly increased 6 years postspill.[35]

In 2003, Dor and colleagues[36] reported the results of their cancer-risk analysis in cleanup workers following the tanker *Erika* oil spill in the Bay of Biscay in 1999 and found increased cancer risks in the crude-oil-exposed cleanup workers. In 2007, Zock and colleagues[37] obtained self-reported questionnaire data from 6,780 fishermen exposed to crude oil and dispersants following the *Prestige* oil spill of the northeast Spanish coast in 2002 and found a significantly higher prevalence of lower respiratory tract symptoms 2 years after oil spill activities with a significant dose–response effect exhibited by the 4,271 higher-exposed oil spill cleanup workers. In 2010, Rodriguez-Trigo and colleagues[38] reported the results of a cross-sectional study among exposed case fishermen ($n = 501$) and unexposed control fishermen ($n = 177$) 2 years following the *Prestige* oil spill in 2002. The authors reported the following results: (1) significantly increased prevalence of persistent lower respiratory tract symptoms in exposed subjects; (2) significantly higher levels of biomarkers of chronic airway injury and repair (8-isoprostane, basic fibroblast growth factor) in nonsmoking exposed cleanup workers; (3) a dose–response effect with greater levels of injury biomarkers reflecting increasing intensity of oil spill cleanup exposures; and (4) a higher proportion of structural chromosomal damage, predominantly unbalanced chromosome alterations, in exposed study subjects.[38]

WHAT'S NEXT?

Chronic Health Predictions Based on Common Genetic Polymorphisms among Oil-Spill-Related Workers and the General Population

Potential health effects might be determine by looking at genetic polymorphisms of potentially effected populations. The more common genetic polymorphisms in exposed oil-spill-related workers and the general population in Louisiana anticipated to have potential chronic health impacts on the populations with the greatest exposures to liquid crude oil, dispersants, weathered crude oil and dispersants, and burning weathered crude oil and dispersants are summarized by mechanisms of toxicity and adverse health effects in **Table 8-14**.[39-46] Many of the genetic polymorphisms compared in Table 8-14 are overrepresented in three minority populations in Louisiana—African Americans AHH deficiency, glucose-6-phosphate dehydrogenase [G6-PD] deficiency), Vietnamese Americans (AHH deficiency, uridine diphosphoglucuronyltransferase [UDP] deficiency, glutathione-S-transferase [GST] deficiency), and Native Americans (acetaldehyde dehydrogenase [AADH] deficiency)—and may represent chronic health disparities.[39-46]

Ecosystem-Related Health Predictions

The longer-term effects of the *Deepwater Horizon* oil spill on ecosystem health will be the hardest to predict given the magnitude of the oil spill disaster; they can only be compared to the prior *Ixtoc I* oil spill disaster in 1979. In August 2010, the U.S. Fish and Wildlife Service's *Deepwater Horizon* Response Consolidated Wildlife Collection Report confirmed the deaths of over 4,000 animals, including 3,902 birds, 517 sea turtles, 71 marine mammals (mostly dolphins), and 1 reptile.[47]

Many natural and man-made events, including agricultural waste runoffs and oil spills, may precipitate subsurface anoxic dead zones and massive surface blooms of red algal phytoplankton in marine ecosystems.[48] A recently described ecosystem phenomenon observed in the Baltic and North Seas, regions of significant deep-sea oil exploration, oil tanker traffic, and occasional oil tanker spills, has been the growth of harmful algal blooms or "red tides."[48] Since the *Deepwater Horizon* oil spill, several red algal blooms have been observed in Louisiana coastal waters and within the Mississippi River delta.

The red algae or dinoflagellates have a symbiotic relationship with nitrogen-fixing cyanobacteria that produce toxins that can bioaccumulate in the marine food chain and in humans.[48] All five groups of cyanobacteria may produce beta-methylamino-L-alanine (BMAA), a neurotoxic amino acid, and the putative causative toxin of a progressive neurodegenerative disorder known as amyotrophic lateral sclerosis/parkinsonism-dementia complex (ALS/PDC).[48-51]

8-14 Common Genetic Polymorphisms Among Oil Spill Workers and the General Population of South Louisiana[39–46]

Genetic Polymorphisms	Hepatic Enzyme Phase	Mechanisms of Adverse Effects	Populations at Risk	Potential Adverse Health Outcomes
Glucose-6-phosphate dehydrogenase deficiency (G6PDD)	Phase 1 G6PDD is an X-linked recessive trait and the most common genetic polymorphism.	Failure to protect RBCs from oxidative stresses imposed by solvents in dispersants and VOCs in crude oil.	Up to 50% of Americans of Southern European ancestry. Up to 40% of Americans of Middle Eastern ancestry. 12% African American males. 4% Asian American males. 4% African American females.	Hemolytic anemia, chronic anemia, gall stones, jaundice, renal insufficiency/failure, cirrhosis, liver failure. [38, 39]
Alcohol dehydrogenases 1B *2 and *3	Phase 1: alcohol dehydrogenase-acetaldehyde dehydrogenase system.	Hyper- versus hypometabolism of ethyl alcohol and related compounds such as the glycols in dispersants: 2-butoxyethanol, propylene glycol.	Native Americans, Asian Americans.	Lactic and metabolic acidosis. Increased risk of fetal alcohol spectrum disorders, including fetal alcohol syndrome. [38, 39]
Cytochrome P1A1 aryl hydrocarbon hydroxylase	Phase 1	Activates carcinogenic benzo-a-pyrenes in PAHs in crude oil, volatilized crude, burning crude, ingested PAHs, and cigarette smoke.	Asian Americans. Also, all populations with high smoking prevalence, including African American and Asian American males.	Increased susceptibility to the following cancers: oral, throat, lung, prostate, colorectal, breast, and skin. [40, 41]
Uridine diphosphoglucuronyltransferase 1A7	Phase 2	Failure to supply adequate amount of glutathione to detoxify PAHs, especially the carcinogenic benzo-a-pyrenes.	Asian Americans. Also, all populations with high smoking prevalence, including African American and Asian American males.	Increased susceptibility to the following cancers: oral, throat, lung, prostate, colorectal, breast, and skin. [42–45]
Glutathione-S-transferase	Phase 2	Failure to detoxify activated PAH-epoxide free radicals, which are cancer promoters.	Up to 40%–50% Asian Americans. Also, all populations with high smoking prevalence, including African American and Asian American males.	Increased susceptibility to the following cancers: oral, throat, lung, prostate, colorectal, breast, and skin. [42–44]

Abbreviations: PAHs, polycyclic aromatic hydrocarbons; RBCs, red blood cells; VOCs, volatile organic compounds.

THE RESOLUTION AND EARLY CONSEQUENCES OF THE DISASTER

After a string of failed efforts to plug a gushing leak in 3.5-mile-deep waters nearly 50 miles off the mouth of the Mississippi River that began on April 20, 2010, BP finally capped the Macondo Prospect wellhead in July, and, for the first time in 86 days, crude oil stopped spilling into the Gulf. In September 2010, nearly 5 months after the blowout, federal regulators declared the well dead after pressure tests confirmed that cement pumped into the base of the well by two relief wells had hardened into an effective plug. Government scientists estimated the total oil spill to be nearly 5 million barrels, far outstripping the 3 million barrels spilled into the Bay of Campeche during the *Ixtoc I* blowout (see Table 8-2).

The long-term ecosystem damage caused by the Gulf oil spill remains unknown for several reasons, including the existence of a deepwater plume of dispersed oil suspended in the Gulf that periodically surfaces and the unprecedented use of subsea dispersants that fragmented spilled oil into chemical compounds small enough to enter the marine food chain. The economic impacts of the disaster also continue to evolve, but are more measurable than the ecosystem impacts.

NOAA has estimated the economic losses to the commercial fishing industries of Louisiana, Mississippi, and Alabama at $2.5 billion.[51] The U.S. Travel Association has estimated the economic impact of the oil spill on the Gulf Coast tourism industry, an industry that supports over 400,000 jobs and generates $34 billion in annual revenues, at $23 billion over 3 years.[18] Hundreds of thousands of people and businesses have filed for emergency payments from the $20 billion BP escrow fund, but Mr. Feinberg had only paid out $2.2 billion as of October 2011.

CONCLUSIONS AND FUTURE RECOMMENDATIONS

The *Deepwater Horizon* oil spill of 2010 was an environmental and economic disaster for the northern Gulf Coast with the potential for longer-term adverse ecosystem and public health impacts. Reliable, stable biomarkers must be selected now and monitored longitudinally over many years to measure the impact of adverse chemical exposures on the ecosystem, on the marine food chain, and on humans.

The NIEHS Gulf Workers' Oil Study grants have now been awarded to academic investigators to study cohorts of highly exposed offshore and onshore cleanup workers and their spouses and children. These studies must account for many confounders to establishing causal outcomes, including smoking, smokeless tobacco use, environmental tobacco smoke exposures, ethnicity, and, especially, genetic poly-morphisms regulating the detoxification of crude oil and dispersants. Respiratory, neurological, and dermal disorders may be anticipated now based on the outcomes of prior exposures to crude oil spills, burning petrochemical fuels, particulates, and VOCs. Screening for adverse mental health outcomes should also begin now and may be predicted to extend to the general population of lesser exposed and nonexposed individuals as a result of economic uncertainly, loss of culture and identity, stress, anxiety, and depression.

Several populations will require special monitoring and longer-term studies, including children of highly exposed cleanup workers and ethnic groups with high prevalence of genetic polymorphisms regulating the metabolism of PAHs and solvents. Lastly, the chronic effects of chemical exposures with prolonged latencies of decades, such as cancer and demyelinating neurological disorders, will need to be assessed frequently in prospective cohorts of exposed and nonexposed subjects with reliable biomarkers of deoxyribonucleic acid (DNA) damage and repair, inflammation and cytokine stimulation, autoimmune effects, immunosuppression and infection, and chromosomal alterations.

As alternative energy sources are developed, the offshore oil industry must continue to meet the nation's energy needs in a more responsible way, with significant changes in company behavior toward aquatic ecosystems, coastal communities, and government regulators. Government oversight of offshore oil exploration must be improved with mandatory oil spill prevention and safety regulations, frequent offshore installation inspections by competent inspectors, greater interagency consultations, and better enforcement procedures. Significant investments must encourage and support research and development of better technologies to prevent oil spills and to improve cleanup operations with less toxic dispersants and more effective containment strategies. Investment funds can come from stiffer penalties on offshore polluters and from congressional legislation establishing an Offshore Oil Spill Superfund with annual liability premium payments made by offshore oil exploration companies. Deepwater drilling for oil and gas is now the latest frontier in the nation's fossil fuel energy supply, and the deepwater ecosystem must be better understood, preserved, and protected.

DISCUSSION QUESTIONS

1. Which competencies described in the Appendix does this case demonstrate?
2. Discuss the major managerial failures on the part of BP and its important subcontractors, such as Halliburton and Transocean, in responding to the *Deepwater Horizon* Gulf oil spill disaster; cite examples of such failures from the case study; and make recommendations on how to avoid repeating such failures in future environmental disasters.
3. Discuss the major regulatory failures committed by federal, state, and local governments in responding to the *Deepwater Horizon* Gulf oil spill disaster; cite examples of such failures from the case study; and make recommendations on how to avoid similar regulatory failures in future environmental disasters.
4. As the incident commander in charge of the national response to the *Deepwater Horizon* Gulf oil spill disaster, discuss the specific steps that you would take to facilitate better communication and collaboration among internal and external emergency response partners.
5. Discuss the benefits of studying the health and ecosystem impacts and the emergency first responses to prior oil spill disasters in avoiding and in planning responses to future oil spill disasters.
6. As the regional state public health director for the impacted coastal areas, how would you initially assess the human health risks and ecosystem impacts of the *Deepwater Horizon* Gulf oil spill disaster for the governor, the secretary of health and hospitals (or equivalent state cabinet officer), the state legislature, the cleanup workers, and the general public? What initial strategies would you recommend to reduce further human injuries, to limit state economic losses, and to communicate timely information on disaster response to the public?

REFERENCES

1. Reproduced from The National Commission on the BP *Deepwater Horizon* oil spill and offshore drilling. Deep water: the Gulf oil disaster and the future of offshore drilling. Report to the President, January 2011. Available from http://www.oilspillcommission.gov/sites/default/files/documents/DEEPWATER_ReporttothePresident_FINAL.pdf.

2. Biello D. One year after BP oil spill, at least 1.1 million barrels still missing—where in the Gulf of Mexico is the oil from the Macondo well blowout? *Scientific American*. April 25, 2011. Available at: http://www.scientificamerican.com /article.cfm?id=one-year-after-bp-oil-spill-millions-of-barrels-oil-missing. Accessed March 16, 2013.

3. Tuckman J. Gulf oil spill: parallels with *Ixtoc* raise fears of impending ecological tipping point. *The Guardian*. June 1, 2010. Available at: http://www .guardian.co.uk/environment/2010/jun/01/gulf-oil-spill-ixtoc-ecological -tipping-point?INTCMP=SRCH. Accessed March 16, 2013.

4. Schrope M. The lost legacy of the last great oil spill. *Scientific American*. July 14, 2010. Available at: http://www.scientificamerican.com/article .cfm?id=the-lost-legacy-Ixtoc-oil. Accessed March 16, 2013.

5. Jernelov A, Linden O. *Ixtoc I*: a case study of the world's largest oil spill. *J Royal Swedish Acad Sci*. 1981;10:299–306.

6. Hayward shares candid views on 2006. *The Daily Telegraph*. December 18, 2006. Available at: http://www.telegraph.co.uk/finance/2952547/Hayward -shares-candid-views-on-2006.html. Accessed March 16, 2013.

7. Stanford Business School. Entrepreneurial spirit needed. May 12, 2009. Available at: http://www.gsb.stanford.edu/news/speakers_vftt.html. Accessed June 8, 2012. Mr. Hayward's entire lecture at Stanford Business School, May 12, 2009 can be viewed at Available at: http://www.youtube.com /watch?v=FwQM00clxgM. Last viewed on March 26, 2013.

8. Swaine J, Winnett R. BP chief Tony Hayward sold shares weeks before oil spill. *The Daily Telegraph*. June 5, 2010. Available at: http://www.telegraph .co.uk/finance/newsbysector/energy/oilandgas/7804922/BP-chief-Tony -Hayward-sold-shares-weeks-before-oil-spill.html. Accessed March 16, 2013.

9. BP oil spill in Gulf of Mexico will have "very modest" environmental impact says firm's CEO [video]. Mr. Hayward's entire interview can be viewed at http://videocafe.crooksandliars.com/scarce/bp-ceo-tony-hayward-oil-spill -impact-very-m. Last viewed on March 26, 2013.

10. BP's Tony Hayward: 'I'd like my life back.' *USA Today*. June 1, 2010. Available at: http://content.usatoday.com/communities/greenhouse/post/06/bp-tony -hayward-apology/1. Accessed March 16, 2013.

11. Quinn J. BP oil spill: Tony Hayward 'will be spliced and diced' by US politicians. *Daily Telegraph*. June 17, 2010. Available at: http://www.telegraph .co.uk/finance/newsbysector/energy/oilandgas/7834475/BP-oil-spill-Tony -Hayward-will-be-spliced-and-diced-by-US-politicians.html. Accessed March 16, 2013.

12. Goldenberg S. 'If he was working for me I'd sack him'—Obama turns up heat on BP boss. *The Guardian*. June 8, 2010. Available at: http://www.guardian.co.uk/ business/2010/jun/08/bp-deepwater-horizon-obama?INTCMP=SRCH. Accessed March 16, 2013.

13. White J. Coast Guard's chief of staff to assist FEMA head Brown. *The Washington Post*. September 7, 2005. Available at: http://www.washingtonpost .com/wp-dyn/content/article/2005/09/06/AR2005090601677.html? referrer=mail. Accessed March 16, 2013.

14. Sherman J. Janet Napolitano defends oil spill response. *Politico*. May 17, 2010. Available at: http://www.politico.com/news/stories/0510/37355.html. Accessed March 16, 2013.

15. Savage C. Sex, drug use and graft cited in Interior Department. *The New York Times*. September 10, 2008. Available at: http://www.nytimes .com/2008/09/11/washington/11royalty.html. Accessed June 8, 2012.

16. Alpert B. Mineral Management Service head resigns. *The Times-Picayune*. May 27, 2010. Available at: http://www.nola.com/news/gulf-oil-spill/index .ssf/2010/05/ap_sources_minerals_management.html. Accessed June 8, 2012.

17. Broder JM. Environmentalists wary of Obama's Interior pick. *The New York Times*. December 17, 2008. Available at: http://www.nytimes .com/2008/12/18/us/politics/18salazarcnd.html. Accessed June 8, 2010.

18. Proctor C. Big price tag for recovery of the Gulf Coast. *Pensacola News Journal*. August 1, 2010. Available at: http://www.pnj.com/article/20100801 /BUSINESS/8010313/Carlton-Proctor-Big-price-tag-for-recovery-of-Gulf -Coast. Accessed June 8, 2012.

19. The Associated Press. OSU's Lubchenko confirmed as head of NOAA. *The Oregonian*. March 19, 2009. Available at: http://www.oregonlive.com /environment/index.ssf/2009/03/osus_lubchenco_confirmed_as_he.html. Accessed March 16, 2013.

20. Hemmer MJ, Barron MG, Greene RM. Comparative toxicity of eight oil dispersant products on two Gulf of Mexico aquatic test species. U.S. Environmental Protection Agency Office of Research and Development. June 30, 2010. Available at: http://www.epa.gov/bpspill/reports/ComparativeToxTest .Final.6.30.10.pdf. Accessed March 26, 2013.

21. Environmental Protection Agency. Science to support EPA's response to the BP oil spill: EPA scientists and engineers are supporting the coordinated response to the *Deepwater Horizon* oil spill. *Science Matters Newsletter*. October 25, 2011. Available at: http://www.epa.gov/sciencematters/june2010/scinews_oil-spill .htm. Accessed June 8, 2012.

22. MS Canyon 252 Oil Spill Surveillance Report, Week 38, From 09/19/2010 70 09/25/2010, pp 1–7. Oil Spill Health Effect Summary. Louisiana Department of Health and Hospitals, Office of Public Health. Section of Environmental Epidemiology and Toxicology. Available from http:// www.dhh.louisiana.gov/assets/docs/SurveillanceReports/OilSpillHealth /_OilSpillSurveillance2010_17.pdf.

23. Gorman RW, Beradinelli SP, Bender TR. *Exxon/Valdez* Alaska oil spill. NIOSH HATA 89-200 and 89-273-2111. May 1991. Available at: http://www .cdc.gov/niosh/hhe/reports/pdfs/1989-0200-2111.pdf. Accessed March 16, 2013.

24. Campbell D, Cox D, Crum J, et al. Initial effects of the grounding of the tanker *Braer* on health in Shetland. *Br Med J*. 1993;307:1251–1255.

25. Campbell D, Cox D, Crum J, et al. Later effects of grounding of tanker *Braer* on health in Shetland. *Br Med J*. 1994;309:773–774.

26. Lyons LA, Temple JM, Evans D, et al. Acute health effects of the *Sea Empress* oil spill. *J Epidemiol Community Health*. 1999;53:306–310.

27. Morita A, Kusaka Y, Deguchi Y, et al. Acute health problems among people engaged in the cleanup of the Nakhodka oil spill. *Environ Res.* 1999;81:185–194.
28. Schvoerer C, Gourier-Fréry C, Ledrans M, et al. *Etude Épidémiologique des Troubles de Santé Survenus à Court Term Chez les Personnes Ayant Participle au Nettoyage des Sites Pollués par le Fioul de l'Erika.* Paris, France: Institut de Veille Sanitaire; 2000.
29. Zock JP, Rodrigez-Trigo G, Pozo-Rodriguez F, Barbera JA. Health effects of oil spills: lessons from the *Prestige. Am J Resp Crit Care Med.* 2011;184:1094–1096.
30. Meo SA, Al-Drees AM, Meo IM, et al. Lung function in subjects exposed to crude oil spill into sea water. *Mar Poll Bull.* 2008;56:88–94.
31. Meo SA, Al-Drees AM, Rasheed S, et al. Effect of duration of exposure to polluted air environment on lung function in subjects exposed to crude oil spill in sea water. *Int J Occup Med Environ Health.* 2009;22:35–41.
32. Lee J, Kim M, Ha M, Chung BC. Urinary metabolic profile of volatile organic compounds in acute exposed volunteers after an oil spill in Republic of Korea. *Biomed Chromatogr.* 2010;24:562–568.
33. Lee CH, Kang YA, Chang KJ, et al. Acute health effects of the *Heibei* oil spill on the residents of Taean, Korea. *Prev Med Public Health.* 2010;43:166–173.
34. O'Neill AK. *Self-Reported Exposures and Health Status Among Workers from the Exxon Valdez Oil Spill: Cleanup* [master's thesis]. New Haven, CT: Yale University; 2003.
35. Palinkas LA, Petterson JS, Russell J, Downs MA. Community patterns of psychiatric disorders after the *Exxon Valdez* oil spill. *Am J Psychiatry.* 1993;150:1517–1523.
36. Dor F, Bonnard R, Gourier-Fréry C, et al. Health risk assessment after decontamination of the beaches polluted by the wrecked ERIKA tanker. *Risk Anal.* 2003;23:1199–1208.
37. Zock JP, Rodriguez-Trigo G, Pozo-Rodriguez F, et al. SEPAR-*Prestige* Study Group. Prolonged respiratory symptoms in cleanup workers of the *Prestige* oil spill. *Am J Resp Crit Care Med.* 2007;176:610–616.
38. Rodriguez-Trigo G, Zock JP, Pozo-Rodriguez F, et al. SEPAR-*Prestige* Study Group. Health changes in fishermen 2 years after cleanup of the *Prestige* oil spill. *Ann Intern Med.* 2010;153:540–541.
39. Haycock PC. Fetal alcohol spectrum disorders: the epigenetic perspective. *Biol Repro.* 2009;81:607–617.
40. Green RF, Stoler JM. Alcohol dehydrogenase 1B genotype and fetal alcohol syndrome: a HuGe minireview. *Am J Obstet Gynecol.* 2007;197:12–25.
41. May PA, Gossage JP, Kalberg WO, et al. Prevalence and epidemiologic characteristics of FASD from various research methods with an emphasis on recent in-school studies. *Dev Disab Res Rev.* 2009;15:176–192.
42. Kiyohara C, Nakanishi Y, Inutsuka S, et al. The relationship between CYP1A1 aryl hydrocarbon hydroxylase activity and lung cancer in a Japanese population. *Pharmacogenetics.* 1998;8:315–323.
43. Kiyohara C, Ohno Y. Role of metabolic polymorphisms in lung carcinogenesis. *Nippon Koshu Eisei Zasshi.* 1999;46:241–249.

44. Wang Y, Duan H, Dai Y, et al. Uridine diphosphoglucuronyltransferase 1A7 gene polymorphism and susceptibility to chromosomal damage among polycyclic aromatic hydrocarbon exposed workers. *J Occ Environ Med.* 2009;51:682–689.

45. Strassburg CP, Vogel A, Kneip S, et al. Polymorphisms of the human UDP-glucuronyltransferase (UGT) 1A7 gene in colorectal cancer. *Gut.* 2002;50:851–856.

46. Chinevere TD, Murray CK, Grant E Jr, et al. Prevalence of glucose-6-phosphate dehydrogenase deficiency in U.S. Army personnel. *Mil Med.* 2006;171:905–907.

47. Merchant B. 4,500 Animals killed in BP spill . . . and counting. *Treehugger.* August 10, 2010. Available at: http://www.treehugger.com/natural-sciences/4500 -animals-killed-in-bp-spill-and-counting.html. Accessed June 8, 2012.

48. Jonasson S, Eriksson J, Berntzon L, et al. Transfer of a cyanobacterial neurotoxin within a temperate aquatic ecosystem suggests pathways for human exposure. *Proceed Nat Acad Sci.* 2010;107:9252–9257.

49. Arnold A, Edgren DC, Palladino VS. Amyotrophic lateral sclerosis: 50 cases observed on Guam. *J Nerv Ment Sia.* 1953;117:517–522.

50. Garruto RM, Yase Y. Neurodegenerative disorders of the western Pacific: the search for mechanisms of pathogenesis. *Trends Neurosci.* 1986;9:368–374.

51. Pablo J, Banack SA, Cox SA, et al. Cyanobacterial neurotoxin BMAA in ALS and Alzheimer's disease. *Acta Neurol Scand.* 2009;20:216–25.

Planning for the Republican National Convention 2004: Findings from the New York City Department of Health and Mental Hygiene

Shadi Chamany

INTRODUCTION

In 2001, after completing medical training as an internal medicine physician in New York City, I moved to Atlanta to become a medical epidemiologist through the Centers for Disease Control and Prevention's (CDC) Epidemic Intelligence Service (EIS). I was motivated by my ongoing interest in population health and methods by which population health can be improved through monitoring, program implementation, and evaluation. I had always intended to do public health at the local level, so following this 2-year program, I returned to postgraduate training as a preventive medicine resident to obtain policy, programmatic, management, and leadership experience to complement my clinical and epidemiology training. One requirement of this program was to complete a practicum year, which I did from July 2004 to June 2005 at the New York City Department of Health and Mental Hygiene (DOHMH). This was an invaluable experience, starting with my first assignment, an evaluation of the planning activities for the 2004 Republican National Convention.

THE ASSIGNMENT

The Republican National Convention (RNC) took place in New York City at Madison Square Garden from August 29, 2004, through September 2, 2004, and was an event for which the DOHMH and other city agencies specifically prepared, given the high-security nature of the event and the potential for harm to the public should a disaster or emergency occur.

DOHMH planning for the RNC began as early as June 2004, utilizing the lessons learned from the World Trade Center attacks on 9/11 as a framework. Planning activities included the following:

1. Identifying specific objectives and the timeline for completion.
2. Assigning individuals to work on those objectives.
3. Determining personnel needs that may arise during an emergency and creating corresponding job action sheets outlining the duties.
4. Creating an on-call roster of staff.
5. Confirming contact information for all essential and senior staff in the event that traditional communication methods fail (e.g., power outage).
6. Ensuring paper versions of all essential documents exist at the home office location and the backup emergency operations

center. Essential documents included, but were not limited to, fact sheets, press release templates, message palettes, protocols and flow sheets, response plans, and case report forms.

As a preventive medicine resident, I was given the task of evaluating the planning and response activities of the DOHMH. There were three components. The first, occurring prior to the RNC, entailed meeting with various DOHMH staff involved in planning activities to document their progress. The second took place during the RNC, at which time I was asked to observe and document any response activities that might occur and could be used by full-time emergency managers in compiling lessons learned. The third part was post-RNC, investigating the series of events around an incident that occurred during the RNC.

It is important to note that while I had some familiarity with emergency response activities, this was from the perspective of assisting in the response activity and not from the planning perspective. During my EIS training between 2001 and 2003, I was deployed three separate times to support the response activities of a local health department or CDC for the following events/outbreaks: (1) World Trade Center attack (DOHMH); (2) 2001 anthrax attacks (DOHMH and New Jersey Department of Health and Senior Services); and (3) SARS outbreak (CDC).

This case study will describe the broad set of planning activities undertaken by the DOHMH for this event; summarize response activities during the RNC, including a response to a nonintentional radiography incident that occurred coincidentally during the RNC; and lessons learned from the perspective of communication and documentation.

INTRODUCTORY MEETINGS

At the time of the RNC, the emergency response structure the DOHMH used, adapted from the incident command system, was called the incident management system (IMS). The IMS consisted of 10 sections: (1) planning, (2) logistics, (3) finance and administration, (4) epidemiology and surveillance, (5) laboratory, (6) mental health, (7) medical/clinical, (8) public and provider information, (9) environmental, and (10) information systems. Over the course of a month, I met with various staff assigned to leadership positions within these sections to gather information about their planning activities. **Table 9-1** outlines activities for each section.

Table	
9-1	**Planning Activities of Each Incident Management System Section of the New York City Department of Health and Mental Hygiene for the Republican National Convention in New York City, August 2004**

Section	Planning Activities
Planning	• Train DOHMH staff in IMS structure and roles during an emergency • Secure emergency operations center (EOC) facilities and stock with backup equipment (e.g., mobile phones, radios, batteries, laptops) • Compile documents for mobile library • Create schedule of core and backup staff • Test the Dialogics communications system (an automated call-down notification system) • Prepare documents for IMS meetings, including action plan forms, fact sheets, and so on
Logistics	• Preposition drivers with vehicles and radios throughout the city • Confirm backup generator at both the main DOHMH and backup EOC
Finance and Administration	• Cross-train staff in tracking unit to work with both personnel and nonpersonnel issues • Identify alternative sites (i.e., workstations) for access to the payroll system • Review emergency protocol for procurement to ensure budget and fiscal units will be able to track expenses on a daily basis • Identify a method to dispense and sign checks in the field
Epidemiology and Surveillance (E&S)	• Enhance existing surveillance systems to meet needs of RNC • Establish temporary surveillance systems during RNC • Develop specific call-up system for rapid mobilization of E&S staff for investigation • Identify staff to prepare reports for daily E&S meeting during RNC • Develop health alerts to be sent to the provider community prior to the event to enhance awareness of need to report syndromes and illness caused by a potential biological threat agent (BTA) • Establish time for daily conference call with hospitals in NYC area

Section	Planning Activities
Laboratory	• Train first responders in BTA specimen handling, collection, packaging, and transport • Train Level A laboratories in BTA response protocols through site visits and distribution of Level A laboratory protocols • Relocate Bioterrorism Response Laboratory (BTRL) to a new Biosafety Level 3 laboratory • Train and cross-train staff to ensure adequate coverage in the event of a surge • Identify backup laboratories for rerouting of specimens if needed during an emergency
Mental Health	• Review emergency protocol with agencies contracted with the Division of Mental Hygiene (DMH), including the possibility of mobilizing staff from these agencies as well as providing operational assistance to agencies • Identify first- and second-tier responders from contract pool • Create DMH provider emergency contact hotline (operations) and inform agencies of this new access line through division personnel
Medical/ Clinical	• Prepare for the assembly of possible point-of-distribution sites (PODS) in midtown Manhattan • Train/drill clinic staff in PODS roles (e.g., greet, triage, evaluation, flow monitoring) • Drill Medical Reserve Corps (MRC)[a] on-call list using Dialogics • Prepare MRC as supplemental personnel for mass prophylaxis, if needed • Identify facilities for PODS and obtain floor plans • Secure supplies from Strategic National Stockpile and place PODS materials at predetermined location for distributor pickup • Preposition training materials at first PODS • Create tracking forms for PODS in coordination with Information Systems (IS) • Preidentify nursing staff to work in shelters requested by American Red Cross
Public and Provider Information	• Identify liaisons to mayor and Office of Emergency Management (OEM) and all members of city and federal joint information centers (JICs) • Develop or gather fact sheets, press release templates, and message palettes, both electronic and paper, into one central location

(continued)

Table	
9-1	*(continued)*

Section	Planning Activities
	• Offer periodic risk communication and media training of DOHMH staff through routine Bureau of Communications activities • Ensure bulk materials accessible (e.g., brochures, fact sheets) in usual and alternative locations • Review preexisting web-based information to ensure up-to-date materials
Environmental	• Determine status of personal protective equipment (PPE) training for relevant staff • Assess pest control efforts at Madison Square Garden (MSG), Pennsylvania Station, and Farley Post Office via follow-up with site consultants to ensure compliance • Schedule weekly baiting of lots around MSG until and through RNC • Identify staff (16 sanitarians, 4 supervisors) to monitor food quality at impacted facilities over the course of the event • Perform routine inventory of equipment and installation of statistical software for environmental epidemiologic analysis on laptops • Create electronic library with draft chemical emergency response plan, fact sheets, flow charts, and so on, in addition to a paper library containing a subset of critical documents listed previously • Identify BioWatch sampling in conjunction with the DOHMH laboratory and relevant external agencies
Information Systems (IS)	• Confirm essential applications on backup server at alternative site • Create infrastructure checklist with names and applications at each DOHMH site that IS supports • Restock inventory of wireless cards for laptops and perform routine maintenance of laptops prior to RNC (e.g., charge batteries) • Obtain approval of prioritized applications by senior staff • Train section chiefs in how to query employee database for their own section • Integrate employee databank, NYC MED[b], and MRC into Dialogics and create scenario groups to activate for certain events • Collaborate with sections to create database templates for various scenarios

[a]The Medical Reserve Corps is a volunteer group of trained health professionals with expertise in numerous health disciplines who are ready to respond to health emergencies.

[b]NYC MED is a web-based portal that allows bidirectional communication and information exchange between the DOHMH and providers.

A SPECIAL CONSIDERATION FOR PLANNING— ENHANCED DISEASE AND ENVIRONMENTAL SURVEILLANCE DURING THE RNC

Disease Surveillance

Given that the RNC was a national event attended by both delegates and demonstrators from across the country, disease surveillance efforts needed to consider these populations. These two populations would not necessarily seek care in the healthcare system that serves New York City residents due to access-to-care issues (e.g., demonstrators who had been arrested) or having already left town by the time of illness onset. Therefore, plans were made to modify the preexisting systems and establish auxiliary systems temporarily (see **Table 9-2**) to ensure early detection of an unusual illness manifestation or a cluster of RNC-related illnesses, including illness related to a biological threat agent or heat.

Table	
9-2	New York City Department of Health and Mental Hygiene Disease Surveillance During the Republican National Convention in New York City, August 2004

Modifications to Existing Disease Surveillance Systems	Description
Traditional Provider-Based Surveillance (medical and veterinary)	A passive system enhanced with (1) health alerts sent to a large provider mailing list 1 week prior to the RNC outlining DOHMH criteria for reporting RNC-associated illness, any suspected bioterrorist disease, or any unusual disease clusters; and (2) daily review by a medical epidemiologist of telephone calls made to the Bureau of Communicable Disease.
Syndromic Surveillance	An electronic system with daily feeds from emergency departments throughout the city was made more sensitive (lower threshold to alarm signal), more geographically focused, and more inclusive (additional syndromes).

(continued)

Table	
9-2	(*continued*)
BioWatch	An environmental surveillance system involving a New York City network of air-sampling units that samples for bioagents that may be used for terrorism surveillance was enhanced with the deployment of additional samplers and more frequent sampling.
Health Emergency Response Data System (HERDS)	A web-based communication and needs assessment tool providing information about hospital resources in 72 acute-care registered hospitals in the New York City area on a weekly basis was enhanced by adding information pertaining to Emergency Department volume, blood supply, admissions, and number of RNC-related visits just prior to and during the RNC. Reporting was daily, and participating hospitals had a daily conference call with DOHMH.
Unusual Death Surveillance	The usual manual review of unexplained deaths in persons aged 1 to 49 years old by a medical epidemiologist was expedited with a faster turnaround during the RNC.
Auxiliary Surveillance Systems	**Description**
Delegates' Hotel Physician Surveillance	Daily tallies of chief complaints during visits in medical practices of physicians serving hotels housing delegates.
Madison Square Garden First-Aid Clinic Surveillance	Daily tallies of number of patients seen and chief complaints during visits to the clinic run by the Fire Department of New York City Emergency Medical Service (FDNY-EMS).
RNC Protest Detainee Surveillance	Daily tallies of specific syndromes and injuries among detainees screened by FDNY-EMS and DOHMH Correctional Health while detained.
RNC Protest Street Medic Surveillance	Daily counts from street medics who tallied chief complaints by major syndrome category (e.g., fever/respiratory, gastrointestinal, heat related, injury).
First Responder Surveillance	Daily tallies of absenteeism and internal clinic visits among law enforcement/first responder agencies by syndrome category.

The plan was to have auxiliary surveillance systems begin prior to and continue throughout the RNC. DOHMH E&S staff met daily during this period as well as during the week after the RNC to review surveillance reports and make recommendations to the leadership, where applicable.

Food Supply and Biologic Air Monitoring

To monitor the food supply, the environmental section assigned 16 sanitarians to 12-hour shifts during the RNC to inspect food delivered to MSG and to monitor food preparation at MSG and the Farley Post Office, where the media was located. These sanitarians worked in conjunction with the U.S. Food and Drug Administration. The laboratory section received environmental specimens around the clock from the BioWatch detectors, in addition to their usual specimen flow.

ACTIVITIES AND EVENTS DURING THE RNC

Emergency Operations Centers

The DOHMH partially activated its own emergency operations center (EOC) over the course of the RNC. In this partially activated state, the incident commander and section chiefs met twice a day on the weekdays, and on each weekend day, the section chiefs called into a morning conference call. Each meeting was limited to 1.5 hours in duration, during which each section chief presented any new updates and follow-up to previous issues. A documentation officer from the planning section was assigned to prepare minutes of each meeting, which were distributed at the end of the day to meeting participants by email. I attended these meetings to directly observe the discussions and decision-making processes and to be ready to respond if there was an incident.

Several other EOCs were established in New York City given the security special event status of the RNC. The New York City Office of Emergency Management (OEM) was fully activated with 24/7 operation over the course of the event. Representatives from federal, state, and local agencies, including the DOHMH, were assigned to work 8- to 12-hour shifts during this time period. Two additional EOCs were specifically created for this event—the federal Multi-Agency Coordinating Center (MACC) and the Weapons of Mass Destruction (WMD) desk—both of which had DOHMH representation under full activation during the RNC.

Enhanced Surveillance

The disease surveillance team conducted seven epidemiological investigations in response to 21 syndromic surveillance signals or provider reports of an unusual illness, none of which yielded true clusters of illnesses. There were no positive samples from BioWatch detectors during the RNC. There were 177 RNC-related visits to area hospitals, reported through HERDS, 7% of which were related to infectious disease syndromes, 30% to trauma, and 63% to other illnesses. The DOHMH did not receive reports of any RNC-related deaths during this time period.

There were 25 RNC-related calls to the delegate hotel physicians, which accounted for 35% of all calls they received during the RNC. There were no concerning patterns of illness among these calls. The first-aid clinic surveillance system transmitted 112 reports, 29 of which were injury related; the rest were mild in nature (e.g., headache, blister). Through the protest street medic system, a rash cluster was reported, which was also reported through the protest detainee surveillance system, the latter also reporting complaints such as headaches, injury, and heat. There were no clusters or changes in visits/absenteeism from baseline reported through the first responder system.

A Radiography Accident

Unrelated to the RNC, on the afternoon of August 29, an independent contractor was performing a routine radiography assessment using a radioactive source to determine the structural integrity of a post office building. During this assessment, the radioactive source of the device was extended beyond its shielded position to expose the film (similar to a clinical radiograph), but the contractor was unable to retract the source back into its shielded position once the radiograph was taken. Because the radiological source contained a significant amount of radioactive material (approximately 65 Curies of Cobalt-60, a radioactive metal that emits both beta particles and gamma radiation), he contacted his radiation safety officer, who then contacted both the manufacturer of the device and the postal police. The New York Police Department (NYPD) began to evacuate the lower floors of the building and secure the perimeter, and the postal police notified the New York City Department of Environmental Protection's Division of Emergency Response and Technical Assessment (DEP-DERTA).

DEP contacted New York City Poison Control to inform them of the incident per the usual on-call system for DOHMH where, during non-business hours, calls to the DOHMH are routed to an on-call manager for environmental concerns. The DOHMH on-call environmental manager subsequently deployed two field staff to the scene and informed the DOHMH Office of Radiological Health (ORH). Within 30 minutes of the Poison Control notification, various DEP representatives at the MACC EOC and the OEM EOC also notified DOHMH representatives at the MACC and OEM EOCs. These DOHMH MACC and OEM EOC representatives both contacted the DOHMH environmental section chief, who subsequently called the DOHMH on-call manager, one of the deployed field staff, and the previously notified ORH staff.

A series of secondary notifications to several other local and state agencies took place, including to those that are required to be notified because of certain regulatory requirements (e.g., the Nuclear Regulatory Commission under the Atomic Energy Act of 1954) and to those that could assist in the response. Throughout the course of the night and following day, indoor and outdoor readings of radiation levels were collected, some of which were below background levels and others that were above, depending on where they were taken. At times, ORH contact with DOHMH field staff was impaired because there was no standard reporting timeline (e.g., every 15 minutes), the field staff was at times in locations without cellular phone reception, or field staff was being called by multiple people.

A mitigation strategy was devised after an on-site interagency meeting and a separate DOHMH conference call among nonfield staff and the device manufacturer took place—lead bricks would be placed around the source to limit exposure until the manufacturer's arrival the following day. With the assistance of the OEM, DOHMH field staff was able to retrieve lead bricks from a truck at the DOHMH public health laboratory and transport them to the site. The bricks were laid over the source between 5:00 and 6:00 AM with postshield readings showing some reduction in levels of radiation. The DOHMH mobile chemical and radiological monitoring van was dispatched to the field at 8:30 AM, and readings were obtained throughout the day along the entire perimeter of the post office building to monitor the situation.

The manufacturer arrived on-site in the early afternoon on August 30 and worked to retract the source over the next several hours. In the meantime, the DOHMH communications staff issued a press release at 1:00 PM,[1] a fact sheet, and a general city hotline (called "311") script response. The radiological source was successfully retracted around

6:30 PM, and it was transported off-site just before 8:00 PM. Five DOHMH physicians were deployed to the incident site and distributed information to individuals in the surrounding area between 7:00 and 8:00 PM. A second press release was disseminated at this time to inform the public of the resolution of the incident.[2]

CONCLUSIONS

Post-RNC: Lessons Learned from the Radiography Incident

Following the RNC, involved parties reviewed the events that took place to identify areas for improvement. One specific area I was tasked with was the creation of a detailed timeline of the DOHMH notifications and response activities. I started by reviewing my notes and minutes from the EOC meetings, but the level of detail requested necessitated a second round of interviews with key responders, as well as review of available response logs and reports from the various agencies, including the DOHMH. One challenge that occurred while creating this timeline was difficulty in getting access to complete records from all involved parties because there was little to no written documentation, the documentation that did exist was incomplete (e.g., no time included), or it was not accessible to me because it belonged to an outside agency. This became even more problematic as time passed and I was relying on participants' recall.

Although there were a series of areas identified for improvement, the most important were communication and documentation. There was a need for timely and nonredundant communication between field staff and the central response team, a rapid and accurate assessment of an incident in the context of a multiagency response where procedures and protocols differ by agency, and a mechanism in place that ensures documentation is adequate for postincident review to identify areas of improvement.

Despite the challenges that arose during this incident, there were many lessons learned that could be applied to any response activity:

1. Response plans should include a reporting protocol that outlines the frequency of reporting from the field to central command (e.g., every 30 minutes), the chain of communication, and the type of information required (e.g., a template for data collection).
2. Field staff should have an on-site team leader to coordinate with multiple agencies so that the field staff is not distracted by reporting and coordinating functions.

3. Information flowing into and out of a section should be coordinated through one point person.
4. Documentation of response activities is a task that should not rest with the responders but rather with a documentation officer and should be done in real time.

What I Learned and How This Experience Shaped My Role at the DOHMH

There were many things I learned through this assignment:

1. Structured reporting and documentation is essential during an emergency response but can be challenging, even if systems are set up a priori.
2. There are limitations to the information a junior-level team member can collect directly from senior-level staff, underscoring the importance of structured documentation.
3. After action reports and lessons learned should be compiled as close to the event as possible to capitalize on response team members' recall.
4. Accept that information collected might not always be complete.
5. Responding to an incident that involves multiple agencies is complex and very stressful. Even if things do not go exactly as they should, staff involved should be acknowledged for their hard work and ability to work under trying circumstances, both during and after the incident.

Since I completed this assignment, I have become increasingly involved with emergency response activities at the DOHMH. These activities include serving as a point-of-distribution site leader for a variety of events, including the H1N1 outbreak in 2009. Currently, I serve in a leadership position for the response group charged with planning for and responding to the distribution of countermeasures (e.g., vaccines, antibiotics). My collective experiences prior to and while at the DOHMH, including the project described in this case study, have been instrumental in my ability to take on these leadership roles over time.

DISCUSSION QUESTIONS

1. Which of the competencies described in the Appendix does this case demonstrate?

2. On which specific content areas should the DOHMH focus for an event like this?
3. What challenges might the preventive medicine resident have faced in completing this assignment?
4. What might be some of the challenges encountered in maintaining surveillance systems to which numerous agencies contribute?
5. What problems might arise from multiple EOCs activated during this time period?
6. How would one set up a communication protocol in the field to ensure that varying field results from different response agencies are handled properly on-site before being communicated back to the various EOCs?
7. What type of messages are important to communicate to the public about the radiography incident and when and how should they be relayed?
8. Since review of response activities and timeline reconstruction are critical to identifying areas for improvement in response activities, what are some processes that can be put in place a priori to facilitate this review?
9. How might the response to the radiography incident have been different if it had not occurred during the RNC? What might have been gained or lost if a different level of city coordination occurred?

ACKNOWLEDGMENTS

I would like to thank Daniel Kass, Marcelle Layton, Elliott Marcus, Jeanine Prudhomme, Erich Giebelhaus, Patricia Yang, and Isaac Weisfuse for their assistance in compiling this case study.

REFERENCES

1. Health Department statement on radiation incident at postal facility at 909 3rd Avenue in Manhattan [press release]. New York, NY: New York City Department of Health and Mental Hygiene; August 30, 2004. Available at: http://www.nyc.gov/html/doh/html/press_archive04/pr112-0830.shtml. Accessed April 10, 2013.
2. Update on radiation incident at 909 3rd Avenue [press release]. New York, NY: New York City Department of Health and Mental Hygiene; August 30, 2004. Available at: http://www.nyc.gov/html/doh/html/press_archive04/pr113-0830.shtml. Accessed April 10, 2013.

10

World Trade Center Attack on September 11, 2001

Robyn Gershon

INTRODUCTION

Each day, an estimated 150,000 to 200,000 people visited or worked in the seven buildings that formed the financial business center known as the World Trade Center (WTC) complex. The centerpieces of the complex were the two iconic WTC towers, referred to as WTC 1 (North Tower) and WTC 2 (South Tower) (see **Figure 10-1**). The complex also included the Marriott WTC Hotel (WTC 3), the U.S. Commodities Exchange (WTC 4), a 9-story office building (WTC 5), the U.S. Customs House (WTC 6), and a 47-story office building (WTC 7), including Salomon Smith Barney as the largest tenant, ITT Hartford, American Express Bank, as well as numerous other tenants such as the Internal Revenue Service regional council, United States Secret Service, and the New York City Office of Emergency Management headquarters. All the buildings were clustered around a five-acre central plaza (see **Figure 10-2**). The complex was located in lower Manhattan, three blocks north of the New York Stock Exchange.

Construction of the twin towers began in 1966, with occupancy beginning in 1970–1971. At 110 stories high, the towers were the

Figure 10-1

World Trade Center complex skyline.

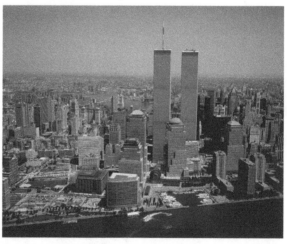

Source: Reproduced from Library of Congress Prints and Photographs Division Washington, Carol M. Highsmith.

Figure 10-2

World Trade Center plaza.

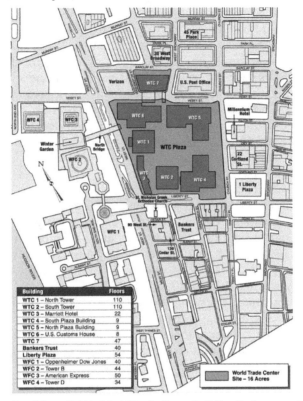

Building	Floors
WTC 1 – North Tower	110
WTC 2 – South Tower	110
WTC 3 – Marriott Hotel	22
WTC 4 – South Plaza Building	9
WTC 5 – North Plaza Building	9
WTC 6 – U.S. Customs House	8
WTC 7	47
Bankers Trust	40
Liberty Plaza	54
WFC 1 – Oppenheimer Dow Jones	40
WFC 2 – Tower B	44
WFC 3 – American Express	50
WFC 4 – Tower D	34

Source: Reproduced from FEMA, World Trade Center Building Performance Study.

tallest buildings in the world at that time. The architectural design was extremely innovative, with a unique external perimeter column structure. On each face of the towers, 59 perimeter columns allowed for unusual structural flexibility, the purpose of which was to allow to the towers to withstand heavy winds. This structure was also less likely to transfer external forces to the core of the buildings. In essence, the cablelike structure served as an exoskeleton for the buildings.

The WTC twin towers were owned and operated by the Port Authority of New York and New Jersey (PANYNJ). There were over 500 leaseholders (employers) leasing space in the more than 10 million square feet of rentable space in the two towers combined.

The towers had so many businesses, they each were designated with their own zip codes. Each tower had approximately 25,000 full-time employees, including facilities management. Each tower also had 99 elevators, including a newly designed express elevator system. Passengers could switch elevators from express to locals at the "sky lobbies," located on the 44th and 78th floors. Other tower employees included a team of on-site elevator repairmen, housekeeping, security, and parking (there were five levels of underground parking). Most of the employees, however, were business-related office workers. Many contract employees also worked in the towers each day (mainly servicemen and women). On the concourse level of the towers, there were dozens of stores and restaurants, with hundreds of employees and an even larger number of patrons.

The observation deck, "The Top of the World," was located on the 107th floor of WTC 2. It was visited daily by roughly 80,000 people and opened each day at 9:30 AM. The observatory provided tourists with 360° views and on a clear day, up to 45 miles in any direction could be observed. An unusual feature of the complex was the vault storage of precious metals; one of the world's largest repositories of gold was stored in the sublevel of WTC 4.

Various mass transit systems were connected to the WTC complex, including the Path trains, which connected New York to New Jersey. This major transit system hub serviced several hundred thousand commuters each day, serving a connection to other transit systems.

Each tower floor had an acre of space, often designed in an open floor plan, with dozens of cubicles. The Morgan Stanley brokerage firm was the largest tenant, with 3,500 workers located in the two towers.

On July 24, 2001, the Port Authority sold the WTC complex to Silverstein Realty, although they remained the managing operators at the WTC and retained their main offices at the South Tower. They had a large workforce of roughly 1,400 employees, including a sizeable police force.

On the morning of September 11, 2001, approximately 58,000 people, including an estimated 200 to 250 pregnant women, were in the WTC complex and concourse (including the subway and train stations). The brand new, multimillion dollar New York City Office of Emergency Management, located in WTC 7, served as the incident command center for all of New York City. In this space, an emergency 6,000-gallon fuel supply for the city was also stored.

THE EMERGENCY PREPAREDNESS PLANNING IN PLACE ON 9/11/2001

The overall emergency management program for the WTC complex was the responsibility of the Port Authority of New York and New Jersey.

Fire Safety and Emergency Features of the Towers

The fire safety system of the towers consisted of suppression systems, detection systems, notification devices, smoke management systems, and passive structural systems, such as compartmentalization and structural protection.[1] Originally, the towers were sprayed with an asbestos-containing film. This was later abated and replaced with asbestos-free mineral fiber spray. In the mid-1990s, the application of additional fireproofing commenced, and by September 11, 2001, a total of 31 floors had received this upgrade. The fire and elevator shafts had two 0.625-inch thick gypsum board layers on the exterior and one 0.625-inch thick layer of gypsum board on the interior surface—these assemblies provided a 2-hour fire rating (that is, they could withstand fire for a 2-hour period).

While the towers did not originally have fire sprinkler protection, it was installed as a retrofit in 1990, and was applied to 100% of both towers. There were standpipes that ran throughout each of the three stairways. Two air-pressurized water extinguishers were also located at each stairway on each floor of both towers. The standpipes had dedicated fire pumps to provide additional pressure. There were several 5,000-gallon water storage tanks to supply the standpipe system.

Smoke management was provided by zoned smoke control systems—this was designed to limit the spread of smoke from the tenants' area to the core of the buildings, thereby assisting the evacuation from an area of smoke. A centralized fire command center for the two towers was located on the concourse level in the operations control center, with additional fire command centers located in the lobbies of each tower.

Fire department telephones were located throughout the towers, but primarily were placed in stairway 3 (on odd floors). The WTC had its own fire brigade, consisting of Port Authority officers specially trained in fire safety. They had access to fire carts located at the concourse and sky lobby levels. The carts contained hoses, nozzles, self-contained breathing apparatus, turnout coats, forcible entry tools, resuscitators, first aid kits, and other emergency equipment. The typical fire or emergency response would result in the emergency brigade setting up operations on the floor below the incident.

Emergency egress was provided by stairways 1, 2, and 3. The three sets of stairways were centrally located and essentially ran from the top to the bottom of each tower. Two sets of fire stairs were 44 inches wide, one set was 56 inches wide. The sets of stairways were not entirely vertical, as they shifted at certain levels, thus requiring the occupants to traverse from one stairway to another through a transfer corridor. There were also internal (dead-end) stairs running between floors located within some areas—essentially serving as convenience stairs for some multifloor businesses. All stairways generally opened onto each floor, however, for security reasons, several floors had a lock-out mechanism. That is, in some cases, you could exit onto the stairs from the hallway, but you could not exit the fire stairways into the hallway and into other office areas. Battery-operated emergency lighting was provided in stairways and retrofitted photoluminescent paint was placed on the edge of the stair treads to provide guidance.

Emergency Training of Occupants

The emergency operations plan called for the evacuation of occupants from the floor of the incident, as well as the occupants from one floor above and one floor below the incident. The training that was provided to occupants by the PANYNJ consisted of semiannual training that took place at the core of each floor, at the elevators.[1] At the training, which was mandatory, each of the three fire stairs were pointed out, but the occupants did not enter the fire stairs. Reportedly, even though training was mandatory, attendance was poor. Additional fire safety training was provided by some of the larger firms, which had their own internal fire and emergency response teams. Persons with disabilities were instructed to let the fire safety team know about their disabilities and any special requirements that they might have in terms of evacuation. There were numerous (an estimated 100) special evacuation chairs that were purchased after the 1993 bombing, but these had been placed in out-of-the-way locations, and few people were aware of their existence or how to use them properly. No full-building evacuation of occupants or special evacuation drills of disabled persons were conducted.

PRIOR EMERGENCY EVENTS AT THE WTC

On numerous occasions, the WTC complex had experienced emergency events.[1] By all accounts, the structural capabilities of the building and the emergency management programs led to positive outcomes. One occurrence, however, the 1993 terrorist bombing, was striking in that there were numerous injuries and six fatalities.

The 1993 Terrorist Bombing of the WTC

At 12:17 PM, February 23, 1993, a bomb exploded in an underground parking garage of the WTC complex. A truck packed with more than 1,500 pounds of urea-nitrate explosives was parked at the B-1 level (first underground) under WTC 1. Ramzi Yousef, an Al-Qaeda trained disciple of Shiek Omar Abdel Rahman, a controversial Muslim cleric, and his coconspirators, planned to destroy WTC 1 and WTC 2 through the bombing. While it did not have its intended effect, the bombing was nonetheless devastating, leading to 6 deaths (most on the B-2 level) and 1,042 injuries, most smoke related. At the peak of the incident, the fire reached 16 alarms and involved more than 700 firefighters (about half of New York City Fire Department [FDNY] on-duty personnel). Roughly 50,000 people in the towers were evacuated, and another 200,000 people from nearby buildings were also evacuated from surrounding areas. The evacuation was hampered by the lack of announcements and suboptimal response by occupants; more than 5 hours after the call for full-building evacuation had been made, firefighters conducting a final sweep through the buildings found occupants sitting at their desks (in the dark and without power). After the 9/11 event, some WTC occupants later told investigators that they had hesitated leaving as previously they had been docked wages when they evacuated the building during the 1993 event.

In the 1993 bombing, the explosion immediately cut off the WTC 1 main electrical line, disabling not only the electrical system but also the emergency lighting system. Thick smoke soon filled the stairwells, making evacuation down the stairways very difficult. Hundreds of people were trapped in the elevators, including a group of 17 kindergartners, who were on their way down from the observation deck when their elevator got stuck for 5 hours between the 35th and 36th floors. A small number of people (less than two dozen) were evacuated (mostly pregnant women) via helicopter from the roof of WTC 1. A rappeller was deployed before this could be effected in order to knock down telecommunication antennas, which covered most of the roof. The telecommunications center on the rooftop was destroyed, and for almost a week, over-the-air broadcast capabilities were lost for most TV stations. Telephone service for much of lower Manhattan was also disrupted. All of the people involved in the bombing were eventually arrested, tried, and convicted, except for one, Abdul Yasin, an Iraqi bomb maker. He soon fled the United States and returned to Iraq; he remains on the FBI's Most Wanted Terrorist List.

The Effect of the 1993 Bombing on the Emergency Preparedness Management of the WTC Complex

The 1993 bombing led to a number of important structural and management changes directed at the emergency operations capabilities of the towers. One of the most important changes made was the upgrading of the buildings' emergency operations infrastructure; more than two million dollars was spent on structural improvements. This included the addition of escalators at the concourse level, new overhead intercom systems installed throughout the buildings, the addition of LED and emergency backup lighting for the stairs, new reflective egress signage, and the installation of photoluminescent tape on stair treads. The implementation of the Fire Warden system, with a greater emphasis on drills, was also made at this time. Many businesses that leased space in the towers similarly increased and improved their emergency readiness plans and hired experienced fire personnel of their own. Unfortunately, some important changes, such as widening stairwells and adding stairways, were not implemented due to cost considerations. At the time of the 2001 attack, the emergency operations and building safety features met or exceeded all pertinent New York City local laws (NYC local law 5) and fire safety codes for high-rise occupancies.

CRISIS BEGINS—8:46 AM, SEPTEMBER 11, 2001

I feel this way about it. World trade means world peace and consequently . . . the World Trade Center is a living symbol of man's dedication to world peace.

—Minoru Yamasaki (1912–1986),
Architect for the WTC, at the 1973 Dedication for the WTC

At 8:46 AM on Tuesday, September 11, 2001, WTC Tower 1 was attacked by terrorists who hijacked an American Airlines Boeing 767 passenger plane (Flight 11) to use as a weapon of mass destruction. The impact occurred on the north elevation of the building between the 94th and 98th floors.

All three stairwells and the elevators were destroyed at the impact zone. All power lines, elevator cables, fire suppression, public announcement, and other infrastructure was immediately destroyed. No occupants above the 91st floor survived. At the time of impact, the airplane was traveling 470 miles per hour and carried an esti-mated 10,000 tons of fuel. The Windows on the World restaurant, above the point of impact, was particularly busy that morning, with more than 150 people attending breakfast meetings.

Seventeen minutes later, at 9:03 AM, terrorists crashed a United Airlines Boeing 767 (Flight 175) into the south elevation of Tower 2 between the 78th and 84th floors, including the sky lobby on the 78th floor.

This plane was traveling 590 miles per hour and also carried an estimated 10,000 gallons of fuel. Two out of three stairwells and all elevators were destroyed at the impact zone. Everyone still remaining in the building above the 78th floor was trapped, unless they could make their way to the one stairway that was still intact. The trajectory of the planes is shown in **Figure 10-3.**

TRAGEDY UNFOLDS[2-7]

Events unfolded rapidly, although many survivors reported that time seemed to be suspended. The timeline of critical events is shown in **Figure 10-4.**

When the first plane was about to hit Tower 1, people already work-ing at their desks in both towers who were facing the north face of the building could see that this was a large jetliner; in fact, some survivors reported that they could see into the cockpit and could see the terror-ists who had taken command of the plane. They knew that this was not an accidental crash. They immediately grasped the implications of the building being under attack, and those that could exit started to do so immediately. The first sign for most occupants was, however, feeling the impact, hearing the noise, and then, shortly thereafter, seeing paper flying through the air (some likened it to "white paper snow"), furnishings, pieces of metal (parts of the plane and office furniture), and other debris. But they could not make sense of what

Figure 10-3

Trajectory of planes.

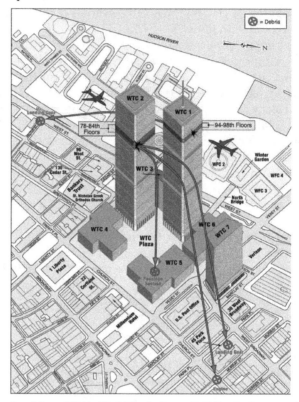

Source: Reproduced from FEMA, World Trade Center Building Performance Study.

they were seeing. They tried to use their phones, but if they had a local phone carrier, their phones were no longer functioning, as many main telecommunication towers were on top of WTC 1. Only those people with cell phone service from outside of the area could make

Figure 10-4

Timeline of critical events.

8:00 AM	8:46 AM	8:55 AM	9:02 AM	9:59 AM	10:28 AM
	Tower 1 (North) hit	PA-Announcement heard in Tower 2 (South)	Tower 2 (South) hit	Tower 2 (South) collapses	Tower 1 (North) collapses

calls, as most of the landlines were damaged, although these continued to function in several areas. The first calls coming out were to 911. Then people started trying to call their families and friends to let them know that they were all right. At Windows on the World restaurant, the first calls made were to 911, then to families; at this point they said they were waiting for help, the stairs were completely in flames and not functional. In fact, at this point, the stairs no longer existed.

As noted, the first input was sensory, something they had seen, felt, smelled, and heard. On the upper floors of Tower 1, those who had survived the initial impact of the plane felt the impact, with some survivors reporting that their office chairs on rollers slid from one end of the room or cubicle to the other, in some cases, moving more than 7 feet. The buildings swayed with the first impact, then swayed back and forth several times. The higher the floor, the greater the swaying effect. People on the upper floors also immediately smelled fuel, although some of them did not know that the fuel was jet fuel. The upper floors also had smoke; some also had flames, debris, walls collapsing, and heavy damage. Water from the sprinkler systems and stand pipes was entering their offices and hallways. On the mid-floors, occupants felt the impact, lost the lights, and heard the blast; shortly after that, they also smelled the fuel as it made its way down the core and elevator shafts. On the lower floors, the swaying was not as noticeable, although survivors at every level said they felt the impact. In the subbasements, the employees heard a terrible crash: it was the sound of the large (50-passenger) elevators dropping to the subbasements. People in the sublevels were blocked by the damage and had to wind through complex spaces to find their way up and out of the building.

The stairwells in Tower 1 were quickly filling with evacuees. Both the buildings were very underpopulated compared to usual mornings. There were several reasons for this: it was the first day of lower school in New York City, it was the mayor's primary election day, it was a beautiful early fall day and people were making their way to work at an unusually easy pace. The estimated number of people who were in the towers at the time of the first plane's impact was 17,000 to 18,000, far short of the typical 25,000 to 50,000. This had enormous implications for the stairway traffic and probably led to many more survivors than would have been predicted based on time/flow studies.

As people from the upper floors (from the 91st floor and below) started to descend, the magnitude of the event was becoming clearer. Many on the stairs from the upper floors were injured; those who were too badly injured to exit on their own were helped or carried by their colleagues, slowly making their way down. The stairways at this point, while intact, were beginning to fill with smoke. The emergency lighting was on, and the photoluminescent tape helped guide their path. All three stairways were used, the two that were only 44 inches wide (built to standard width in 1970) became especially crowded.

On the midlevel and lower floors, people in WTC 1 were spending precious time on gathering things, attempting to shut down their computers, attempting to make phone calls, and looking for others. Since few people were already at work, those that were there started looking throughout their workspace for someone familiar; they began to move into the hallways, looking for someone they knew and to try and find out what had happened, and importantly, what they should do. Some people, especially new or very junior employees, reported that they were seeking out a supervisor to get permission to exit the building. Others hesitated because they were docked pay when they self-evacuated the building in 1993, prior to the order from the fire department to evacuate. People visiting the building for business meetings said that they waited until their host decided what to do—in any case, they were unfamiliar with the building and could not effect an evacuation without direction. Other people said they delayed the start of their evacuation because they did not know where the three stairways were located; some did not even know that there were, in fact, three stairways.

Others were not sure if they would get locked inside the stairwells, or where the stairs ended, and this made them hesitate to enter them. People were anxiously seeking out someone to tell them what to do—they wanted leadership. In some cases, people with some type of emergency experience (e.g., military, fire [volunteer], policing, facilities, or boy scouts) took charge of the group they were with and encouraged them to rapidly start their exit via the stairways. People who took charge tended to have a calm, take-charge demeanor, often using a loud, low voice to organize the cluster of people in their group.

Some people had momentary panic attacks in the hallways and in some of the stairwells. When this happened, others around them quickly calmed them down, in some cases carrying them if they were frozen, and in other cases holding them tightly. Afterward, those that calmed others down said they did so because they were afraid panic would spread. Many survivors reported that they pretended to be calm for the same reason; they did not want to set off panic within the crowd.

In WTC 1, as people were making their way to the stairs or were actually on the stairs, disaster was about to strike in Tower 2, as the second plane neared for the attack. By this time, people on the streets below were milling about outside, emergency operations had called a general emergency, and all operations were focused on Tower 1. Hundreds of emergency responders and heavy response equipment were converging on the WTC complex. In the stairways in Tower 1, occupants were starting to see firemen begin their long ascent to the upper floors.

During the 1993 bombing, it took firemen more than 2 hours to reach the upper floors. Firemen on the stairs, which were getting hotter every minute, were carrying a great deal of heavy equipment. Their presence was calming to those in the stairwells, and they encouraged people to keep moving down and out. As the emergency responders made their way up the stairs, they served as a counter-flow to the traffic coming down, especially in the narrower 44-inch stairways. People reported having to move sideways down the stairs. Some people attempted to leave the stairs to search out a less crowded stairway, but doors to some floors were reportedly locked. People who had descended from much higher floors were getting tired, especially older, less fit evacuees. These people were frequently stopping at various floors to rest, get a drink of water, try to phone their family, or simply to catch their breath. Women reported that they had to stop to rest their feet or to remove their high heels, which were then lost during the descent. This became problematic as they made their way to the concourse and lobby, where there was a great deal of broken glass—many reported that they suffered cuts at this point and had trouble walking away from the area.

People with disabilities had a difficult time. One man made it down from a high floor with the help of his sure-footed guide dog— the presence of the dog also reportedly had a calming effect on other people in the stairwells. Other disabled people were not so fortunate; at one point people were taking their coworkers, who were in wheel-chairs, to elevator lobbies, in order to await the arrival of firemen. All of these people are believed to have perished. Others were helped down the entire way by large groups of colleagues who took turns carrying the people in wheelchairs. In one instance, eight people rotated four at a time to carry down an estimated combined weight of 600 pounds (equipment plus person), as this disabled person used complex wheelchair equipment that helped him to breathe.

Generally in the stairwells, the atmosphere, though tense, remained calm and purposeful. People reported counting in unison (counting out the floors), chanting, praying, singing, and behaving in supportive, adaptive, and prosocial ways. People urged each other on, assisted them when they tripped, and tried to stay on task. People tried to stay with the group they were with when they first entered the stairwell, but they were often separated. They then quickly became part of another group walking down the stairs. One thing everyone reported afterward was that no one wanted to be alone. As groups formed and new people joined, information about what had happened was shared. In some cases, people had information that they had obtained from family members (via cell phones), who were watching the disaster unfold at this point on the television. But for many people, there remained a serious lack of situational awareness, and almost no one thought, at least out loud in the stairwells, that the buildings could ever collapse. This lack of information had a beneficial effect, helping to prevent panic in the increasingly crowded WTC 1 stairwells.

Inside the WTC 1 building space, conditions continued to worsen for those left behind. Most people in elevators whose cables had been cut were killed instantly, except in two rare instances. In one elevator, the emergency brakes worked, and this halted the elevator car 10 feet above the lobby level, and another elevator was stranded at the lobby level. From these two elevators, there were some people who managed to survive.

EVENTS IN WTC 2—9:02 AM

Before the second plane attacked, several people above the point of impact in Tower 2 had seen the plane hit Tower 1. Therefore they knew that this was not an accident. Most of these people took steps to begin exiting immediately, many of them taking the elevators down.

Shortly after WTC 1 was hit, at 8:55 AM, an announcement from security came on over the PA system in Tower 2 that said, "Stay at your desks to await further information." The incident at WTC 1 was causing a lot of debris to fall on the plaza and it was dangerous to be outside. Many people nonetheless started to egress, and many also took to the stairs. Some of the people who were in the stairs at the time of the announcement went out and took an elevator back to their offices, and some of these people with offices on the higher floors likely perished. Still, many remained committed to evacuating the building and they continued down the stairs. People as high as the 103rd floor made their way down via the stairs. Those in the stairs at the time of the WTC 2 impact heard the sound of the impact and they experienced many of the same sensory impacts as the occupants in Tower 1. Those on the lower 70s and 60s also reported smoke, debris, and water.

Some elevator cables in WTC 2 were cut, and in one case, the elevator was stuck between floors. In this elevator, a group of people clawed their way out onto the 50th floor using the most rudimentary of tools (a window washer).

In Tower 2, 16 employees who escaped from areas above the crash followed the lead and advice of an occupant who said he had volunteer firefighting experience; another group that attempted to leave via the roof followed a high-ranking businessperson. The people who escaped were able to do so because one stairwell remained intact. However, because this stairwell was filled with smoke above the point of impact, many frightened occupants ascended to the roof only to find their egress blocked by locked and damaged doors. In any case, the roof was obstructed by smoke and flames and covered with communication antennae that would have prohibited helicopter rescue efforts. The workers were unaware that the smoke obscured only two or three floors in the impact area. All of the occupants who ascended the smoke-filled stairwell perished. All 16 people who pushed through the smoky stairs survived.

CONDITIONS WORSEN

WTC 1 conditions continued to worsen as the upper floors became entrained with thick dark-gray and black smoke, and the fires spread. Those trapped above the impact zone were getting desperate.

This was the beginning of suicide jumpers leaping from inaccessible areas. People had frantically broken out the heavy windows in order to let in air, but the smoke and flames only grew worse. In the restaurant, groups of people huddled together. Those with phone service let others use their phones to say good-bye to loved ones. Reports from families who had spoken with restaurant victims said that it was quiet and somber in the restaurant, with people staying in their functional roles until the end. The manager continued to make calls for help, and was repeatedly told that help was on its way, however, there was no possibility of escape from this totally inaccessible floor. All of these people perished, along with the restaurant employees who were on duty. One young employee was on the 57th floor when the plane hit WTC 1, as he was delivering a fruit basket; he is the only known survivor of the Windows on the World workforce on duty that day.

EMERGENCY RESPONSE: PROBLEMS WITH COMMUNICATIONS

The initial fire incident command post was set up shortly after the first impact in the ground floor lobby of Tower 1 (North) by the first battalion chief from FDNY to arrive (this is the third-highest position in FDNY). Within minutes of the initial attack, hundreds of firefighters, EMTs, and police forces flooded to the site. The FDNY chief arrived on the scene shortly before the South Tower was hit, and he assumed the role of incident commander. The command center had, at this point, relocated to the South Tower. The mayor at the time, Rudolph Giuliani, responded to the site and immediately ordered a full evacuation of lower Manhattan. He issued constant news releases urging citizens to remain calm. The FDNY radios did not communicate with NYPD radios or Emergency Medical Services (EMS) dispatchers, and there was hardly any interagency coordination at this point. This was especially problematic as the Office of Emergency Management (OEM) was located in WTC 7, but because of worsening conditions at the complex, they had to evacuate roughly 30 minutes after the initial event. The OEM incident command center was disabled.

DISASTER UNFOLDS

Transportation infrastructure in New York City was quickly impacted. Many subway lines were shut and buses were diverted to other areas off their route. People were leaving the city any way they could. Long Island Rail Road, New Jersey Transit, and Amtrak all shut down. As soon as the government realized it was a terrorist attack, all of the bridges and tunnels (at 9:21 AM) were shut off to all but emergency vehicles. Lower Manhattan was cordoned off and people were not allowed to enter. Schools in the immediate vicinity were evacuated and school officials tried to reach parents. Parents tried desperately to find their children.

Meanwhile, events unfolded, with the Pentagon attacked at 9:37 AM. Authorities realized that at least one other plane was unaccounted for, resulting in an unprecedented decision made by the secretary of transportation, Norman Mineta, to ground all civilian aircraft. At the time (9:32 AM), there were 4,546 airplanes in the air. People were stranded at airports as flights were cancelled. The WTC complex and surrounding areas were chaotic. Numerous fire departments and other emergency responders from throughout the greater metropolitan area rushed to the scene.

WTC 2 COLLAPSES—9:59 AM

Suddenly, with people watching, both on the street and on television, the unimaginable happened—the collapse of WTC 2. A mere 56 minutes after impact, the second tower to be attacked, WTC 2, collapsed. The collapse was recorded by Columbia's Lamont-Dougherty laboratory as a level 0.8 on the Richter scale, the equivalent of a very small earthquake. But on the ground, there was colossal destruction. Starting at the top, with progressive collapse of each floor beneath it, the tower came down in under 10 seconds.

On the street, chaos ensued. People ran to find any shelter they could, even crawling under cars, to get away from the terrible cloud plume. Once the South Tower collapsed, the incident command center in the North Tower issued a general evacuation order of the entire North Tower (firefighters could not hear the order as their radios were not working). With the collapse of WTC 2 (South Tower) at 9:59 AM, the immediate and surrounding area of the WTC complex entered a new phase of an acute environmental disaster of enormous magnitude. People in the process of exiting the towers and other buildings in the WTC complex and surrounding buildings were swept up in the dust cloud (see **Figure** 10-5). So were emergency response personnel and people in the area. The collapse sparked a wider evacuation of lower Manhattan as the smoke and choking debris covered the entire lower tip of Manhattan, an area of approximately half a square mile.

WTC 1 COLLAPSES—10:28 AM

Inside WTC 1, people were continuing their descent, unaware of the nearby catastrophic collapse of WTC 2, although many heard the thunderous roar of the collapse. There were several hundred people still making their way out even minutes before the collapse. The lower levels were filling with the dust cloud caused by the collapse of WTC 2 and stairwells at the bottom became clogged with dust and debris. People continued to make their way down and out of the building, some running if they could. Some people reported that

Figure 10-5

People caught up in the dust cloud.

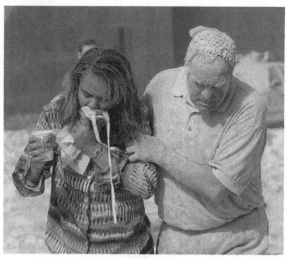

Source: Library of Congress Prints and Photographs Division Washington, Don Halasy.

they were confused once they reached the lower levels; their normal workday routine involved entering and exiting the building in the same location, and using the same elevators. Coming out of unfamiliar stairways, they were disoriented. Most were unfamiliar with most of the massive building's architecture. Once out on the street they were not sure where they were, even those that left the area before the dust cloud hit, and many were not sure where to go next. They were amazed at the scene on the street and tried to make sense of it. Still, people continued to exit, including a few who escaped only seconds before the North Tower collapsed.

At 10:28 AM, less than 1 hour after the collapse of WTC 2, the North Tower, WTC 1, collapsed. Again, it registered as a level 0.8 on the Richter scale and again it only took 10 seconds to collapse. The FDNY chief, who was the incident commander at the scene, was killed from falling debris when the North Tower fell. A final distress call went out to all responders in the building to immediately evacuate the North Tower shortly before it fell, but many firemen in the North Tower did not hear the order as the radios were not working (the boosting antennas were located on the top of the South Tower, which had already collapsed). Also many off-duty firemen had responded—without their radios. The command post was relocated to a firehouse in Greenwich Village.

ENVIRONMENTAL CONDITIONS WORSEN

Hundreds of tons of concrete, steel, and other materials from the buildings (including asbestos, glass fibers, polychlorinated biphenyls, dioxins, and other chemicals) quickly filled the air. The dust was highly alkaline (ph 9.0–11.0). Eventually an estimated 1.8 million tons of debris were removed from the disaster site. All seven buildings in the complex came down or were destroyed in the next few days. The fires burned for several days before finally going out. As the dust cloud flooded the area and spread out over Manhattan, people tried to escape any way they could. Most left on foot, taking to the bridges and tunnels that were now empty of vehicular traffic.

MEDICAL RESPONSE

EMS arrived within 10 minutes of the initial impact, and they quickly set up a staging area outside of the North Tower. Eventually, as more EMS arrived, five triage sites were set up (see **Figure 10-6**). 911 call centers

Figure 10-6

Medical triage station.

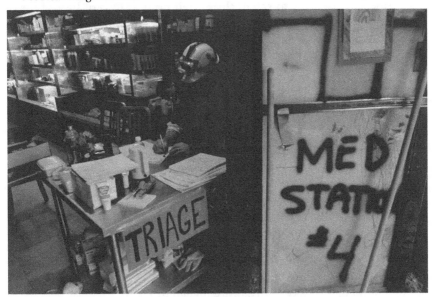

Source: FEMA, Andrea Booher.

were overwhelmed; dispatchers did not have situational awareness, unlike most people watching the unfolding disaster on television. By 11:00 AM, EMS, with volunteer registered nurses and doctors, set up triage centers at Chelsea Piers and the Staten Island Ferry Terminal. They attended to the arrival of mass casualties, but by 5:00 PM, the centers were closed as it became clear that there would likely be no more survivors from the rubble (eventually 11 people were rescued from the rubble).

Hospitals were forced to develop crowd control measures. By late that same month, the greater New York Hospital Association (representing 91 metropolitan hospitals) reported that ER treatment had been provided to about 6,000 victims of the attack, roughly 900 were admitted.

Victims were also treated by many other hospitals—covering three states—also many were treated outside of acute-care settings. Within 6 hours after the attacks, the New York City Department of Health and Mental Hygiene (DOHMH) began to accumulate statistics on the number and type of injury treated at five key hospitals in lower Manhattan. Shortly after the event, people rushed to the nearest hospitals to see if they could volunteer in any way and to give blood. DOHMH staff monitored food and water quality at Ground Zero (as it became known), as many organizations (e.g., restaurants) and individuals delivered food to the site. Many abandoned area restaurants had to be cleaned out to prevent outbreaks of rodents.

DOHMH held news conferences on the air quality. They prepared guidance documents for people living in the downtown area—especially on how to safely clean their homes. Tens of thousands of indoor and outdoor air samples were tested. The levels of contaminants dropped over time and distance. Fibrous glass and asbestos were identified in indoor dust samples near Ground Zero. DOHMH recognized early on that recovery site workers, especially those deployed early on after the event and those who worked at the site for extended periods, were the most highly exposed to toxic dust. Their health continues to be monitored; some have become gravely incapacitated by their exposure. DOHMH mental health identified three priorities early on. First, DOHMH provided crisis intervention for bereaved families and friends, survivors, workers, and the general public. DOHMH instituted a mental health hotline for telephone counseling in nine languages. Family assistance centers were established (filing death certificates, DNA sampling, counseling, etc.). Second, the DOHMH helped found Project Liberty, providing support services at 68 agencies in 120 sites. Third, DOHMH needed to augment the public mental health system. This was accomplished by funding more than 1,000 agencies to care for 300,000 New Yorkers with mental illness or disability related to the 9/11 event.

IMPACT ON SURVIVORS AND THE COMMUNITY

Within hours, maybe minutes, of the disaster, family and friends of people who worked in the towers tried desperately to contact them. Because most cell phone service was disrupted and landlines were quickly overwhelmed, people could not connect. By early evening, people went from hospital to hospital searching for their missing relatives. Within a very short time, people started posting photos of those missing. Studies of New York City residents after the event indicated an increase in mental health disorders. One of the factors correlated with this was the number of hours spent watching newscasts of the event. Communication and other problems in the towers, and, of course, the experience of the event itself (many evacuees reported feeling as if they were victims of attempted murder), may have served to heighten the traumatic stress of the event and may have led to adverse outcomes in surviving evacuees. Studies on drug and alcohol use in New York City residents soon after the 9/11 attack showed significant increases in smoking, alcohol use, and drug abuse.

It took some people many hours to let their families know that they had survived, and in some cases it took several days until they were finally reunited. When it became clear that there were many who had died, and were not just missing, the city collectively started to mourn.

Apartments located near Battery Park were evacuated, and in some cases residents were not allowed back in for extended periods. All of these displaced persons became part of the fabric of shared loss in the city. For some, their apartments were completely uninhabitable; for others, it was not until months later that they were allowed to return, after heavy decontamination had taken place.

DEAD AND INJURED

With 2,749 people listed as missing or dead following the 2001 WTC attack (as of 2012), including 147 individuals on the 2 airplanes, this was the worst terrorist attack in our nation's history (the Pearl Harbor death toll stands at 2,403). The Fire Department lost 343 firefighters and EMTs. The NYPD lost 23 officers. The Port Authority Police lost 37 officers. Data collection on injuries and fatalities began within hours of the WTC attack, and the Centers for Disease Control and Prevention's review of victims' injuries found that of 810 individuals treated at 5 local hospitals after the attack, 16% required hospitalization and 0.4% died receiving emergency care. Although 14% of the patients suffered noninjury conditions (e.g., cardiac, respiratory, psychiatric), most victims suffered from exposure to smoke, dust, debris, and fumes. Other common injuries included burns, fracture, head injuries, and crush injuries. The percentage of WTC inhabitants treated was much lower than that in some other terrorist attacks, such as the Oklahoma City bombing, because most WTC victims either escaped or died. The survival of any employee or rescue worker remaining in the buildings at the time of collapse was nearly impossible.

PUBLIC HEALTH RESPONSE

Thirty-two minutes after the first plane crashed, the DOHMH activated its own incident command center. Twenty percent of the DOHMH workforce worked in lower Manhattan, and they were all evacuated. But by that afternoon, they joined with the Red Cross to staff 10 emergency shelters and to transport medical supplies. By the next day, they had moved the central office staff to a new location and had reestablished their information system. Within days, efforts were focused on surveillance. Four surveillance systems were put into place: rapid assessment of injuries, hospital needs assessment, a reporting system for injuries among rescue and recovery workers, and syndromic surveillance for monitoring symptoms (biological or otherwise). Fifteen Centers for Disease Control and Prevention (CDC) Epidemic Intelligence Service (EIS) officers were assigned to hospital emergency rooms. An equal priority was to maintain routine DOHMH functions. By nightfall, a CDC plane was allowed to fly to an undisclosed location near New York City. It was delivering one of the "push-packs," the CDC's emergency set of supplies in case of a public health emergency. The push-pack contained vaccines and drugs—including therapeutics for treatment of bioterrorism diseases.

THE CLEANUP

For 8.5 months, cleanup and recovery at the site continued for 24 hours a day and involved thousands of workers. The massive pile of debris smoked and smoldered for 99 days. The cleanup crew experienced acute, then chronic cough (WTC cough) and other health problems. The dust problem was compounded by the EPA shortly after 9/11 stating that the air was safe. Respiratory protection was inadequate in the beginning of the cleanup and was not well enforced.

LONG-TERM IMPACT: BUILDING AND FIRE SAFETY CODES

One of the most important changes that occurred after the WTC disaster was the change in high-rise fire safety codes. These changes ensured that high-rise buildings would be better able to protect their occupants from severe conditions (e.g., events requiring full and rapid building evacuation, shelter-in-place, partial evacuation, and in-building relocation) and that the chief fire safety director would be trained to serve as the incident commander until such time as a higher-ranking authority took over the command function.

GOING FORWARD

The master plan for the new Freedom Tower (1,776 feet) designed by Daniel Libeskind is slated for completion in 2013. A new WTC 7 office building opened in 2006. Five other new office towers are planned for the site. New York City has rebounded from the financial and psychological impact of the 9/11 disaster. A new memorial is now operational, providing a focus for the survivors and grieving families and friends.

DISCUSSION QUESTIONS

1. Which of the competencies described in the Appendix does this case demonstrate?
2. What were the best aspects of the communications on September 11, 2001, and what strategies were not effective (inside the towers and elsewhere)?
3. Immediately after the first plane struck Tower 1, all power was lost, including the public announcement system. Most cell phones (local numbers) did not work. However, some businesses had backup generators, and some computers, televisions, and radios were still working. What communications strategies would you have used to communicate what was happening and what steps to take? How would that differ from strategies you would and could use today?
4. The incident command post at the WTC was chaotic. What were the most obvious difficulties you identified, and what were the not so obvious ones?

5. What do you think are the key elements of a workforce emergency preparedness program? Should ALL employees receive this type of training? Should only new employees be provided this training? Should it be mandatory? Why?

6. Does the type of workplace matter with respect to emergency preparedness training? For instance, should only high-rise worksites or large worksites receive this type of training?

7. Knowing a little bit about the layout of WTC 1 and WTC 2 and the complex itself, what aspects of this work environment do you think presented challenges in terms of (1) training the workforce, and (2) developing and implementing an emergency preparedness plan?

8. What type of specialized training do you think might be needed for workers with disabilities? Describe how you envision this type of training program.

REFERENCES

1. Averill J, Mileti D, Peacock R, et al. *Occupant Behavior, Egress, and Emergency Communication. Federal Building and Fire Safety Investigation of the World Trade Center Disaster.* NIST, Technology Administration, U.S. Department of Commerce; 2005.

2. Gershon RRM, Magda LA, Riley HEM, Sherman MF. The World Trade Center evacuation study: factors associated with initiation and length of time for evacuation. *Fire and Materials.* 2011.

3. Sherman MF, Peyrot M, Magda LA, Gershon RRM. Modeling pre-evacuation delay by evacuees in World Trade Center Towers 1 and 2 on September 11th, 2001: a revisit using regression analysis. *Fire Safety Journal.* 2011;46(7):414–424.

4. Gershon RRM, Rubin MS, Qureshi KA, Canton AN, Matzner FJ. Participatory action research methodology in disaster research: results from the World Trade Center evacuation study. *Disaster Medicine and Public Health Preparedness.* 2008;2(3):142–149.

5. Qureshi KA, Gershon RRM, Smailes E, et al. A roadmap for the protection of disaster research participants: findings from the WTC evacuation study. *Prehospital and Disaster Medicine.* 2007;22(6):484–489.

6. Gershon RRM, Qureshi KA, Rubin MS, Raveis VH. Factors associated with high-rise evacuation: qualitative results from the World Trade Center evacuation study. *Prehosp Disaster Med.* 2007;22(3):165–173.

7. Gershon RRM, Hogan E, Qureshi KA, Doll L. Preliminary results from the World Trade Center evacuation study—New York City, 2003. *MMWR.* 2004;53(35):815–816.

11 Addressing the Mental Well-Being of New Yorkers in the Aftermath of the 9/11 and Bioterror Attacks

Neal L. Cohen

INTRODUCTION

Just before 9:00 AM on the morning of September 11, 2001, I received a call from the New York City Health Department that an airplane had crashed into the North Tower of the World Trade Center (WTC). I immediately sped to the WTC complex to take a seat at the New York City's state-of-the-art emergency operations center (located at WTC 7). Serving as commissioner of both the New York City Department of Health and the Department of Mental Health since 1998, I had participated in a number of desktop and real-time drills that were conducted by the New York City Office of Emergency Management (OEM), and knew the protocol to participate in the response to potential large-scale disasters. Upon arriving, however, I was unable to enter WTC 7, as it had become the site of fuel oil fires that would lead to the building's collapse by late afternoon. Mayor Giuliani and several of his senior cabinet members were also at the site, and I joined them in establishing a makeshift outpost at 75 Barclay Street, from which the mayor contacted the White House, confirmed that the nation was under attack, and sought military air cover to protect New York City from further attack. After about 15 minutes, at 9:59 AM, we heard a loud rumbling. Someone shouted, "It's coming down! Hit the deck!" and a dark cloud seemed to cover the windows as the building trembled. After encountering several locked doors, we were led out through a smoke-filled basement maze to exit onto Church Street into a throng of ghostly, ash-caked pedestrians who were struggling to get away from the storm of debris raining down after the collapse of the first tower.

With cell phones disabled and landline phones not working, we trooped north for about 15 blocks before finding a firehouse with working communications equipment. The immediate focus after the attack was on assessing the health impact and mobilizing the resources needed to handle the public health and medical emergency that would emerge from the tragedy.[1] With the collapse of two office towers that could each accommodate 25,000 people on a busy workday, we expected large numbers of injuries that would strain the surge capacity of the healthcare system throughout the metropolitan area. However, in fact, relatively small numbers of people with life-threatening injuries came to the city's emergency departments; nevertheless, about 8,000 people were seen over the next several days throughout the tri-state area (New York, New Jersey, Connecticut) for injuries, both physical and emotional, sustained on 9/11. One immediate lesson to be learned from this civilian response is that terrorism may create health impacts that reach far beyond the immediate boundaries of a disastrous event, as people will, whenever possible, seek to leave the immediate area and return to their homes. Consequently, planning for the management of a terrorist event must always be regional in approach, not local.

An additional public health focus of immediate concern was the secondary environmental issues, especially asbestos, dust, smoke, and chemical inhalation. The public health response was further complicated by the fact that, at Ground Zero, fires continued to burn for many weeks, with the ongoing release of particulate matter into the air. Public health surveillance was also prioritized to monitor the potential illnesses that might emerge from the disruption of the physical infrastructure (e.g., food- and waterborne diseases). With hundreds of restaurants losing power, rotting food and pest control also needed to be addressed.

While situated at the firehouse for several hours, we were able to turn on a small television set to view the reports of the chain of events as the mayor was communicating with both government and media. The videos of the planes hitting the towers and the subsequent explosions and fires were shown repeatedly that morning. Watching the broadcasts as we prepared to move city government to a more secure site, I sensed that these images were signaling the potential emergence of a looming mental health crisis that would require an unprecedented public health response.

THE MENTAL HEALTH RESPONSE

Later that day, when I was able to speak to my own staff, I asked them to review the literature on the sequelae of the Oklahoma City terrorism bombing. I knew that the bombing had triggered an important series of studies on the development of posttraumatic stress disorder (PTSD) as a consequence of terrorism and might provide a framework for crafting the public health response that would be needed in New York. I recalled that PTSD was diagnosed in approximately one-third of direct bombing survivors.[2] Similarly, I knew that disaster rescue workers in traumatic events were also reported to be susceptible to PTSD and other psychiatric sequelae.[3]

Initially, we responded to mental health needs with the model of crisis counseling and support we had used in the 1990s, through prior management of the psychological impacts of mass violence and terrorism. An arson that killed dozens of people in a Bronx dance club in 1990 led to the creation of a Division of Crisis Intervention Services at the Department of Mental Health (DMH). We began to build a series of crisis teams that could provide crisis intervention services throughout the city with a mobile outreach capacity. Furthermore, the WTC bombing in 1993 and two airline crash disasters in the late 1990s gave us experience in mobilizing large numbers of volunteer mental health professionals to support the needs of survivors and family members of victims.[4]

We began to prioritize our interventions by identifying categories of higher risk, medium, and lower risk individuals to be addressed. At highest risk were those evacuees from the towers, rescue workers, family members of the deceased, as well as the residents in the immediate area of Ground Zero. Over the first several days it became clear that the rescue efforts at the Ground Zero "pile," directed principally by New York City firefighters and police, were emotionally very highly charged, as their close friends and coworkers were among those caught in the collapse of the WTC buildings.

There were some unique challenges to mobilizing the social support networks of families and surviving coworkers. Despite the enormous grief and emotional needs that would follow the death of 343 firefighters that day, we learned from Fire Department and Police Department leadership that the uniformed services workers do not readily trust or welcome outsiders with their personal and family matters. The Fire Department had its own established counseling programs; our response was to adapt a model by which we paired a peer counselor (a current or retired firefighter with training in counseling services) with a licensed mental health professional well-credentialed and trained in disaster mental health and bereavement.

The mayor called for the establishment of a family assistance center to provide a site for family members to gather to receive information, concrete services, crisis counseling, and support for their bereavement. However, family members often followed a slow course in accepting the finality of their loss. All New Yorkers witnessed the missing persons posters that were placed throughout the city with images of lost loved ones and requests for information on their whereabouts. Family members learned that survival for up to 2 weeks might be possible under optimal conditions; consequently, the formal progression from a rescue to a recovery operation moved slowly and unevenly as many families held onto the hope that loved ones might still be rescued. Sensitive to the trauma of New Yorkers, particularly to the victims' family members, Mayor Giuliani asked me to bring in experts in mass bereavement and trauma who could provide guidance on how best to speak of the tragedy with healing words while respecting the bereavement process of the victims' families.

As a psychiatrist, I had been appointed commissioner of the DMH in 1996. My appointment in 1998 as commissioner of the Department of Health was made with the expectation of merging the two public health agencies to facilitate a model of public health that would integrate mental health issues into the mainstream of the public health agenda. Wearing both public health commissioner hats helped to facilitate the inclusion of mental health activities in the larger public health responses post-9/11. The public mental health response included (1) prioritizing populations into higher and lower risk categories as a consequence of the directness of the 9/11 impact (e.g., survivors, family members of victims, witnesses, residents of lower Manhattan), (2) mobilizing the social support networks of families of victims and surviving coworkers, and (3) recognizing that all New Yorkers were affected to some degree and would benefit from healing and help-promoting messages as part of a public education and community outreach campaign.

The large-scale public health response required of the city's DMH meant serving a citywide constituency much broader than that traditionally served by the public mental health system. Historically, the priority focus of the New York City DMH had been on the serious and chronically mentally ill who were struggling to live in communities outside of mental institutions in the post-deinstitutionalization era. Over the prior 40 years, the DMH had evolved into a "contract agency" that planned, funded, and monitored the large network of community-based programs that were serving about 300,000 New Yorkers yearly. Despite weaknesses in public health resources (e.g., surveillance systems, epidemiology trained staff, and evidence-based models for broad population-based mental illness prevention and mental health promotion), the DMH could call upon the assets of a well-developed, community-based network of mental health programs and agencies that were very well connected to the communities and to the special populations they served.

In the days following 9/11, some groups with national experience in disaster and stress debriefing met with me and offered to take the lead in bringing counselors from their organization into New York City. But the DMH oversaw a large service provider network of 230 agencies that offered a total of nearly 1,000 discrete mental health programs. Consequently, drawing on the abundance of local expertise and resources (community-based agencies, academic health centers, medical schools, and training institutes) seemed a better way to go. This decision was influenced by my awareness that we could attempt to rapidly mobilize the city's large mental health service sector through the assistance of its well-established advocacy organizations for hospital-based mental health providers (Greater NY Hospital Association) and community-based mental health providers (Coalition of Voluntary Mental Health Agencies). We proceeded to bring the leadership of the mental health services system together and provided them consultation with national mental health experts.

Working with the Mental Health Association of New York City, the city expanded the role of LIFENET, its 24/7 mental health hotline, to answer the public's questions and to make referrals. LIFENET had been designed for a culturally diverse population and provided direct assistance in English, Spanish, Cantonese, and Mandarin.

The declaration by President Bush of New York City as a federal disaster area allowed for federal funding for postdisaster mental health services through the crisis counseling program funded by Federal Emergency Management Agency (FEMA). This care model emphasizes outreach and public education, crisis intervention, supportive counseling, and referrals for more in-depth psychological care when necessary. Consequently, mobilizing the service delivery system required a much different approach and intervention effort than standard clinical practice. *Project Liberty* was the name given to the array of immediate and longer-term mental health services.[5] The New York City Department of Mental Health, Mental Retardation, and Alcoholism Services developed the response plan and engaged local mental health agencies in the service model. The New York State Office of Mental Health took the lead in setting up training of mental health professionals, emphasizing key concepts of disaster mental health, including survivor needs and reactions, disaster counseling skills, and determining the need for referral for more intensive mental health services.

We created a series of subway and bus posters that provided messages from New Yorkers describing those activities that were helping them to better cope with the tragic consequences of the 9/11 attacks. Under the theme of "New York Needs Us Strong," the posters depicted advice from everyday citizens to others providing a destigmatized framework for recognizing one's own sense of grief and the measures that may promote resiliency. Examples of the advice included the following:

What's Helping

- Talked with my coworkers about everything.
- I'm trying to stay in constant communication with my brother, a NYC police officer.

- Went to three sessions with a therapist to talk with other men about our feelings.
- Spend quality time with my wife, going places and doing things together, dinner out, shopping.

—William, 35, Brooklyn

What I've Been Doing to Cope

- I spent that first weekend with my daughter and her family; they were worried about me being alone.
- I work with senior citizens and they've seen it all. That helps my perspective.
- I've started calling my children more often; I want them to know how much I love them.
- I've been spending time with my friends. We've created our own support network.

—Maria, 63, Bronx

The assumptions underlying this broad-based response strategy are that most people's stress reactions, although personally disturbing, constitute normal responses to a traumatic event and will be short-term in duration. Personal and community resiliency remain powerful factors even in the aftermath of a major disaster. Thus, the corresponding interventions should emphasize helping people identify their responses to trauma, understand those responses as normal reactions, and reconnect with preexisting social supports.

Researchers at the New York Academy of Medicine (NYAM) carried out pivotal research on the incidence of PTSD, depression, and substance use in the New York metropolitan area following the 9/11 events.[6-7] Using random-digit telephone surveys of approximately 1,000 adult New Yorkers living in Manhattan at intervals of 5–8 weeks, 4–5 months, and 6–9 months following the attacks, NYAM investigators were able to track the trends in probable and subsyndromal PTSD prevalence. The studies found that at the 5–8 week interval, 7.5% reported symptoms consistent with a diagnosis of current PTSD related to the attacks, and 9.7% reported symptoms consistent with current depression. Living close to the World Trade Center was associated with a prevalence of 20%.[7] The follow-up studies at 4-month and 6-month intervals found a sharp decline in prevalence of possible PTSD related to the attacks in the New York City population, with probable PTSD prevalence 2.3% at 4–5 months and 1.5% at 6–9 months postattack.[8] Despite the rapid decline of probable PTSD in the general New York City population over the first 6 months, the NYAM studies found that subsyndromal PTSD remained elevated, with 4.8% at 4–5 months and 5.3% at the 6–9-month follow-up interval.[9]

Although it is not possible to make clinical diagnoses from the telephone surveys, even subsyndromal PTSD is associated with significant functional impairment and disability including elevated rates of suicidality.[10,11] Of note is that the calls to the LIFENET telephone hotline increased each month for up to 1 year, with the majority of calls made by or on behalf of persons with no prior history of psychological treatment. These data suggest that the Project Liberty public education campaign may have enabled a population significantly affected by the 9/11 tragedy to recognize a need for and a potential benefit from professional mental health care providing some mitigation of the emotional impacts.

BIOTERRORISM

While recovery efforts were ongoing at Ground Zero, and the city was healing from the physical and emotional wounds of the attacks, the confirmation of a case of inhalational anthrax in a Florida man on October 4, 2001, created a new challenge for New Yorkers' health and mental well-being. For a number of years, there was a great deal of media attention that focused on the Office of Emergency Management bunker, a complex, multimillion dollar telecommunications facility that was located at 7 WTC. The siting of the OEM at the WTC site was expected to facilitate opportunities for city, state, and federal agencies to gather together for emergency management planning and response, including the threat of bioterrorism. Health Department personnel had participated in a number of practices and drills, including biological, chemical, and terrorist attack scenarios under an incident command structure. In fact, a point of distribution (POD) exercise had been scheduled for September 12, 2001, at Pier 92 on the Hudson River, with about 1,000 police and fire recruits scheduled to act as civilians who had been exposed to a bioterrorism release event and awaiting receipt of antibiotic prophylaxis. Ironically, 4 days following the 9/11 attacks, the city moved its new emergency operations center to Pier 92.

Within 24 hours of the 9/11 attack, and with bioterrorism still a concern, I had requested the Centers for Disease Control and Prevention (CDC) to assist the city in the syndromic surveillance of 15 hospital emergency departments in addition to the city's prior established monitoring of 911 ambulance dispatch calls. Syndromic surveillance involves the tracking of any unexpected clustering of symptoms or disease that might be an early warning sign of an intentional release of agents of biological terrorism. Within a few weeks the process was computerized, with 29 hospitals sending a daily log of patients seen along with a breakdown by symptom categories such as respiratory, gastrointestinal, neurological, and so on. The report on October 4, 2001 of a case of inhalational anthrax in Florida triggered our Health Department's enhanced active surveillance with daily calls made to intensive care units, infectious disease physicians, and laboratories.

The first anthrax-positive laboratory result in New York City was reported in the early hours on October 12, 2001, of an NBC employee following biopsy of a skin lesion. It set in motion a new threat that was to expand as a national crisis—despite the focus on Washington, DC, and New York, and the subsequent impact on postal workers in the northeast corridor. After being notified early that morning by the CDC of anthrax in the biopsy of the NBC assistant to newscaster Tom Brokaw, I met with the mayor at 7:00 AM. We placed a call to CDC director Jeffrey Koplan, who told the mayor that the tests were compatible with a diagnosis of anthrax, and a press conference was held within hours.

Over the next few days additional highly suspect cutaneous anthrax cases were reported at other media outlets: ABC, CBC, and the New York Post offices. The mayor, myself, and Health Department staff went to each of these outlets and met with their staff to explain the nature of the investigations (both public health and criminal investigations) that were going to take place (e.g., chronological review; environmental testing; clinical assessment with nasopharyngeal swabs for epidemiological purposes, and antibiotic prophylaxis for those at risk). The public health and epidemiological investigation needed to be carried out jointly with law enforcement (New York City Police Department and Federal Bureau of Investigation), and environmental testing of office spaces and mailrooms soon followed. The psychological terror of the WTC bombing had occurred only weeks before, and the onset of new incidents of bioterror created a fear of further and more devastating attacks.

The terror felt by the public was manifested in a huge demand for testing of powders of all kinds, greatly overwhelming the resources of public health laboratories nationwide. Surgeon General Satcher, speaking in the last weeks of his tenure, stated that the CDC laboratories were antiquated, inadequate, and constituted a national disgrace. The truth needed to be acknowledged by a public health leader of Dr. Satcher's stature.

With my long-standing interest in a more integrated public health model, I was particularly proud of the performance of our two public health agencies and the clinics they set up at the media outlets that received the anthrax letters—with nurses, physicians, and medical epidemiologists working side by side with mental health professionals who were offering support and crisis counseling to the employees in a very open and destigmatizing fashion. Vulnerable New Yorkers benefited from the implementation of the integrated public health vision for which we had been advocating.

AFTER THE ATTACKS

For several years following the 9/11 attacks, new government priorities provided an infusion of significant funding for CDC infrastructure and enhanced laboratory capacity in state public health labs. But we remain challenged by the historical schism between public health and clinical medicine with widespread underreporting of diseases. The detection of West Nile virus (WNV) in the summer of 1999 was made possible by the report of a community physician to the city Health Department of 2 patients in a Queens hospital with atypical clinical presentations of encephalitis; but, as it turned out, there were already 17 patients in hospital beds with WNV by the time we learned of these cases.

Even with new funding, rebuilding the public health infrastructure requires a commitment to meaningful working partnerships and changes in medical school curricula that will influence the thinking and practice of the next generation of physicians and other healthcare professionals about preventive medicine practices. For this to happen, we will need leaders in public health and clinical medicine committed to bridging the cultural chasm between public health and clinical medicine. Leaders will need to lend their voices and prestige to changing the dynamic so that the nation benefits from a health system that fully integrates the population-based concerns of public health professionals with consistently good clinical practice.

Lastly, one of the strengths of New York City's response to 9/11 and the anthrax attack was the effort made in providing timely communication with the public as well as with the medical community. Our assistant commissioner for communicable disease, Dr. Marci Layton, provided frequent public health alerts throughout the crisis that were widely disseminated regionally and nationally at a time when such information was greatly needed by public health and healthcare communities. In contrast, on the national scene, there was inconsistency and a lack of an authoritative and reliable voice to communicate the real nature of the threat.

In response to the anthrax attacks, there was no textbook experience to guide a response. Regrettably, a number of assumptions about the virulence and pathogenesis of anthrax infectivity were proven to be incorrect. For example, the CDC did not believe that sealed mail handled by postal workers posed a health threat; that lethal inhalational anthrax would occur following exposure to a relatively small number of anthrax spores through the handling of cross-contaminated mail, as is thought to have occurred with an elderly Connecticut woman and a Bronx hospital worker; or that aggressive treatment would lead to a survival rate of 60% compared to the 15% to 20% previously reported.

Nevertheless, a spirit of resiliency and rebound was taking place in the city, with a government leader willing and able to provide a public narrative that moved the trauma of the attack and personal loss toward a vision of recovery for the larger community. Much has been written about Mayor Rudolph Giuliani's leadership during and after the 9/11 attacks. Jonathan Alter wrote in *Newsweek* that the Mayor "inhabited the role of wartime leader with a fine mixture of brisk compassion and a gritty command presence."[12] On a daily basis he held press conferences with new information as it came along, but always in the context of looking forward to the next steps in the city's recovery.

The public health field's understanding of ways to maximize positive outcomes in response to stress and adversities benefits from a risk and protective factor conceptual framework. While we have limited ability to predict outcomes from any set of specific and known risk and protective factors, the concept of resilience informs a number of relevant research areas, including the field's search for preventive interventions. Using a consensus definition of resilience as "the process of, capacity for, or outcome of successful adaptation after trauma or severe stress," Norris and colleagues.[13] describe the unique characteristics of the trajectory toward good mental health following exposure to traumatic events among resilient individuals. The authors posit that different response trajectories can be measured and studied across stressors and settings, allowing for the potential implementation of relevant interventions to enhance resiliency and recovery.

Wearing two hats, as commissioner of both the Department of Health and the Department of Mental Health in New York City, enabled my greater focus and integration of efforts to address mental well-being as a major component of disaster response efforts. Prior tragedies in New York City (e.g., massive fires, airplane crashes) had fueled the development of mental health crisis response teams and programs. New York City's creation of an Office of Emergency Management in 1996 provided the organizational structure and leadership to convene citywide drills to improve responses to a wide range of possible threats; mental health was usually "at the table."

Despite efforts to formalize the role of mental health into the city's public health responses through a merger of the two agencies into one integrated public health agency, political bickering between the mayor and city council representatives stymied the ability to alter the existing agency structure legislatively. Following the events of 9/11, the popularity of Mayor Giuliani enabled a public referendum on this merger to pass on election day 2001; consequently, an integrated Department of Health and Mental Hygiene (DOHMH) was launched in the early months of 2002.

The following decade saw the emergence of mental health as a more widely recognized public health priority in New York City. For example, the DOHMH issued *Take Care New York*, a widely disseminated comprehensive health policy setting ambitious goals in each of 10 priority areas that included 3 behavioral health targets: tobacco use, alcohol and drug dependence, and depression. The Epidemiology Division now routinely makes data available from its biannual Community Health Survey and Youth Risk Behavior Surveillance Survey, which includes questions on frequent mental distress, nonspecific psychological distress, depression in the past 12 months or by history, and suicidal thoughts or gestures. Furthermore, programs that address the interrelationship of health and mental health have been launched, including depression screening in primary care, a focus on metabolic syndrome in psychiatric patients, and smoking cessation initiatives. Certainly, expanded programming and policy initiatives addressing both mental and physical well-being are needed to gain greater traction for more integrative public health practice in the 21st century.

The experience of leading both health and mental health New York City agencies during the crises of 9/11 and bioterrorism affirmed my belief in the value of integrated public health approaches in the core areas of training, research, and practice. Those events provided clear evidence for the need for emergency preparedness to address the mental well-being of the population in an integrated public health framework of surveillance, community health education, health promotion, and illness prevention. The growing evidence for the enormous burden of mental disorders to society in terms of both human suffering and economic hardship[14-17] underscores the need for applying the tools and strategies of public health practice into an integrated health and mental health agenda that extends well beyond preparation to respond to terrorist threats. An eminent public health leader, Surgeon General David Satcher, became a leading voice for the mainstreaming of mental health into the larger public health landscape with the publication of the first of three reports, *Mental Health: A Report of the Surgeon General*, in which he stated, "Mental health is fundamental to health and human functioning. Yet much more is known about mental illness than about mental health."[18(p. 453)]

While encouraging individuals to seek treatment when experiencing disturbances to their mental well-being, the surgeon general's message also advocated moving the mental health/mental illness focus into the core priorities of our nation's public health agenda. As a follow-up to the message of this first report, additional reports on suicide prevention[19] and children's mental health[20] further developed the framework for applying the tools and strategies of public health practice to the challenges of mental illness prevention and mental health promotion.

With the publication of two major Institute of Medicine reports in 2009,[21,22] the field of practice for the prevention of mental disorders has received critical support as a mainstream public health priority. Over the past few decades, significant advances in mental health epidemiology have provided opportunities to recognize the associated factors that place people at risk for illness and those factors that confer some protection against those risks. With multiple risk factors affecting both physical and mental well-being, 21st-century public health practice is discovering models of integrated health and mental health focus that carry promise to synergistically extend the reach of preventive interventions toward a more holistic conceptualization of health.

Translating the prevention science into community-level interventions that reduce risk exposures and promote safer and more nurturing physical environments will require an infrastructure for community engagement and participation involving numerous stakeholders. The inclusion of mental health concerns, mental health promotion, and mental illness prevention into an integrated public health model that fully recognizes the interrelationships of physical and mental well-being will be key to advancing effective and cost-effective interventions for greatest societal benefit.

DISCUSION QUESTIONS

1. Which of the competencies described in the Appendix does this case demonstrate?
2. What are some of the approaches that can best establish a role for mental heath focus as a component of emergency preparedness and response to public health emergencies?
3. What are some of the challenges to addressing mental health needs and issues with the emergency response groups (e.g., police, firefighters)?
4. What are some ways to get the word out to communities that one's mental health is often affected by traumatic events and may need to be addressed by mental health professionals?
5. How might messages to the public about mental health issues avoid the stigma associated with mental illness?
6. How can a municipality prepare its mental health provider community to respond to emergency events?

REFERENCES

1. Cohen NL. Reflections on the public health and mental health response to 9/11. In: Danieli Y, Dingman R, eds. *On the Ground After September 11: Mental Health Responses and Practical Knowledge Gained.* New York, NY: Haworth Press; 2005:24–28.
2. North CS, Nixon SJ, Shariat S, et al. Psychiatric disorders among survivors of the Oklahoma City bombing. *JAMA.* 1999;282(8):755–762.
3. Ursano RJ, Fullerton CS, Vance K, Kao TC. Posttraumatic stress disorder and identification in disaster workers. *Am J Psychiatry.* 1999;156(3):353–359.
4. Cohen NL. Lessons learned from providing disaster counseling after TWA Flight 800. *Psychiatr Serv.* 1997;48(4):461–474.
5. Felton CJ. Project Liberty: a public health response to New Yorkers' mental health needs arising from the World Trade Center terrorist attacks. *J Urban Health.* 2002;79(3):429–433.
6. Boscarino JA, Galea S, Adams RE, Ahern J, Resnick H, Vlahov D. Mental health service and medication use in New York City after the September 11, 2001 terrorist attack. *Psychiatr Serv.* 2004;55(3):274–283.

7. Galea S, Ahern J, Resnick H, et al. Psychological sequelae of the September 11 terrorist attacks in New York City. *N Engl J Med*. 2002;346:982–987.

8. Galea S, Resnick H, Ahern J, et al. Posttraumatic stress disorder in Manhattan, New York City, after the September 11th terrorist attacks. *J Urban Health*. 2002;79(3): 340–351.

9. Galea S, Vlahov D, Resnick H, et al. Trends of probable post-traumatic stress disorder in New York City after the September 11 terrorist attacks. *Am J Epidemiol*. 2003;158(6):514–524.

10. Marshall RD, Olfson M, Hellman F, Blanco C, Guardino M, Streuning EL. Comorbidity, impairment, and suicidality in subthreshold PTSD. *Am J Psychiatry*. 2001;158(9):1467–1473.

11. Stein MB, Walker JR, Hazen AL, Forde DR. Full and partial post-traumatic stress disorders: findings from a community survey. *Am J Psychiatry*. 1997;154:1114–1119.

12. Alter J. Grit, guts and Rudy Giuliani: on the front lines, grieving more than the public knew, the mayor guides his city through hell. *Newsweek*. September 24, 2001; 53.

13. Norris FH, Tracy M, Galea S. Looking for resilience: understanding the longitudinal trajectories of responses to stress. *Soc Sci Med*. 2009;68:2190–2198.

14. Druss B, Marcus S, Olson M, Pincus HA. The most expensive medical conditions in America. *Health Aff*. 2002;21(4):105–111.

15. Eaton WW, Martins SS, Nestadt G, Bienvenu OJ, Clarke D, Alexandre P. The burden of mental disorders. *Epidemiol Rev*. 2008;30:1–14.

16. Ustun TB. The global burden of mental disorders. *Am J Public Health*. 1999;89(9):1315–1318.

17. Cohen NL, Galea S. 21st century public health practice: preventing mental illness and promoting mental health. In: Cohen NL, Galea S, eds. *Population Mental Health: Evidence, Policy, and Public Health Practice*. London, England: Routledge; 2011:341–357.

18. U.S. Public Health Service. *Mental Health: A Report of the Surgeon General*. Washington, DC: U.S. Department of Health and Human Services; 1999.

19. U.S. Public Health Service. *The Surgeon General's Call to Action to Prevent Suicide*. Washington, DC: U.S. Department of Health and Human Services; 1999.

20. U.S. Public Health Service. *The Surgeon General's Conference on Children's Mental Health: A National Action Agenda*. Washington, DC: U.S. Department of Health and Human Services; 2000.

21. Institute of Medicine. *Preventing Mental, Emotional, and Behavioral Disorders Among Young People: Progress and Possibilities*. Washington, DC: National Academy Press; 2009.

22. Institute of Medicine. *Depression in Parents, Parenting, and Children: Opportunities to Improve Identification, Treatment, and Prevention*. Washington, DC: National Academy Press; 2009.

Section

III

Emerging Infections

12 Gastrointestinal Anthrax Associated with a Drumming Circle in New Hampshire

Chris N. Mangal, Christine L. Bean, and Scott J. Becker

BACKGROUND

The anthrax events of October 2001 killed five Americans, terrorized millions more, and caused substantial financial damage to America's health and homeland security sectors. Prior to that series of events, a select group of leaders had the foresight to envision a network of laboratories that could respond to public health emergencies. In 1999, this group of leaders, comprising representatives from the Centers for Disease Control and Prevention (CDC), the Association of Public Health Laboratories (APHL), and the Federal Bureau of Investigation (FBI) articulated the vision for what is now known as the Laboratory Response Network (LRN). This network was constructed to align local, state, and federal laboratory assets to provide a rapid and robust response to biological threats, such as anthrax, plague, botulism, and smallpox. Since its inception in 1999, communities across the United States have made daily use of the LRN. The network played a crucial role in responding to the anthrax events of 2001 and continues to be a vital asset for public health and national security. In 2009, the network was instrumental in responding to a case involving gastrointestinal anthrax.

THE LABORATORY RESPONSE NETWORK

Formed by the CDC, APHL, and FBI, the Laboratory Response Network has been the nation's premier system for identifying, testing, and characterizing potential agents of biological and chemical terrorism. The original objective of the LRN was to create a highly effective and united national laboratory infrastructure to respond to bioterror threats. Early emphasis was placed on rapidly developing and distributing detection and confirmatory assays and reagents, training to develop proficiency in laboratory staff and managers, and improving the public health laboratory system in the identification and handling of biological agents used in terrorism. Today, the LRN maintains an integrated national and international network of laboratories that can quickly respond to acts of chemical or biological terrorism, emerging infectious diseases, and other public health threats.[1]

The LRN leverages a systems approach, building upon the foundation of sentinel, or clinical, laboratories (those based in hospitals or stand-alone centers in the community) and their ability to rapidly move suspect specimens into reference laboratories, typically the state and large local public health laboratories (PHL). The value of this network was demonstrated in 2001 when anthrax-contaminated letters were sent through the mail to public figures in New York City and Washington, DC. That mailing resulted in LRN laboratories in every state being inundated with blood and white powder samples needing analysis to rule out anthrax. The LRN was able to confirm the method of exposure (letters) and quickly test thousands of samples for possible contamination. Since that time, the LRN has broadened its role to focus on improving laboratory capacity in response to a full range of threats beyond bioterrorism.

The types of laboratories within the LRN system are organized by levels of capability and responsibility. Currently, there are three tiers of laboratories: sentinel, reference, and national (see **Figure 12-1**). Each of the three types of laboratories has distinct tasks. Sentinel laboratories typically have biosafety level 2 (BSL-2) practices in place. Biosafety levels, the containment procedures necessary to safely work

Figure 12-1

The LRN for biological terrorism preparedness and response.

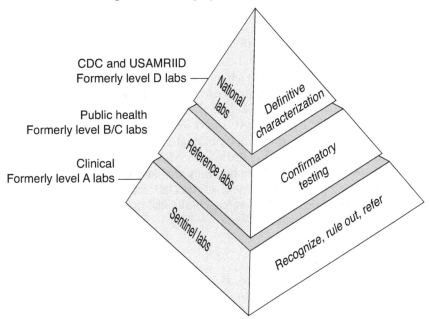

Source: Reproduced from the Centers for Disease Control and Prevention. The Laboratory Response Network: Partners in Preparedness. 2013. Available at http://www.bt.cdc.gov /lrn/ Accessed March 26, 2013.

with infectious organisms, vary depending on the nature of the work and the organism. The majority of reference laboratories have BSL-3 practices in place and the national laboratories have BSL-3 and BSL-4 practices in place. BSL-4 is the most stringent containment standard.

According to the CDC publication *Biosafety in Microbiological and Biomedical Laboratories,*

> The term 'containment' is used in describing safe methods, facilities and equipment for managing infectious materials in the laboratory environment where they are being handled or maintained. The purpose of containment is to reduce or eliminate exposure of laboratory workers, other persons, and the outside environment to potentially hazardous agents. The use of vaccines may provide an increased level of personal protection. The risk assessment of the work to be done with a specific agent will determine the appropriate combination of these elements.[2]

Sentinel Laboratories

Sentinel laboratories rule out and refer any specimens that test positive for biological threat agents such as *Bacillus anthracis* (anthrax) and *Yersinia pestis* (plague) to their associated LRN reference laboratories. When a sentinel, or clinical, laboratory receives a specimen that may be suspected of containing a biological threat agent, they perform testing following the American Society for Microbiology (ASM) *Sentinel Level Clinical Microbiology Laboratory Guidelines for Suspected Agents of Bioterrorism and Emerging Infectious Diseases.* These guidelines offer standardized methods to aid microbiologists in ruling out threat agents and to refer specimens to LRN reference laboratories for further testing for biological threats. Given that they are likely the first laboratories to encounter a patient's specimen, sentinel laboratories play a critical role in providing the initial alert that a biological threat agent is suspected.

Reference Laboratories

Those test sites designated as reference laboratories include state, local, and federal public health laboratories, military installations, and selected international laboratories that can conduct specialized tests with high confidence in the results. A high level of confidence can be the basis for both public health and law enforcement intervention. The reference laboratories conduct testing of clinical specimens (e.g., human blood), food and environmental samples (e.g., white powders, water), and are affiliated with state and local health departments and federal agencies. The state and local public health laboratories total approximately 70% of the 165 LRN reference-level laboratories.

Generally, the reference laboratories, with standards of BSL-3,[2] use federally approved equipment and standardized validated methods for testing of clinical and environmental samples. Using BSL-3 practices, facilities, and standardized technologies, the reference labs can test several sample matrices for agents such as *Bacillus anthracis*, *Brucella* species, and *Francisella tularensis*. Reference laboratories also maintain established linkages with law enforcement agencies, including the FBI. When working on samples that may be evidence of a potential crime, the reference labs utilize established chain-of-custody and LRN-approved testing protocols that are consistent with legal evidentiary requirements.

National Laboratories

National laboratories, including those operated by the CDC and the U.S. Army Medical Research Institute for Infectious Diseases (USAMRIID), perform all testing done by reference laboratories as well as additional specialized tests. These include definitive characterization of agents, strain typing, susceptibility testing, and bioforensics. The CDC and USAMRIID are equipped with BSL-4 facilities to safely handle highly infectious biological organisms.

HISTORICAL PERSPECTIVE ON ANTHRAX IN THE UNITED STATES

Bacillus anthracis, the cause of anthrax, is a zoonotic disease in domestic animals and was first isolated by Dr. Robert Koch in 1877.[3] The name *anthrax* comes from the Greek word for coal, because of the black skin lesions developed by victims with a cutaneous anthrax infection. Goats, cattle, sheep, and other grass-grazing animals become infected when they ingest soil-borne spores. In turn, humans may become infected through contact with infected animals or by handling contaminated animal products such as wool, hair, and hides.[4] In August 2000, a case of cutaneous anthrax was linked to an outbreak among livestock in North Dakota, resulting in the quarantine of 32 farms and the death of 157 animals.[5] The incidence of human infection with *B. anthracis* cannot be accurately determined due to unreliable reporting; however, it is more common in regions where agriculture is predominant and the control of anthrax among animals is poor.[6] Regions where disease is more common include South and Central America, Southern and Eastern Europe, Asia, Africa, the Caribbean, and the Middle East.[7] Within the United States, anthrax is rare, with an average of only one to two cases of cutaneous disease a year.[8]

In 1925, the American Public Health Association (APHA) committee on anthrax began recording the number of anthrax cases, as states reported the incidence to them. One of the first and most deadly outbreaks associated with occupational exposure in the United States occurred in 1957. A total of nine individuals became ill while working with black goat hair at the Arms Textile Mill located in Manchester, New Hampshire.[9] Four out of five individuals who were exposed by inhalation developed "anthrax pneumonia" and died thereafter.[10] During this time, that mill and three other facilities that processed raw, imported goat hair participated in the first study to evaluate the effectiveness of an anthrax vaccine.[11] The vaccine was first developed for use in humans in 1954, but none of the nine individuals who became ill in the Manchester mill received the study vaccine. Since then, the anthrax vaccine has been improved, with increased protective antigenicity and stability.[12]

Events that occurred in October 2001 illustrated the true dangers of *B. anthracis* and how the organism could be used as a weapon. Anthrax spores were mailed to four public figures in the United States. Two of the envelopes were postmarked September 18, 2001. One was addressed to Tom Brokaw, NBC news anchor; the other to the editor of the *New York Post*.[13] The remaining two letters were postmarked October 9, 2001, and addressed to U.S. senators Tom Daschle and Patrick Leahy.[13] Twenty-two individuals exposed to these letters became infected with anthrax. Of the 22 exposures, 11 were confirmed with inhalation anthrax and the remaining 11 were identified as having cutaneous anthrax with 7 confirmed.[14] Five of the inhalation cases resulted in death.[15] Antimicrobial prophylaxis was prescribed to 32,000 individuals as a result of the investigation, and 10,300 received medical recommendations to complete a 60-day course.[13] During this bioterrorism event, public health laboratories from around the country that were part of the LRN tested more than 125,000 clinical specimens and an estimated 1 million environmental samples.[15]

Since the 2001 bioterrorism event, additional cases of non-bioterrorism-related anthrax continued to emerge sporadically. A case of inhalation anthrax was reported by the Pennsylvania Department of Health in February 2006. In another case, investigation determined that the source of infection in a New York City man was his exposure to dried goat and cowhides imported from Africa. The man would scrape the hair off the animal hides before using them to make traditional African drums.[16] In August 2007, the Connecticut Department of Health reported cutaneous anthrax cases in a drum maker and his 8-year-old child. The drum maker was reported to have been working with untreated African goat hides from Guinea.[17]

INFECTION CAUSED BY *B. ANTHRACIS*

Human infection can occur via three routes: (1) exposure through abrasions in the skin; (2) inhaling airborne spores; or (3) ingesting contaminated food.[8] Cutaneous anthrax causes black necrotizing lesions primarily on the hands, forearms, and head. During the industrial age it was known as "woolsorter's disease" because of its association with individuals who worked with wool or animal hair in textile mills.[4]

Inhalation anthrax occurs when spores are inhaled and lodge into the alveoli. Phagocytes then transport the spores to the thoracic lymph nodes, where they germinate, multiply, and begin producing edema and lethal toxin. These toxins are responsible for hemorrhagic inflammation of the thoracic lymph nodes, edema, and necrosis.[7]

Causes of gastrointestinal anthrax are often attributed to the ingestion of contaminated food, primarily meat from an infected animal. The spectrum of disease ranges from no symptoms to death by shock or sepsis. There are two clinical manifestations of gastrointestinal anthrax: oropharyngeal and intestinal. Characteristics of oropharyngeal anthrax include body temperature greater than 102°F (39°C), ulcers in the oropharynx, sore throat, difficulty swallowing, regionally located swollen lymph nodes, and marked neck swelling.[17] Symptoms of intestinal anthrax are progressive and usually begin with nausea, vomiting, anorexia, a temperature greater than 102°F (39°C), and can advance to severe abdominal pain, vomiting of blood, and bloody diarrhea.[17,18] Spores may produce lesions in the stomach, esophagus, jejunum, ileum, and cecum, and these lesions may hemorrhage. The mucosa and regional lymph nodes of the intestinal tract are always implicated, and other complications such as the accumulation of serous fluid in the peritoneal cavity, shock, and sepsis may occur.[17] Severe gastrointestinal and pulmonary infections are more often fatal. However, any form of infection can lead to death if not identified and treated promptly.[7]

THE NEW HAMPSHIRE PUBLIC HEALTH LABORATORIES

The mission of the New Hampshire (NH) Public Health Laboratories is to protect the state's public health through responsive, unbiased, quality laboratory testing; to actively participate in national and international surveillance networks; and to improve the quality of health and laboratory services in both the public and private sector.[19] The NH PHL fulfills its mission through five core functions. The laboratory responds to critical incidents, which include disease outbreaks, radiological emergencies, chemical contamination or tampering of a product, and environmental water testing. To ensure that foods are safe, laboratories conduct microbiological testing of dairy products, shellfish, and other food products. Labs also test for metals in fish and other food products. Laboratory services for infectious disease control include testing for tuberculosis, rabies, sexually transmitted diseases, arboviral disease, and parasites. Testing of samples is also performed to assess occupational and environmental health hazards, such as arsenic levels in well water and radiological surveillance of environmental samples in dairy milk and air. To ensure quality and continuing education, laboratories conduct training for clinical laboratories and other partners, internships, and technology transfer (e.g., developing methods and guidance and sharing this information with partners) for laboratorians as well as coordination of the New Hampshire Laboratory Response Network.

THE ASSOCIATION OF PUBLIC HEALTH LABORATORIES AND PUBLIC HEALTH PREPAREDNESS AND RESPONSE

The Association of Public Health Laboratories (APHL) is a national nonprofit organization located in Silver Spring, Maryland, that is dedicated to strengthening the ability of laboratories to carry out their public health mandate. The association's members include state and local public health laboratories, state environmental and agricultural laboratories, and other government laboratories that conduct testing of samples with public health significance. Individuals with an interest in public health laboratory science and practice also participate in the association. The APHL strives to provide its member laboratories with the resources and infrastructure needed to protect the health of U.S. residents and to prevent and control disease globally. To achieve its mission, the APHL works closely with a number of partners, including the federal CDC and the Department of Homeland Security (DHS).

Through its Public Health Preparedness and Response (PHPR) program, the APHL works collaboratively with the CDC and other partners to strengthen the capability and capacity of public health laboratories. By building partnerships among public health laboratories, the CDC, the DHS, the Environmental Protection Agency (EPA), the FBI, other federal and state agencies, and the broader health community, laboratories are better able to prepare for, respond to, and recover from all public health emergencies. The APHL improves laboratory capacity and capability by training and providing technical and scientific guidance on laboratory assays and performance data, regulations, data messaging, surge capacity, continuity of operations plans, and other programs to assist members in responding to all-hazard threats, as well as providing operational support for public health laboratories in the LRN. The APHL works with the CDC to coordinate planning activities, such as proficiency testing for LRN reference and national laboratories to ensure that laboratories meet the LRN standards and laboratorians are competent to perform highly specialized methods and report results. During an event involving biological threats, such as anthrax, the APHL works with the CDC to coordinate the response by convening partners, identifying laboratories to provide surge capacity support, and providing scientific guidance to the laboratories and to the CDC.

UNKNOWN ILLNESS

On December 5, 2009, a 24-year-old woman began experiencing minor sweating and myalgias that progressed to back pain. Within a week, symptoms of nausea and vomiting had developed, and by December 15, she was admitted to a local New Hampshire hospital.[20] Blood was drawn to be cultured and the patient underwent an exploratory laparotomy where necrosis of the terminal ileum was noted.[21]

She was transferred to a tertiary-level academic medical center hospital in Massachusetts for further evaluation.

When the laboratory at the New Hampshire hospital read the blood culture tests on December 15, they found that the culture broth signaled that bacteria was growing, and they subcultured onto plates of Sheep Blood Agar (SBA) and Chocolate Agar to determine the type of bacterial organism growing in the broth. By the next day, December 16, the culture media grew visible organisms that were gram stained and shown to be gram-positive, spore-forming bacilli in chains. The isolate was nonhemolytic on the SBA and nonmotile, and originally thought to be a possible skin contaminant.

As described by the ASM, the conditions for sending isolates to an LRN reference laboratory to rule out or confirm *Bacillus anthracis* are catalase positive, nonhemolytic, nonmotile, gram-positive, spore-forming bacilli.[22] Based on the findings of the New Hampshire hospital's laboratory, the isolate should have been submitted to the NH PHL. However, a laboratory technologist who only occasionally rotated through the microbiology department performed the work in the supervisor's absence and was not familiar with the protocol. Not knowing that additional action was required, the technologist did not notify the supervisor and the hospital did not consult with the NH PHL about the isolate.

The infectious disease practitioner at the New Hampshire hospital, believing that the isolate was a contaminant, also did not follow through on the protocol for suspected agents. It is routine that three sets of blood cultures are drawn at separate time points in order to increase the likelihood of recovering a pathogen and also to aid in determining if growth is a contaminant or a cause of septicemia. The second and third sets of blood cultures drawn on this patient were negative, as was a culture of ascites fluid.

By the time the isolate was received at the Massachusetts hospital, evaluated, referred to the Massachusetts Public Health Laboratory, and confirmed as *B. anthracis*, more than 1 week had passed, and the patient remained in critical condition in that hospital. When the culture plates were sent to the reference laboratory in Massachusetts, that lab consulted with the infectious disease practitioner at the New Hampshire hospital and learned why no further action had been taken there.

In Massachusetts, a separate investigation was carried out. When the patient was transferred to the academic medical center in Massachusetts, blood specimens were sent to the William A. Hinton State Laboratory Institute, the LRN reference laboratory operated by the Massachusetts Department of Public Health. On December 24, the laboratory staff at the Reference Laboratory identified *Bacillus anthracis* in the patient's blood culture, which led to the patient being diagnosed with gastrointestinal anthrax. That day, following the LRN protocols established by the CDC, the reference laboratory quickly notified the New Hampshire Department of Health and Human Services (DHHS), the CDC, and the FBI, informing them that they had identified and diagnosed a case of gastrointestinal anthrax in the 24-year-old woman.

It was Christmas Eve and Elizabeth Talbot, the deputy state epidemiologist for New Hampshire, was on call. Upon receiving the phone call about the positive lab result, she activated the DHHS emergency management team to conduct a rapid assessment. Dr. Talbot called the public health nurses designated to conduct the investigation. In addition, the protocol prompts a series of notifications of those "with a need to know." A call was placed to the CDC's special pathogen group and the FBI was contacted. Within 24 hours, the team conducted multiple phone calls to sketch out a plan for the investigation.

EPIDEMIOLOGICAL INVESTIGATION

The investigative team considered the patient's risk factors and identified several leads. Given the patient's participation in an African drumming circle within the known incubation period for anthrax, state and federal officials quarantined the campus ministry building of the patient's university, where the drumming circle had occurred. As a consequence of the threat and the circumstances, a decision to quarantine and evacuate the building was the safest action while the investigation proceeded. Although the people who owned the building and the university where it was located were stakeholders, the authority to quarantine rested with the DHHS. They explained the decision to the stakeholders, who were fully cooperative throughout the process. The building was quarantined and evacuated and then the investigation progressed.

The resulting investigation involved numerous local, state, and federal agencies, including the New Hampshire Department of Environmental Services and Civil Support Team (CST), officials working with hazardous materials, local fire and other town officials, the CDC Select Agent (SA) Program, University of New Hampshire (UNH) officials, a CDC Epidemic Intelligence Service officer, the New Hampshire Department of Homeland Security, the EPA, and the New Hampshire DHHS. In New Hampshire, the CST is called to duty by the governor in an emergency event to assist with the state's response. In this case, they supported the response by driving their mobile laboratory van to the site to perform screening and testing.

The investigation was coordinated by the New Hampshire DHHS. The DHHS notified surrounding states that a case of anthrax was diagnosed and an epidemiological assessment had begun. The investigative team included epidemiologists from the state and local health departments, public health nurses, and experts from the CDC who were deployed to New Hampshire to assist in the response. The objectives of the investigation were to serve as a liaison with the appropriate federal authorities, determine if the case was naturally occurring or an intentional act, characterize the risk factors for illness, and identify the mode of transmission in order to prevent subsequent spread. Following the quarantine, the team focused on identifying the source of the infection, the patient's risk factors, how she contracted the anthrax, finding others who were potentially exposed, and then determining how to prevent further illness in other potentially exposed individuals.

The New Hampshire DHHS's Health Alert Network (HAN) and the LRN list serve, overseen by a designated coordinator in the PHL, were used to communicate with the New Hampshire LRN laboratories, the hospitals, and healthcare providers via email messages and faxes. These messages described the situation and asked the LRN partners to conduct a retrospective review of their infection control logs to see if there could have been other *Bacillus* cultures missed. The New Hampshire DHHS used statewide surveillance, including the Automated Hospital Emergency Department Data System and Vital Records Death Data, to attempt to identify other possible cases by querying for patients who presented for care with clinical symptoms similar to those of anthrax. Hospital laboratories, as members of the New Hampshire LRN, were asked to review 3 months of bacterial culture records and report any gram-positive rods that were not identified. No additional anthrax cases were identified through the retrospective study.

The New Hampshire DHHS investigation team interviewed the woman's friends and family to obtain information about possible risk factors. Exploring the patient's lifestyle was an important factor in understanding how this had happened. As possible modes of transmission varied, investigators considered what foods she had been exposed to, sources of water exposure, and aerosolization. The

Figure 12-2

Timeline of events.

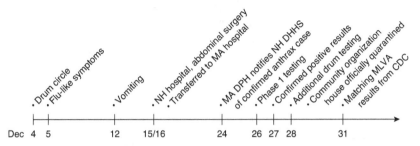

Source: Prepared by the Division of Public Health Services, New Hampshire Department of Health and Human Services.

FBI assessed the risk that the anthrax was released through an intentional act. Investigators asked questions about her drug use, food habits, and overall health. Looking at events starting on October 1, 2009, the investigation focused on the time period approximately 60 days before and after her exposure (see **Figure 12-2**).

The Investigation

The woman who developed anthrax was a vegan who had worked on an organic farm 3 months prior to her developing the disease. While a potential cause, possible links to organic farming were too remote, as this route of exposure occurred during the summer months and into September, so investigators did not pursue that possibility. In addition, she had participated in an event involving African drums held on December 4. The drumming circle, where a group of people got together to play drums and/or observe, took place at the United Campus Ministry House (Ministry House) located at the University of New Hampshire in Durham, New Hampshire. Drums were also stored in the basement of the facility.

As part of the investigation, the National Guard's 12th Civil Support Team collected environmental samples from both the Ministry House and the woman's residence to determine the source of infection. Given that no threats had been made to the campus ministry organization, it did not appear to be an event involving terrorism. The building layout was examined physically and pictures of the event and attendees' locations in the building were examined in an attempt to understand why this young woman was exposed and not others who also attended the event. Given that the drumming event took place at the Ministry House and the drums were stored in the basement, samples were not collected from any other buildings on the university campus.

The investigators hypothesized that during the drum circle, a brief aerosolization of anthrax spores located on the drum skin led to one of three scenarios. They theorized that (1) anthrax spores were deposited into the woman's gastrointestinal tract because she was either drumming or close enough to the drumming to be exposed and then ate food without washing her hands, (2) she inhaled anthrax spores through her oropharynx, or (3) she ingested the spores from either contaminated bread or a water bottle that was in the pathway of released spores during the event. Investigators learned that the ill woman had been a drummer.

B. Anthracis Found

Forty drums and six environmental samples were collected. Using LRN protocols, the samples were tested by the NH PHL for the presence of B. anthracis. Of the 46 samples tested, B. anthracis was isolated and grew in three samples—two from drums and one pooled sample of electrical outlets. Isolates from both the woman who became ill and the drums were submitted to the CDC for a test called the multiple-locus variable-number tandem repeat analysis (MLVA), a method used to discriminate or compare different B. anthracis isolates. This method employs the amplification of eight different variable-number tandem repeat loci by polymerase chain reaction (PCR), a test used to detect specific targets on the genome of the bacteria. The markers, specific known DNA sequences that can be found and quantitated, are then detected and measured using a DNA sequencer. Results from the isolates indicated that the loci were identical. With matching loci, investigators received confirmation that the isolate found in the blood sample from the woman who became ill and the isolate from the environmental sample matched, and thus the exposure occurred at this location. As a result, state and federal officials determined that 84 individuals who either worked, used, walked into, or lived in the building or participated in the drumming event were considered exposed. The EPA, New Hampshire DHHS, New Hampshire CST, New Hampshire Department of Environmental Services (DES), and CDC were all involved in this decision.

Determining Exposure Pathways

A second phase of the investigation sought to better characterize how the woman was exposed by studying any surfaces in the environment where the drumming event took place that may have become contaminated by the anthrax. The goal was also to look for any additional drums that were harboring anthrax spores. The NH PHL worked closely with the New Hampshire Department of Environmental Services, EPA, National Institute for Occupational Safety and Health (NIOSH), CDC, and New Hampshire DHHS to develop a sampling and testing plan. The NH PHL used a CDC method that had not previously been shared with the state labs.

Over 2 days, January 7 to 8, 2010, the second phase of samples was obtained from the Ministry House for a semiquantitative analysis, to detect and quantify the number of *Bacillus anthracis* spores present in the environmental sample. The CDC estimated that one lab could only process 10 to 20 samples per day. Due to the 10-fold volume of samples and the extensive processing time, the NH PHL requested assistance from other LRN reference laboratories, including New York City; Connecticut; Virginia, which had previous experience with testing for anthrax; and Tennessee, which had a drum hide that was present at the New Hampshire event. With the additional resources, it took a day or two and results were available.

With the results from all of the LRN reference laboratories, the investigative team determined that levels of *B. anthracis* spore contamination, while spread within the campus ministry facility, were low. Of the 85 additional samples processed, *B. anthracis* was isolated from only 6 samples, including 2 drums that had previously tested positive, a baseboard heater, the top surface of a kitchen cabinet, a computer screen, and desktop computer, all in two rooms adjacent to each other. Results were reported to the EPA, DES, DHHS director, and the CDC LRN. **Table 12-1** reflects results from both phases of testing. These findings resulted in the hiring of a professional cleaner to decontaminate the building.

CONCLUSION AND CHANGES IN PRACTICE

With appropriate treatment and a lengthy stay at the academic medical center in Massachusetts, the woman survived. The investigation lasted months before the DHHS could mitigate, as it took time before they had confidence in the processes proposed and used. Given the

Table	
12-1	**Summary of Testing of Nonclinical Samples**

Date	Total Samples Tested	Positive Samples	Total CFUs
Phase 1: Qualitative			
12/26/2009	40 drums from United Campus Ministry House	2 drums	NA
	6 environmental samples	1 electrical outlet	NA
12/28/2009	10 drums from drum teacher	None	NA
Phase 2: Semiquantitative			
1/7/2010	2 drums from United Campus Ministry House	Previous positives	300 and 171
	72 environmental samples	1 baseboard heater of event room	44
		1 upper surface of cabinet in adjacent kitchen	20
		1 computer screen in community area	20
		1 computer tower in community area	20
1/8/2010	11 drums from community brought to event	None	NA

Abbreviations: CFU, colony-forming units; NA, not applicable. 20 CFU/sample is at the limit of detection for this test.

active public health threat, the process involved waiting for both results and confirmatory results before the building could be restored to full use. The thorough investigation included searching for other people who may have fallen ill, but no one else was found who became infected and none of the other people deemed exposed became sick. Potentially exposed persons were offered postexposure prophylaxis for anthrax, consisting of antimicrobial agents (oral doxycycline or ciprofloxacin for 60 days from the last potential respiratory exposure) and anthrax vaccine adsorbed. Some chose to be treated and some declined treatment.

The NH PHL hosts quarterly LRN meetings to update labs and review issues in laboratory practice. At the next quarterly meeting, the New Hampshire hospital where the patient was originally admitted reported what they had learned to the other clinical laboratories. As a result of this experience, a change in practice was implemented. All clinical laboratories were required to immediately send cultures with suspect isolates to the New Hampshire Public Health Laboratory so that the reference lab could rule out or confirm that threat agents were present. This new protocol was issued in a memorandum to those attending the LRN meeting and through an LRN message via the HAN Communicator Notification System. In the memorandum, the New Hampshire PHL stressed that any test where the results indicate a suspect isolate be sent without hesitation.

At this quarterly meeting, New Hampshire laboratorians also discussed policy changes that would require all hospital staff who rotate through any of the microbiology departments to attend hands-on wet laboratory trainings and to participate in the College of American Pathologists' Laboratory Preparedness Surveys. Such training prepares lab personnel to identify and rule out bioterrorism agents by giving them experience with organisms that pose such a dangerous public health threat. In addition, the LRN partners were to attend wet lab trainings offered by the New Hampshire PHL at least once annually. Given workforce shortages and lack of funding, it has been difficult to implement these policy changes. In response, the New Hampshire PHL explored alternative educational modes to enable all laboratorians across the state to receive the training. Now, LRN wet lab trainings are offered twice yearly to provide options and increase access for those required to attend.

At the meeting, the hospital also discussed the difficulty of communicating effectively with the numerous agencies involved in the response. The process of HAN messaging was discussed to determine the best method of communicating with all of the stakeholders. It was decided that a message on the HAN is more likely to be received in a timely manner if at least two people per LRN site receive alerts from the HAN. The bioterrorism coordinator at the state's public health laboratory was designated to maintain up-to-date communication systems and to look at ways to enhance communications and partnerships with healthcare providers and other laboratorians across the state, despite budgetary constraints. Communication drills have been conducted since this event and will continue to be conducted annually, with results reported to the LRN partners at quarterly meetings.

DISCUSSION QUESTIONS

1. Which competencies described in the Appendix does this case demonstrate?
2. Describe the Laboratory Response Network. What are the pros and cons of a standardized system?
3. How does the role of a public health laboratory differ from the role of a clinical diagnostic laboratory such as a hospital laboratory?
4. Discuss the sustainability of multiple public health laboratories in one state.
5. Looking at the response timeline (see Figure 12-2) for this case, are there points where different decisions could have been made?
6. Should laboratorians working with potentially deadly microorganisms such as *Bacillus anthracis* be vaccinated? What are some of the policy issues that require resolution with mandatory vaccination of laboratory employees?
7. Thinking of the current technologies used for detecting biothreat agents, would you institute new technologies at point-of-care locations (e.g., physician's office, hospital) to confirm the presence of a biothreat agent?

REFERENCES

1. Centers for Disease Control and Prevention. The Laboratory Response Network: partners in preparedness. 2013. Available at: http://www.bt.cdc .gov/lrn/. Accessed March 26, 2013.
2. Chosewood LC, Wilson DE, eds. *Biosafety in Microbiological and Biomedical Laboratories*. 5th ed. HHS publication No. (CDC) 21-1112. 2009. Available at: http://www.cdc.gov/biosafety/publications/bmbl5/BMBL.pdf. Accessed September 16, 2011.
3. Karlen A. *Man and Microbes: Disease and Plagues in History and Modern Times*. New York, NY: Simon and Schuster; 1995:166.
4. Bollet AJ. *Plagues and Poxes: The Impact of Human History on Epidemic Disease*. New York, NY: Demos Medical Publishing; 2004:205–213.
5. Centers for Disease Control and Prevention. Human anthrax associated with an epizootic among livestock—North Dakota, 2000. *MMWR*. 2001;50:677–680.

6. Advisory Committee on Immunization Practices. Use of anthrax vaccine in the United States. *MMWR Recomm Rep.* 2000;49:1–20.
7. World Health Organization. *Anthrax in Humans and Animals.* 4th ed. Geneva, Switzerland: Author; 2008. Available at: http://whqlibdoc .who.int/publications/2008/9789241547536_eng.pdf. Accessed March 26, 2013.
8. Centers for Disease Control and Prevention. The National Center for Zoonotic, Vector Borne, and Enteric Diseases: anthrax, technical information. Available at: www.cdc.gov/nczved/divisions/dfbmd/diseases/anthrax /technical.html. Accessed August 26, 2011.
9. Wattiau P, Govaerts M, Frangoulidis D, et al. Immunologic response of unvaccinated workers exposed to anthrax, Belgium. *Emerg Infect Dis.* 2009;15:1637–1640.
10. Brachman PS, Gold H, Plotkin SA, et al. Field evaluation of a human anthrax vaccine. *Nations Health.* 1962;52:632–645.
11. Belluck P. Anthrax outbreak of '57 felled a mill but yielded answers. *The New York Times.* October 27, 2001. Available at: http://www.nytimes.com/2001/10 /27/us/nation-challenged-epidemic-anthrax-outbreak-57-felled-mill-but -yielded-answers.html?n=Top%2fReference%2fTimes%20Topics% 2fSubjects%2fT%2fTextiles. Accessed March 26, 2013.
12. Puziss M, Wright GG. Studies on immunity in anthrax. X. Gel-adsorbed protective antigen for immunization of man. *J Bacteriol.* 1963;85:230–236.
13. Jernigan DB, Raghunathan PL, Bell BP, et al. Investigation of bioterrorism-related anthrax, United States, 2001: epidemiologic findings. *Emerg Infect Dis.* 2002;8:1019–1028.
14. Dewan PK, Fry AM, Laserson K, et al. Inhalational anthrax outbreak among postal workers, Washington, DC, 2001. *Emerg Infect Dis.* 2002;8:1066–1072.
15. Centers for Disease Control and Prevention (CDC). Update: investigation of bioterrorism-related anthrax, 2001. *MMWR.* 2001;50:1008–1010.
16. Centers for Disease Control and Prevention (CDC). Inhalation anthrax associated with dried animal hides—Pennsylvania and New York City, 2006. *MMWR.* 2006;55:280–282.
17. Centers for Disease Control and Prevention (CDC). Cutaneous anthrax associated with drum making using goat hides from West Africa—Connecticut, 2007. *MMWR.* 2008;57:628–631.
18. Centers for Disease Control and Prevention, American Society for Microbiology, Association for Public Health Laboratories. Basic diagnostic testing protocols for level A laboratories for the presumptive identification of *Bacillus anthracis.* March 2002. Available at: https://www.premierinc.com /safety/topics/disaster_readiness/downloads/06-lab-protocol-bacillusanthracis .pdf. Accessed August 26, 2011.
19. Public health laboratories. New Hampshire Department of Health and Human Services website. Available at: http://www.dhhs.state.nh.us/dphs /lab/index.htm. Accessed August 26, 2011.
20. Lamothe W. Gastrointestinal anthrax in New Hampshire: a 2009 case report. *Lab Medicine.* 2010; 42:363–368.

21. Centers for Disease Control and Prevention (CDC).Gastrointestinal anthrax after an animal-hide drumming event—New Hampshire and Massachusetts, 2009. *MMWR*. 2010;59:872–877.

22. American Society for Microbiology (ASM). Sentinel level clinical microbiology laboratory guidelines for suspected agents of bioterrorism and emerging infectious diseases, *Bacillus anthracis*. May 6, 2010. Available at: http://www.asm.org/images/pdf/Clinical/Protocols/anthrax.pdf. Accessed August 31, 2011.

13

Surveillance in Emergency Preparedness: The 2009 H1N1 Pandemic Response

Michael A. Jhung

INTRODUCTION

In 1997, the first human case of H5N1 avian influenza was identified in a 3-year-old boy in Hong Kong. Within a few months, several more cases of human infection with avian influenza A (H5N1) in Hong Kong were confirmed, and public health officials began a fervent investigation to determine whether these cases were the start of a global influenza pandemic. In due course, the investigation revealed that this influenza virus was not transmitted efficiently from person to person, and that most of these cases had exposure to a live poultry market, where they likely became infected. This, as it turned out, was not the start of a pandemic, but it did mark the beginning of a period of time that saw unprecedented funding, effort, and attention directed toward preparing for what many people thought would be the next global public health disaster.

By 2009, more than 400 cases of H5N1 infection had been reported, and the case fatality ratio exceeded 60%.[1,2] Most of these cases were in Asia (China, Indonesia, Thailand, and Vietnam, among other countries), but by 2005 to 2006, the virus had spread, and Africa, Europe and the Middle East had seen their first cases as well.[3] Public health officials around the world were keenly aware of the threat posed by avian influenza and were preparing for the worst. Their biggest fear was that we would see another pandemic like the 1918 disaster, which caused up to 100 million deaths worldwide.[4] Pandemic planning had become an important part of the influenza agenda—all signs were pointing to some form of avian flu as the likely cause, and the expectation was that it would start somewhere in Africa or Asia. The U.S. government developed a comprehensive national pandemic response plan that, although broad in scope, identified H5N1 avian influenza as the greatest pandemic threat.[5] As it turned out, the next pandemic would start in neither Africa nor Asia, and would come from a different animal as well.

A STEEP LEARNING CURVE INDEED

At the time of the Hong Kong outbreak of H5N1, I was busy applying to medical school 12 time zones away, and it took a while for news of these events to catch up with me—but when they did, I was riveted by accounts of how a team of epidemiologists from the Centers for Disease Control and Prevention (CDC) flew to Hong Kong from Atlanta to investigate the outbreak. I remember thinking at the time— this sounds like something I would really like to do! After medical school, I completed residency training in preventive medicine and public health and then joined CDC's Epidemic Intelligence Service (EIS) program in 2005[6] as an officer with a group responsible for hospital-acquired infections. In August 2009, I transitioned from the hospital infections group at the CDC to the Influenza Division. As we will soon see, this was about 4 months into the 2009 pandemic, right before the start of the second wave in the United States. So, after spending 4 years studying hospital infections (which, by the way, rarely include influenza), I had a lot of catching up to do and little time in which to do it.

Of course, I was not the only one at the CDC making changes, and the adjustments made in the very early phases of the pandemic were a little unexpected. As the nation's premier public health agency, it fell to the CDC to lead the scientific response to the first influenza pandemic in over 40 years. Throughout the rest of this case study, we will see what this entailed and discuss how the clinical, laboratory, and epidemiologic data the CDC collected were used to help guide the public health response. For now, it is interesting to note that much of the early effort in the response was spent revising our pandemic plans, which were based on the 1997 outbreak of avian influenza in Hong Kong, an outbreak that had much greater clinical severity than what the 2009 H1N1 pandemic ultimately showed. Toby Crafton, chief of staff during the 2009 H1N1 pandemic response at the CDC, puts it this way:

> We had to make huge modifications because the assumptions in our planning process were based around an H5N1 kind of response, and it starting somewhere else. Basically, what happened was it was not an H5N1, and it started here—actually in Mexico. But it came here real quick, and what we were expecting was it would start somewhere in Asia and we would have several weeks before it came to the United States, and that's not what happened at all. And of course most of our planning was around a real severe pandemic H5N1, where the mortality rate is up around 60% for that virus. This particular pandemic was not anywhere near that severe, so we need to do more planning around general scenarios and general principles as opposed to specific viruses, and a lot of our planning in the past was done around a specific virus.[7]

IT'S JUST A COLD, RIGHT?

Most people know enough about influenza to realize that, for the most part, it causes relatively mild illness.[8] In fact, if you are one of the 15 to 60 million people who get the flu every year, you might be tempted to ask what the fuss is all about. First, although the majority of influenza cases are mild and self-limiting, complications can occur. The primary complication of influenza is pneumonia, and each year hundreds of thousands of people in the United States are hospitalized with,[9] and 3,000 to 49,000 people die from influenza.[10] Most of the really severe diseases occur in the elderly (people over 65 years of age), but children younger than 5 years of age, pregnant women, and people with underlying medical conditions are also at increased risk for hospitalization or death.[11] Along with this characteristic age distribution, seasonal influenza epidemics in the Northern Hemisphere also follow a predictable time course, with activity typically beginning in October, ending in May of the following year, and peaking sometime between February and March.

Most experts think that flu viruses are spread mainly by respiratory droplets made when people with the flu cough or sneeze. That means people with influenza can spread it to others up to about 6 feet away. These respiratory droplets can land in the mouths or noses of people who are nearby or possibly be inhaled into the lungs. Less often, a person might also get influenza by touching a surface or object that has virus on it and then touching his or her own mouth or nose. Most healthy adults may be able to infect others beginning 1 day before symptoms develop and up to 5–7 days after becoming sick. Children may pass the virus for longer than 7 days. Symptoms start 1–4 days after the virus enters the body. Some persons can be infected with the influenza virus but have no symptoms. During this time, those persons may still spread the virus to others.[8]

Vaccination is the best method for preventing influenza and its complications, but it must be given every year, and it works best when the vaccine strain matches the circulating virus (see **Figure 13-1**). Antiviral medications can also reduce serious morbidity and mortality related to influenza, but there is growing concern that circulating virus strains will become resistant to the few antiviral medicines that we currently have.

Figure 13-1

Artist's rendering of influenza A virus.

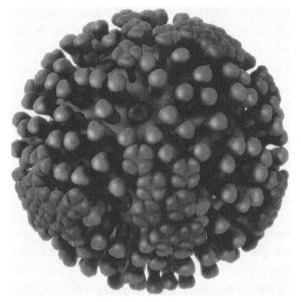

Source: Dan Higgins, CDC.

THE VIRUSES, THEY ARE A-CHANGING

This brings us to the second reason why you should care so much about influenza. Unlike many other organisms, the influenza virus is *always* changing, and changes in the virus, whether they are big or small, lead to the two things people worry about the most—resistance to antiviral medications and emergence of a novel influenza strain. Novel influenza strains are what cause pandemics. Small changes within the genetic material of influenza viruses occur frequently. This genetic drift does not lead to emergence of a new virus with pandemic potential, but can cause changes in virulence or transmissibility that can make influenza vaccines and antiviral medications less effective.

Without getting too bogged down with details, influenza viruses come in three flavors: types A, B, and C. Of the three, type A is the most alarming because it can infect both animals and humans, and thereby initiate a big change—an antigenic shift. An antigenic shift occurs when different influenza viruses exchange genetic material, resulting in major changes in viral surface proteins. When a single host cell is coinfected by two different influenza viruses, their genome segments can undergo reassortment and create an entirely new influenza virus. Pigs are thought to be a common mixing vessel for reassortment of avian, swine, and human influenza strains, and although relatively uncommon, human infections with reassortant swine viruses do occur.[12] These new viruses quickly die out, however, unless they retain the ability to replicate well in humans and are transmissible among humans. Prior to 2009, this had only happened three times in the last century, leading to influenza pandemics in 1918, 1957, and 1968. The worst of these pandemics (and some argue, the worst public health disaster of any kind) occurred in 1918, when up to 100 million people died from influenza.[4] By 2009, it had been over 40 years since the last pandemic, and there was growing concern that a new influenza virus might soon emerge and become efficiently transmitted among humans. This concern was justified, as the next global pandemic turned out to be right around the corner.

THE OUTBREAK: SERENDIPITOUS TESTING

On April 15, 2009, the first case of the 2009 pandemic was identified in a 10-year-old boy in Southern California; two days later, a second case of infection with the same pH1N1 virus was confirmed in a 9-year-old girl in an adjacent county in California.[13] The story of how these viruses were discovered is an interesting one and one of the first great successes of the pandemic response.

The diagnostic test used to identify influenza by most public health laboratories in the United States employs a molecular technique called reverse-transcription polymerase chain reaction (RT-PCR). Using RT-PCR, scientists can take a small amount of an unknown influenza virus and amplify its genetic material (in this case, RNA) until they have enough to "match" it against samples of virus whose identity they already know and have cataloged. In this way, they are able to describe influenza virus *type* (either A, B, or C) and *subtype*—a combination of letters and numbers that describes the composition of two important viral proteins (hemagglutinin and neuraminidase). A fully characterized influenza virus includes both descriptors, although only type A viruses are subtyped (e.g., influenza A H3N2, a common virus seen in seasonal epidemics). Although type B influenza viruses are composed of the same genetic material as type A viruses, they do not exhibit enough antigenic variation to warrant classification into subtypes.

When specimens from the two California cases were first tested, the results were unusual: influenza A, no recognizable subtype. The reason for this is that the RT-PCR test that was initially used to identify these cases included only avian (influenza A/H5) and seasonal (influenza A/H1 and A/H3) subtypes in its matching catalog. Because pH1N1 originated in swine, the RT-PCR test essentially could not recognize it. All human infections with influenza viruses of unknown subtypes are events of public health importance because these viruses all have pandemic potential. In fact, they are considered so important that they must be reported to the global public health community as a public health emergency of international concern (PHEIC) within 24 hours of identification.[14]

Human infections with swine flu viruses are rare and usually limited to people who have had contact with pigs (e.g., children who show pigs at a state fair). From 2005 until just before the start of the pandemic, only 11 sporadic cases of human infection with swine influenza (H1) had been reported to the CDC.[12] To ensure that these occasional cases did not become a bigger problem, the CDC was developing the ability to recognize swine viruses in its RT-PCR testing kits. In fact, they had a working model of this RT-PCR test ready just before the first two pandemic cases were reported.[15] Dr. Stephen Lindstrom, one of the CDC scientists who helped develop the new test, recalls its first application:

> It was very odd timing. Luckily, we had an assay almost ready, and it was designed to let us know if there was a novel virus emerging. This was a situation where our advanced work on swine really helped—if we had needed to start from scratch, it would have taken another two weeks to develop.[7]

At first it was not clear whether the California cases were just a few more isolated cases of swine flu. But what caught Lindstrom's attention (along with everybody else at the CDC) was the fact that neither California case had had any contact with pigs, or with each other. Lindstrom notes, "That was a pretty big red flag."

Over the next 2 weeks, additional cases of infection with this new virus were detected in Mexico, California, Texas, and other states.[16,17] When a case of human infection with novel A influenza is identified, the CDC undertakes a complex and comprehensive set of laboratory, epidemiologic, and communications measures to determine the extent and severity of each incident (see **Figure 13-2**).

Figure 13-2

Flow chart showing essential steps in an investigation of human infection with a novel A influenza virus.

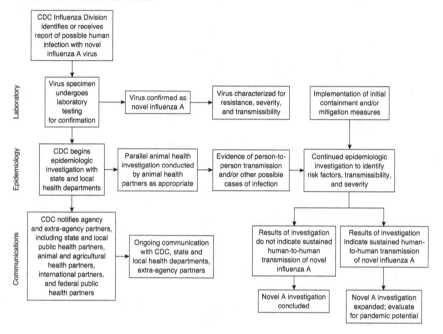

At this point, the CDC still did not really know what it had—clearly *something* was happening, as there were multiple infections with a novel influenza A virus in people that were unlikely to have been exposed to the same animal. Dr. Lyn Finelli, the CDC lead epidemiologist during the response, puts it best:

> On April 15, when we heard about the first case, we thought that that this would be a typical swine flu investigation, and it wasn't obvious to me that it would be as unusual as it turned out to be. It wasn't until two days later, when we heard about the second case, that I realized this might be very different from the novel A investigations we had done before. Within a few days, the parents of both children in California had been interviewed many times, and we just couldn't link the kids to any swine exposure. Now, about three weeks before all this happened, we had started to hear about outbreaks of severe respiratory disease in villages and small towns in Mexico where some people were hospitalized. So when we heard about two cases in Texas, another state bordering Mexico, I became

really alarmed. We thought that this was a big outbreak, potentially a very big one, involving multiple states and Mexico, but we weren't quite sure whether it was the pandemic or not. Over the next week, we very sincerely asked each other many times during the day—do you think this could be a pandemic? We really didn't know.[7]

FOURTEEN MONTHS IN THE SUBBASEMENT

By late April, however, there were dozens of confirmed cases in the United States, and the public health response had begun in earnest. The CDC quickly deployed six field investigation teams to California, Texas, Mexico, and other areas, and activated its Emergency Operations Center to help manage the rapidly increasing amount of data and requests for information that came pouring in.

What We Needed to Know #1

The public health questions surrounding pandemic influenza are not fundamentally different from those of seasonal influenza—at the beginning of the pandemic, we had the same two questions we ask during every influenza season: How big will this get (i.e., questions regarding geographic spread and burden of illness), and how bad will this be (i.e., questions regarding severity of illness)?

But the difference between pandemic and seasonal influenza is that a pandemic suggests widespread circulation of a *novel* virus, which means that pH1N1 characteristics such as its transmission properties, clinical spectrum, and antiviral resistance profile were largely unknown (see **Figure 13-3**). We also needed to know the answers to these questions quickly—much more quickly than for seasonal epidemics. Only certain pieces of information describing a new virus, however, are available early in its emergence, and this created tremendous tension between a need for careful and deliberate collection of information and the desire to take immediate action.

What We Needed to Know #2

It was also critical to describe the epidemiology and transmission of pH1N1 to make accurate recommendations to clinicians on how to protect themselves and treat their patients, and to make good

Figure 13-3

Diagram of surveillance data elements and relative timing of their availability in a pandemic.

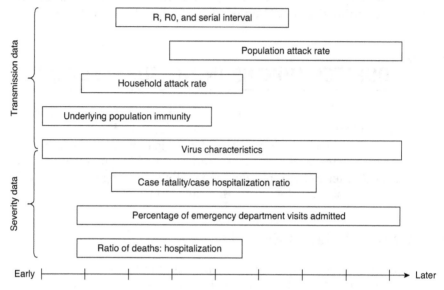

decisions on nonpharmaceutical interventions such as restricting travel and closing schools.

Every year, the CDC's Advisory Committee on Immunization Practices (ACIP) makes recommendations about the use of influenza vaccine and antiviral medications to prevent and control influenza.[11,18] These recommendations include priority groups for whom vaccine is especially important due to increased risk of severe complications from infection. The literature describing the epidemiology of seasonal influenza is quite extensive, and this allows the ACIP to be confident in prioritizing certain persons (e.g., the very young, the elderly, and people with underlying medical conditions) for vaccination and antiviral treatment. But there was no guarantee that pH1N1 would affect the population in the same way as seasonal influenza viruses. It was therefore very important to describe the epidemiology of pH1N1 accurately and quickly in order to identify priority groups for H1N1 vaccine, which initially was available in limited supply. Martin Meltzer, a senior health economist at the CDC who was extensively involved in the response, describes it well:

We knew vaccine production would take time. Who gets the first doses off the production line? Who goes to the front of the line? We've been discussing this for a number of years, and one of the most critical decisions was the ACIP recommendations about who should be vaccinated first. The ACIP as you know, gave a list of people who should be vaccinated first, but they also had another list within that list of what if there is a shortage of vaccine—who is the most important to vaccinate first? And that was the most critical decision in our response as far as I am concerned, because that then defined the whole nature of the vaccine-related response. The other critical decision was the use of antivirals. So those basic decisions upfront about what to do with the response resources in terms of vaccine and antivirals—who should get it—clearly defined the rest of the response. Everything about the response from then on led from this primary decision.[7]

WHAT WE DID

Activate the Emergency Operations Center and Create Regional Surveillance Teams

Almost immediately, the CDC activated its Emergency Operations Center (EOC) to help handle the increased information flow due to the pandemic response (see **Figure 13-4**). The EOC serves as the CDC's central public health incident management center for coordinating and supporting staff, information, communication, and security issues associated with a response to public health disasters, emergencies, disease outbreaks, and investigations. The EOC incident manager relies on a team of experts from across the CDC to staff the EOC during an event. This team determines the level of response required for each incident, depending on the information provided and analysis of each situation. The level of public health response also determines how many personnel will be needed to work in the CDC EOC during events. When asked how big the 2009 pandemic response was, Chief of Staff Toby Crafton had this to say:

It ended up being close to $2 billion that we got from the federal government to respond to H1N1. At the end when it was all said and done here, there were a little over 3,000 people that had in some way participated in the response. So it started off as probably 20 people, and it grew from there.[7]

Figure 13-4

A typical day in the Centers for Disease Control and Prevention's Emergency Operations Center in Atlanta, GA during the 2009 H1N1 pandemic response.

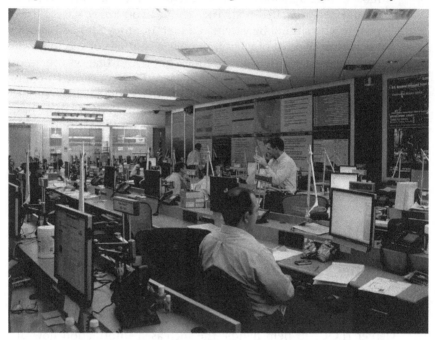

Source: Mark Fletcher, CDC.

Throughout the pandemic, the EOC served as the information center of the response and provided a means to collect and disseminate data to the hundreds of international, federal, state, and local public health partners involved. In the United States, regional surveillance officers were based in the EOC to maintain daily contact with state and territorial public health departments in order to gather information, impressions, and concerns that were not reflected by formal surveillance systems (see **Figure 13-5**). The regular and frequent contact between this team and state responders provided an avenue for quick exchange of very specific information, and information from the regional surveillance team was used to identify patterns of influenza severity and distribution manifesting in individuals or small clusters. Under the structure of the CDC's pandemic epidemiology and surveillance team, regional surveillance officers were tasked with gathering information about unusual or particularly severe clinical presentations, institutional clusters (such as in prisons or schools),

Figure 13-5

A team of regional surveillance officers at work in the Centers for Disease Control and Prevention's Emergency Operations Center in Atlanta, GA during the 2009 H1N1 pandemic response.

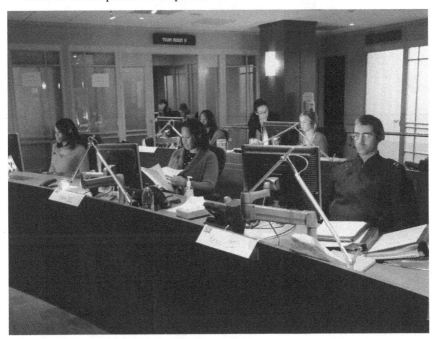

Source: Mark Fletcher, CDC.

and cases in vulnerable groups such as pregnant women or healthcare workers. Regional officers were also identified as a primary point of contact for state and local health departments to exchange information with the CDC regarding diagnostic laboratory testing during the pandemic and for questions about other CDC surveillance systems. The information gathered by the regional surveillance team proved valuable for many reasons; notably, it was often the initial impetus for launching a field investigation, and it was also used to provide situational awareness of the pandemic to senior leadership at the CDC.

What this meant for me was that the first "office" I had in my new position with the Influenza Division was a giant room I shared with 40 to 50 other people, the majority of whom rotated through about every 2 to 4 weeks. I spent the first 14 months of my new job in the CDC's secondary EOC (which happened to be in the subbasement of the oldest building on campus—not in the main EOC on the third

Figure 13-6

The author at work during the 2009 H1N1 pandemic response.

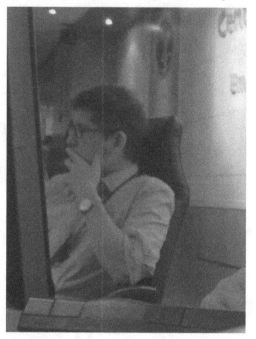

Source: Mark Fletcher, CDC.

floor of a brand new building), supervising the regional surveillance officers, managing one of our new influenza national surveillance systems, and sifting through incoming data for anomalies that would trigger a field investigation. I was often the first person in the building (usually before 6:00 AM), but was almost never the last to leave, even though I typically left after 7:00 PM every night—people in the Influenza Division were routinely working 12 to 16 hours a day, and everybody was focused on the pandemic (see **Figure 13-6**). Professionally, it was one of the most rewarding times of my life.

Rely on Existing Surveillance Systems

As pH1N1 activity accelerated throughout the United States, national influenza surveillance systems began to accumulate more data that confirmed findings from early investigations and case studies. In fact, the bulk of the robust epidemiologic data available during the 2009 pandemic were collected largely from preexisting local, state, and federal influenza surveillance systems. Influenza surveillance in the United States is composed of many systems that provide data on the location, timing, severity, and viral characteristics of influenza each season.[19] These systems have three primary goals: (1) to detect and characterize influenza viruses through determination of antigenic and genetic changes over time; (2) to determine the burden, epidemiology, and clinical characteristics of influenza and influenza-like illness (ILI); and (3) to detect the onset, duration, and geographic spread of disease caused by seasonal and other influenza viruses.

A fundamental responsibility of national influenza surveillance systems is to conduct laboratory surveillance for influenza viruses. In the United States, all state public health laboratories collaborate with the CDC and the World Health Organization (WHO) as do some county and city public health laboratories, as well as some large tertiary care or academic medical centers. This consists of approximately 80 laboratories that report the total number of human specimens received for respiratory virus testing and the number positive for influenza types A and B each week to the CDC; influenza A subtype, when known, is also reported. There are 70 National Respiratory and Enteric Virus Surveillance System (NREVSS) laboratories that report the total number of respiratory specimens tested and the number positive for influenza types A and B each week to the CDC. Most NREVSS laboratories participating in influenza surveillance are hospital laboratories; some have the ability to perform and report influenza A subtyping. During the 2009 pandemic, WHO/NREVSS laboratories provided influenza diagnostic test result data on more than 900,000 clinical specimens (see **Figure 13-7**).

In 2007, the Council of State and Territorial Epidemiologists (CSTE) and the CDC designated human infection with novel influenza A viruses as a nationally notifiable disease. Since that time, local, state, and territorial epidemiologists have worked alongside public health laboratories to report suspected novel influenza A infections in humans to the CDC Influenza Division. This arrangement worked as designed in April 2009 when the CDC Diagnostics and Strain Surveillance Branch rapidly confirmed the identification of two cases of pH1N1 infection in children from Southern California, marking the beginning of the 2009 pandemic.

Another component of U.S. national surveillance is responsible for influenza-associated hospitalizations. FluSurv-NET is a collaborative network with participants from the CDC, state and local health departments, and academic institutions. In 2004, surveillance for

Figure 13-7

Graph of laboratory specimens tested for influenza by WHO/NREVSS laboratories and at the Centers for Disease Control and Prevention.

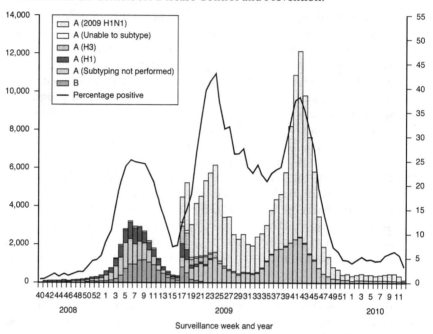

Source: The Epidemiology and Prevention Branch, Centers for Disease Control and Prevention.

laboratory-confirmed influenza resulting in hospitalization among children less than 18 years of age was initiated in nine Emerging Infections Program (EIP) sites; surveillance was expanded in 2005 and 2006 to include hospitalized adults, and an additional site was included. In September 2009, six new sites were added to FluSurv-NET, and this network of population-based sites in 16 states now represents approximately 7 million children and 21 million adults. FluSurv-NET's main goals are to characterize the incidence of, and risk factors for, laboratory-confirmed influenza resulting in hospitalization. During the pandemic, FluSurv-NET collected detailed information describing the epidemiology of over 7,000 patients hospitalized with influenza and was critical in assessing the severity of illness associated with the pH1N1 virus.

The U.S. Outpatient Influenza-Like Illness Surveillance Network (ILINet) conducts surveillance for outpatient healthcare encounters for influenza-like illness (ILI is defined as fever [temperature >

100°F /37.8°C] with cough or sore throat). In this collaborative network, data regarding ILI among outpatients are collected by healthcare providers recruited and coordinated by local, state, and territorial health departments. Each week, the providers report directly to the CDC Influenza Division their total number of office visits and the number of visits for ILI. The integrated data provide regional and national views of current influenza activity. The network functions year-round and currently has approximately 4,000 providers enrolled in 50 states, covering approximately 30 million patient visits per year. Due in part to the relatively mild illness associated with many pH1N1 infections, most of the estimated 61 million pandemic cases in the United States did not result in hospitalization or death,[20] and the only opportunity to conduct surveillance for these cases was during an outpatient healthcare encounter. The CDC, therefore, relied upon ILINet to track the temporal and geographic distribution of the vast majority of all influenza activity during the pandemic, and the network rapidly became the most important routine surveillance system in use during the pandemic.

Two national surveillance systems monitor mortality related to influenza. The 122 Cities Mortality Reporting System collects reports each week from vital statistics offices representing 122 cities and metropolitan areas. This system identifies, by age group, the proportion of filed death certificates that include a diagnosis of pneumonia or influenza. These data are used to define a baseline and epidemic threshold for mortality due to pneumonia and influenza and provide a means to compare mortality from year to year. The Influenza-Associated Pediatric Mortality Reporting System was initiated in 2003, when the CDC began requesting voluntary reporting of all deaths among children less than 18 years of age due to laboratory-confirmed influenza. In 2004, the CSTE designated influenza-associated pediatric mortality a nationally notifiable disease for public health surveillance.

The final component of the national system is the State and Territorial Epidemiologists' Report, which is responsible for detecting the onset, duration, and geographic spread of disease caused by seasonal and other influenza viruses. Each week, the CDC receives reports from state, territorial, or regional epidemiologists estimating their region's overall level of influenza activity. The epidemiologists' estimates are based on data obtained from several surveillance sources within their jurisdictions, including ILINet, 122 Cities Mortality Reporting System, and local reports of school absenteeism.

Enhancements to existing influenza surveillance systems were ongoing prior to the 2009 pandemic and included activities such as increasing the number of ILINet providers, particularly the number of sites that could submit electronically gathered data; establishing electronic laboratory reporting between public health laboratories and the CDC; and encouraging electronic reporting of influenza-associated mortality. Existing influenza surveillance systems were further augmented early in the pandemic to improve timeliness and geographic coverage to meet the special needs of the response. These modifications included increasing the frequency of ILI, laboratory, and mortality reporting from a subset of surveillance sites as well as the addition of new sites collecting population-based hospitalization rates.

These systems were relied upon heavily during the pandemic, and they provided two important benefits for the response, in addition to the information they gathered during the course of the pandemic. First, because they had been in continuous operation and had longstanding infrastructure in place, they could accommodate a rapid surge in activity when the pandemic began. Second, they provided a seasonal influenza baseline against which to compare pandemic illness burden and clinical severity.

Although not dedicated solely to influenza surveillance, the CDC's national automated biosurveillance system, BioSense, was also used extensively during the pandemic. BioSense receives primarily syndromic health data from U.S. civilian hospitals, Department of Defense and Veterans Affairs hospitals, emergency departments, and outpatient clinics.[21] Since 2007, BioSense has included a special influenza module that summarizes data from three sources within the National Influenza Surveillance System: chief complaint and International Classification of Diseases, Ninth Revision, Clinical Modification (ICD-9-CM) discharge diagnosis data from emergency departments, diagnosis data from outpatient clinics, and third-party payer electronic prescriptions for influenza antiviral medications.[22] The Distribute project was implemented in 2006 by the International Society for Disease Surveillance to assist with national monitoring of ILI reported from state and local health departments. The network was designed to aggregate ILI reports from existing emergency department syndromic surveillance systems and, as such, is closely related to the BioSense system in both purpose and operation. Distribute, in fact, incorporates some BioSense reports into its data stream. Originally developed as a proof-of-concept system, Distribute was rapidly expanded during the pandemic, and by November 2010, the systems participating in Distribute represented approximately one-third of the emergency department visits in the United States. Although syndromic surveillance likely overestimated influenza illness due to a nonspecific case definition, BioSense and Distribute generated reports on a daily basis, making them two of the most timely systems providing data to the CDC during the pandemic.

Outbreak Investigations and Special Studies

Early in the pandemic, case reports, field investigations, and case series were instrumental in answering several key questions surrounding the newly emerged pH1N1 virus (see **Figure 13-8**). Knowledge of community and household attack rates, reproductive rate, and generation time was crucial for understanding the epidemiology of the pandemic and informing control measures. Field investigations also provided critical data that helped shape early pandemic response efforts. Dr. David Swerdlow, one of the leads for the epidemiology and laboratory task force during the the response, tells us how these investigations got started:

> The epidemiologic investigations team was manned with EIS Officers or staff. When we heard about a cluster or an outbreak the team would send people or sometimes just give advice to the state epidemiologist and others at the state level. I actually called my friends in Foodborne Diseases who've had a lot of experience with this kind of outbreak, and they helped tremendously with investigations and with setting up a system for states to report cases to us. We were able to get that system up and running in 12 hours, and it was identical to systems that we had used for food-borne disease outbreaks. So that was one of the things that we did. It was sort of just nice that we had friends. I had come from Foodborne Diseases not that long ago, and we had friends there, and we were able to use their expertise.[7]

ILI attack rates were estimated in a household survey in a heavily affected Chicago community following an outbreak of

Figure 13-8

Surveillance at the beginning of the pandemic, showing an early transition from case-based reporting to aggregate surveillance for severe outcomes.

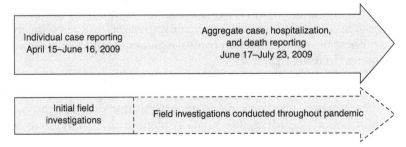

laboratory-confirmed pH1N1 at a neighborhood elementary school.[23,24] Attack rates, risk factors, and the effect of nonpharmaceutical interventions were the focus of an investigation of the first reported U.S. university pH1N1 outbreak, which occurred in Delaware during April 2009.[25,26] The secondary household attack rate following introduction by an index patient with influenza is an important indicator of the overall transmissibility of an newly emerged influenza virus.[27]

Secondary household ILI attack rates were estimated during field investigations in Texas, California, and New York City. In San Antonio, Texas, one of the first affected areas in the United States, transmission and the effect of nonpharmaceutical interventions was investigated in 77 households between April 15 and May 8, 2009, in which at least one person in the household had laboratory-confirmed pH1N1 infection.[28] In New York City, following the first large laboratory-confirmed pH1N1 school outbreak in the United States, 222 households of high school students with ILI were evaluated.[29] In San Diego County, California, 117 contacts in 38 households in which at least one person had laboratory-confirmed influenza were investigated at the onset of the pandemic (CDC unpublished data). Finally, 216 index cases with laboratory-confirmed pH1N1 and 600 household members reported to the CDC from April 2009 to June 11, 2009, were described in a study to estimate the secondary attack rate of pH1N1 to be at the lower range of that seen for seasonal influenza (10%–40%) and lower than that reported during previous pandemics.[30]

In May, the CDC investigated a cluster of approximately 50 cases of pH1N1 infections in a Chicago hospital in order to help characterize virus transmission.[31] At this time, the public health community was still struggling with personal protective equipment (PPE) recommendations, and it was thought that an outbreak in a healthcare facility might present a unique opportunity to determine whether surgical masks or N-95 respirators were needed to protect healthcare workers against pH1N1 transmission. Although results were inconclusive, this was an especially exciting investigation for me, as it was my first contribution to the pandemic response effort, allowing me to combine my recent infection control experience with a long-standing interest in influenza.

Data from seven focused epidemiologic studies and field investigations conducted from April through June 2009 were used to estimate infectiousness of ill individuals, an analysis that provided important information regarding the duration of time that individuals with

ILI should remain isolated to reduce spread of the pH1N1 virus.[32] Finally, a description of an outbreak at an elementary school in rural Pennsylvania at the outset of the pandemic provided insight into the dynamics of school outbreaks and transmission within schools.[33,34]

Early field investigations also provided information used to determine the basic reproductive number and the generation time (serial interval) for pH1N1 infection. The basic reproductive number R_0 is defined as the average number of secondary cases per typical case in a susceptible population.[35] Data from early cases were used to estimate the reproductive number of pH1N1 to be between 2.2 and 2.3,[35] although estimates decreased to 1.7–1.8 after adjustment for increased case ascertainment during the initial pandemic period. In a sensitivity analysis making use of previous estimates of the mean serial interval, the reproductive number was estimated to be between 1.5 and 3.1.[35] Cases from the initial outbreak in Mexico were used to estimate R_0 in the range of 1.2–1.6,[36] and reported case clusters in the United States estimated R_0 to be 1.3–1.7.[37] Most estimates of R_0 for pH1N1, therefore, have indicated that the virus was at the low end of transmissibility compared with the strains that caused the 1918 pandemic, and comparable, or slightly lower than the 1957 and 1968 pandemics. The time period between successive generations of infected persons can be measured indirectly by using the serial interval (the time between onset of symptoms in successive generations) and incubation period (the time between exposure and onset of symptoms) associated with a disease.[38,39] The serial interval for pH1N1 was estimated to be between 2.2 and 3.2 days,[30,35,37] less than that of seasonal influenza,[40,41] possibly due to higher proportions of susceptible persons. The distribution of the serial interval determines, along with R_0, the rate at which an epidemic can spread and can inform recommendations for control measures such as school closure, isolation of infected persons, and use of other nonpharmaceutical interventions.[30,35]

Several case series were also initiated early in the pandemic to help define the clinical spectrum of pH1N1 illness, identify populations at risk for severe disease, and assess the overall burden of disease. Two hospitalized case series[42,43] and one death case series[44] were conducted to help define the clinical spectrum of illness and identify risk factors for severe illness associated with pH1N1. In addition, serological studies were conducted to assess the level of preexisting immunity in the population and estimate infection rates at the conclusion of the pandemic.[45,46] Finally, several focused investigations were conducted to assess the impact of pH1N1 on important groups thought to represent at-risk populations. These included pH1N1 among persons infected with HIV,[47] Alaskan Natives and Pacific Islanders,[48,49] and healthcare personnel in the United States.[50,51]

Through rapid response activities like these, public health practitioners were able to confirm quickly that human-to-human transmission of pH1N1 virus was sustainable, describe the efficiency of transmission as approximately equivalent to that of seasonal influenza, and identify a broad clinical spectrum of pH1N1 illness whose severity was largely less than previous pandemics and similar to that of seasonal influenza. This, of course, is not the whole story of the pandemic, and it was partly through the use of influenza surveillance systems described in the forthcoming sections that public health identified a key feature of pH1N1—the relative sparing of health impact on older adults compared to both seasonal influenza and prior pandemics, and its disproportionate impact on children.

Modify Existing Surveillance Systems and Create New Ones

New methods to track pH1N1 and better understand its epidemiology were employed during the pandemic to fill critical knowledge gaps. Case-based reporting by state health departments, as described in the previous section, allowed tracking of detailed data and trends in severe disease with greater geographic representativeness than would have been possible with existing systems alone. As the pandemic evolved, however, case-based reporting rapidly became unmanageable, and the CDC began to encourage aggregate reporting of severe influenza outcomes (see Figure 13-8). In September 2009, the CDC and the Council of State and Territorial Epidemiologists formalized this sentiment by implementing a new influenza surveillance system to supplement available data from established systems, improve surveillance timeliness, and expand geographic coverage to meet the needs of the pandemic response. The Aggregate Hospitalization and Death Reporting Activity (AHDRA) was part of an overall national influenza surveillance strategy that was intended to provide timely and representative notification of severe outcomes associated with pH1N1. Objectives of this new system included the ability to (1) track severe disease within states and territories in order to better capture the focal nature of the pandemic, (2) track disease trends over brief units of time in order to respond rapidly to changes in pH1N1 epidemiology, and (3) accommodate variation in resources by providing a simple, flexible method to allow reliable reporting by all states and territories without overwhelming health departments during the course of the pandemic response. From August 30, 2009, through April 6, 2010, the CDC requested weekly reporting of influenza-associated hospitalizations and deaths from all 50 states and 6 U.S. territories. States and territories were asked to identify hospitalizations and deaths in their jurisdictions according to either a laboratory-confirmed or syndromic surveillance definition and could use either definition to report hospitalizations or deaths. Jurisdictions were instructed to submit aggregate weekly counts, by age group, to a secure website. Laboratory-confirmed reports from AHDRA were used to estimate weekly ratios, which were age-group specific, of influenza-associated deaths relative to influenza—associated hospitalizations. These values were also incorporated into a model used to estimate the national illness burden of influenza-associated cases, hospitalizations, and deaths during the pandemic, accounting for variation in medical care–seeking, laboratory practice and detection capability, and underreporting of confirmed cases.[20] Data collected by AHDRA helped characterize the epidemiology of pH1N1-associated influenza hospitalizations and deaths in the United States, revealing a time course and illness distribution for pH1N1 that were substantially different from those seen in seasonal influenza epidemics.[9,52–54] Although the total AHDRA laboratory-confirmed hospitalization and death counts likely substantially underestimated the total number of pH1N1-associated hospitalizations and deaths, they were helpful in monitoring trends in the distribution of illness and age groups over time in specific jurisdictions. The AHDRA data helped define the beginning and end of the 2009–2010 influenza season and accurately depicted the second wave of pH1N1 illness seen in the fall of 2009; similar double-wave patterns have been seen in previous pandemics.[55–57] AHDRA was also instrumental in the detection of and response to a minor third wave of pH1N1 activity in the southeastern United States in early 2010.[58] Although also useful in monitoring trends within jurisdictions, the AHDRA syndromic reports were less effective, as these data were complicated by limited representativeness and a low specificity for detecting influenza-attributable hospitalizations and deaths among those associated with respiratory illness. Because the system was implemented within a few weeks, AHDRA may prove particularly useful as a model for a national influenza pandemic surveillance system that needs to be implemented quickly and efficiently.

Dr. Nancy Cox, Influenza Division director at the CDC, provides some important perspective on the work done at the CDC during the 14-month-long response:

> I think that the rewarding thing about the public health mission working on the H1N1 response is that every day mattered. What you did at work every day mattered. That's the way most of us feel who work at the CDC anyway. But this was a response where you knew that you were going to have to work very hard every single day of the response, and that you would be making decisions or helping make decisions that would make a difference in saving lives and helping people.[7]

I WISH THAT I KNEW THEN WHAT I KNOW NOW

Since the pandemic was declared over by the World Health Organization in June 2010, many in the public health community have reflected upon lessons learned from this first pandemic of the 21st century. In the United States, demands of the response were met using different public health systems, depending on the timing and nature of disease activity—as the course of the pandemic evolved, response efforts evolved as well. By its end, a tremendous amount of information was available to describe the scope, magnitude, and severity of the pandemic. In fact, more data describing the epidemiology of influenza was collected, analyzed (some are still being analyzed!), and disseminated during the pandemic than at any time previously. This information was collected by thousands of public health practitioners using a combination of existing influenza surveillance systems, enhancements to these existing systems, new influenza surveillance systems created to address pandemic needs, outbreak investigations, and special studies. As post-H1N1 assessments continue and preparations for the next pandemic begin, we would do well to remember some of the most important lessons learned during 2009 and 2010.

The Importance of Strong Public Health Partnerships

In planning for and responding to influenza pandemics and other public health emergencies, collaboration with public health partners is essential. The response to the 2009 pandemic was successful largely thanks to teamwork among public health partners in state and local health departments, schools, and businesses. The comprehensive public health response to the pandemic would not have been possible without creating, maintaining, and refining partnerships inside and outside the public health community. The design and implementation of measures to prevent and control disease transmission relied upon a similar network of partners to inform and engage communities. Vaccination and antiviral therapy, in particular, are effective interventions that are less useful without the infrastructure to distribute them and a public notion that they offer protection from infection and illness. Success in the control of pandemic influenza, as with any public health threat, required awareness of the necessary partnerships to make surveillance and interventions useful. The 2009 pandemic response also required active engagement of the public, and for that, collaboration between public health and community partners was essential.

The Value of Having a Wide Range of Resources Available

We were fortunate in that when the pandemic began in 2009, the CDC was already operating multiple surveillance systems for influenza, each of which added information to what we knew about pH1N1. Because many of these systems had been in operation for years, (decades for some), there was infrastructure and experience in place that allowed us to scale surveillance up or down as needed, depending on the severity and timing of the pandemic. While it was initially difficult to forecast the course or duration of this pandemic, we suspected that there would likely be defined periods between the onset of pandemic activity, the peak of disease transmission, and the resolution of disease (this turned out to be true). These time points would dictate which surveillance systems and response strategies would be appropriate. As communities, regions, territories, and states were affected by pandemic influenza at different levels of intensity and at different times, regional public health authorities were able to implement surveillance and response strategies asynchronously and focus efforts on communities as they were affected. The multiple influenza surveillance systems used during the response worked very well to provide a comprehensive picture of the pandemic. In addition, although the bulk of information came via long-standing disease surveillance systems, other "surveillance" activities such as outbreak investigations and case studies were important in understanding pH1N1 transmission, clinical severity, and risk groups for illness.

The Value of Preparedness Planning

Although the timing, nature, and severity of a pandemic may be difficult to predict, it is imperative that preparedness planning occur to mitigate the impact of influenza. Regardless of its extent and severity, a pandemic can be expected to strain local, state, and federal resources, and without suitable planning, it may overwhelm them. The pandemic influenza plan in the United States [5] includes aggressive surveillance for novel influenza virus strains, comprehensive seasonal influenza surveillance, and enhanced virologic and disease surveillance once sustained human-to-human transmission is documented.

Prior to the 2009 H1N1 pandemic, the Department of Health and Human Service (DHHS) and the CDC were engaged in a broad array of surveillance activities with multiple public health partners to prepare for an influenza pandemic. These included efforts to expand geographic coverage of sentinel disease-reporting sites, improve the timeliness of influenza-related reporting to public health officials, develop clinical and epidemiological assessment tools, and establish rapid outbreak identification for both domestic and international events. One of the most important surveillance modifications occurred in 2007 when human infection with a novel influenza A virus became a nationally notifiable health condition. This new reporting requirement was preceded by an increase in diagnostic capacity at state public health laboratories, improving their ability to detect unusual influenza viruses. Together these activities enhanced a system that in April 2009 did exactly what it was designed to do—identify and report novel influenza A infections with pandemic potential.

Finally, the importance of practicing should not be overlooked. In the 5 years prior to April 2009, the CDC had conducted five functional pandemic exercises, each designed to simulate the response to an actual influenza pandemic. Functional exercises are complex events, usually lasting several days, that allow participants to learn and practice response plans while facilitating review and refinement of response strategies. Toby Crafton, chief of staff during the 2009 pandemic, commented on the value of pandemic exercises:

> Instituting pandemic exercise programs was probably the best thing we ever did. People complained, but after about the first month or two of the actual response, you heard them say, "Well it was a good thing we did those exercises." It really, really helped. The exercises we did were against a completely different scenario,

but it didn't matter. It was the processes and the procedures and the things that you learn, and how you interact and communicate during those exercises that I think was real important. And it doesn't matter what the disease is. It can be anything.[7]

Despite these achievements, there were some aspects of the response that should have gone better. Although years of pandemic planning left the United States with a public health infrastructure well-prepared to respond to the 2009 pandemic, there is no question that unanticipated gaps in the response existed.

THE ROAD AHEAD

Rapid and Ongoing Impact Assessment

One of the most-requested pieces of information about the pandemic revolved around the question of public health impact. Historically, the severity of influenza pandemics have been described using estimates of the case fatality ratio (CFR),[59] but this approach is limited because it does not account for the effect of virus transmissibility or for vulnerable population subgroups (e.g., children, the elderly, people with chronic medical conditions). Using the CFR to estimate severity was thought to be particularly ineffective in 2009 because information describing deaths from pH1N1 would not be available until weeks after the pandemic began, too late to inform recommendations for evidence-based public health interventions, and because initial reports suggested that this pandemic caused predominantly mild illness, resulting in too few fatalities to estimate an accurate CFR.

Rather than rely on the CFR as a sole measure of pandemic impact, the CDC developed an impact assessment framework based on five measures of transmission and three measures of severity, including community, school, and workplace attack rates; secondary household attack rates; the basic reproductive number (R_0); the case-hospitalization ratio; and a death-to-hospitalization ratio in addition to the CFR. Many of these measures will be available earlier in a pandemic than would data to estimate the CFR, and because the framework is designed to accept multiple inputs, it has flexibility to accommodate more (or fewer) measures as additional data become available (or if anticipated data are delayed). Although it has only been tested on historical data, this new approach shows promise for making pandemic impact assessment a more accurate and timely process.

A Nimble Way to Visualize and Access Data

Integrating, sharing, and disseminating information among public health partners were important parts of the pandemic that were moderately successful throughout the response. However, there are two groups in particular that would benefit from a more nimble way to visualize and access available data—decision makers and the public. Clear, concise, and easily accessible information would help speed decision making and facilitate a common understanding of issues among all contributing stakeholders.

To address this issue, the DHHS/CDC is adopting a technique used by the military to visualize positions, identify emerging and existing threats, manage available resources, and command troops in battle. A common operating picture (COP) can be defined as a single identical display of relevant information describing an event. At its simplest level the COP identifies *what* is *where*, but as more information is compiled and portrayed, the COP can give stakeholders greater situational understanding and allow decision makers to be more proactive in application of resources. Because the COP approach is also used by many U.S. government sister agencies, it should help synchronize reporting and data sharing among the CDC's external partners.

Additionally, displaying information in a clear, intuitive, and accessible manner would allow the nonscientific public to better understand the scope and severity of the pandemic and make better personal decisions regarding vaccination, social distancing, and other prevention strategies. Easily accessible information also has the added benefit of alleviating some of the public health resource burden of trying to answer each request for information individually. During the pandemic, the CDC assessed its communication strategies for epidemiologic and surveillance data with a goal to improve visualization of important public health data at FluView, its main influenza information site (http://www.cdc.gov/flu/weekly/); two recent modifications have been made. The first is the addition of a state-specific activity level indicator to the U.S. Outpatient Influenza-Like Illness Surveillance Network to facilitate a better understanding of how much ILI is being treated in outpatient clinics and doctor's offices (see **Figure 13-9**).

The second is a change in the way FluSurv-NET influenza-associated hospitalization data are displayed (see **Figure 13-10**). Both of these changes incorporate an interactive element and allow the user to tailor the way data are displayed. FluView is updated every week during the normal influenza season and is a very useful tool for learning about influenza and its associated complications—if you have not accessed it yet, I encourage you to give it a try.

Figure 13-9a

Screenshot of FluView, showing recent modification allowing state-specific visualization of influenza-like illness each week.

Influenza season week 12 ending October 22, 2011

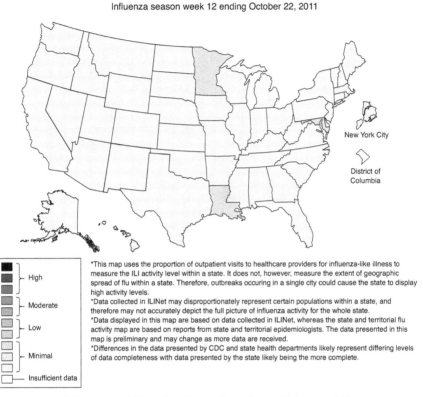

High

Moderate

Low

Minimal

Insufficient data

*This map uses the proportion of outpatient visits to healthcare providers for influenza-like illness to measure the ILI activity level within a state. It does not, however, measure the extent of geographic spread of flu within a state. Therefore, outbreaks occuring in a single city could cause the state to display high activity levels.
*Data collected in ILINet may disproportionately represent certain populations within a state, and therefore may not accurately depict the full picture of influenza activity for the whole state.
*Data displayed in this map are based on data collected in ILINet, whereas the state and territorial flu activity map are based on reports from state and territorial epidemiologists. The data presented in this map is preliminary and may change as more data are received.
*Differences in the data presented by CDC and state health departments likely represent differing levels of data completeness with data presented by the state likely being the more complete.

Source: CDC's FluView. Available at: http://www.cdc.gov/flu/weekly/. Accessed May 5, 2013.

Better Use of Electronic and Automated Data Sources

New electronic data sources for influenza surveillance were introduced during the pandemic to supplement existing national systems. These sources generally fell into one of three categories: (1) syndromic data that monitored aggregate ILI occurrence, (2) administrative data (e.g., ICD-9-CM discharge diagnosis codes), and (3) information from patient electronic medical records (EMRs) that provided deidentified patient-specific data from outpatient and inpatient healthcare encounters. Early in the pandemic, it was

Figure 13-9b

Screenshot of FluView, CDC's weekly online influenza information site showing percent of outpatient influenza-like illness each week.

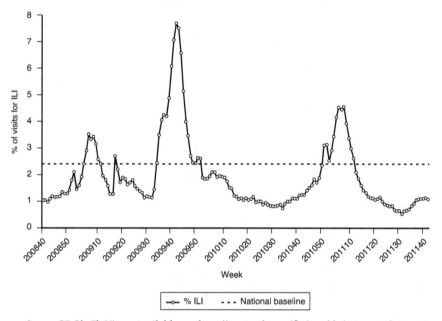

Percentage of visits for influenza-like illness (ILI) reported by
the U.S. Outpatient Influenza-like Illness Surveillance Network (ILINet), Weekly
National summary, September 28, 2008–October 22, 2011

Source: CDC's FluView. Available at: http://www.cdc.gov/flu/weekly/. Accessed May 5, 2013.

thought that electronic data streams could be incorporated into national surveillance for influenza quickly and efficiently. By the end of the pandemic, however, it was clear that none of the available electronic data sources evaluated by the CDC could be utilized without additional substantial time and resource expenditures. Fundamentally, these data were encumbered by a lack of experience at the vendors supplying them and the infectious disease epidemiologists at the CDC trying to validate and incorporate them into traditional influenza surveillance reports.

Difficulties encountered with electronic surveillance data included a lack of timeliness in receiving reports, limited representativeness for some sources, and the inability to obtain consistently valid and

Figure 13-10a

Screenshots of FluView, showing old depiction of influenza-associated hospitalization rates (Figure 13-10a) and recent modification (Figure 13-10b), which allows user to change display modes.

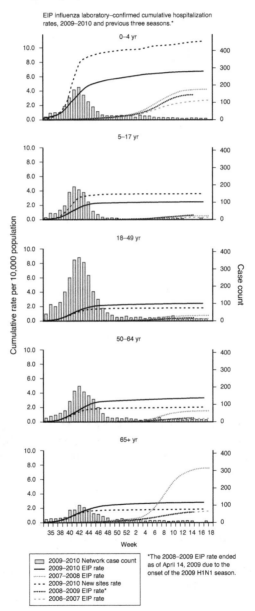

Source: CDC's FluView. Available at: http://www.cdc.gov/flu/weekly/. Accessed May 5, 2013.

Figure 13-10b

Screenshots of Fluview, showing old depiction of influenza-associated hospitalization rates (Figure 13-10a) and recent modification (Figure 13-10b), which allows user to change display modes.

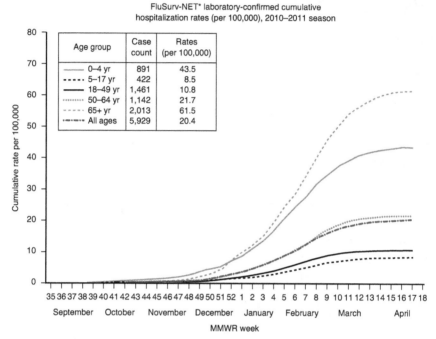

FluSurv-NET* laboratory-confirmed cumulative hospitalization rates (per 100,000), 2010–2011 season

Age group	Case count	Rates (per 100,000)
0–4 yr	891	43.5
5–17 yr	422	8.5
18–49 yr	1,461	10.8
50–64 yr	1,142	21.7
65+ yr	2,013	61.5
All ages	5,929	20.4

*FluSurv-NET results include surveillance at EP sites and at sites in six additional states (ID, MI, OH, OK, RI, UT)

Source: CDC's FluView. Available at: http://www.cdc.gov/flu/weekly/. Accessed May 5, 2013.

complete data. Of the three categories of data sources, syndromic data were the most timely and the easiest to implement. Although syndromic data streams did not provide much additional information over what was already being captured by existing surveillance systems, their application during the pandemic can be considered a success as they were indeed more timely and represented a higher volume of illness activity for the areas they covered. EMR data likely have the most potential for contributing to pandemic and influenza surveillance, and may prove to be a rich source of information for conducting scientific studies to describe influenza illness. However, issues of data storage and management and compatibility of data will need to be resolved before EMRs can be relied upon as an accurate and timely information source for surveillance purposes. The extent to which electronic data may eventually enhance traditional influenza surveillance remains to be seen, but limitations are likely to persist because administrative data and EMRs were not designed for surveillance purposes; instead, their primary roles lie in remuneration and provision of clinical care. Thus, system attributes such as data quality, representativeness, and sensitivity, which are critical to the successful operation of surveillance systems,[60] may not be priorities for vendors providing these data.

Estimating the Influenza Burden Better

One of the most frequently asked questions throughout the pandemic was, "How many people will become ill?" Early in the response, the CDC was able to answer only partially—we could provide very good estimates of the number of people who would become hospitalized or die with pH1N1 because we had very good surveillance systems monitoring those events. But that did not satisfy the demand for the number of cases overall, and we initially struggled to provide an estimate because (1) all of our established surveillance systems were set up such that they monitored people who had a healthcare encounter for influenza, and (2) most people who get influenza do not end up seeing a doctor for their illness. In other words, we were unable to capture as broad a spectrum of illness as we would have liked in order to estimate the burden of the pandemic—our surveillance was missing most of the people who get infected with influenza, and we needed some way to measure disease outside the healthcare system (see **Figure 13-11**).

During the pandemic, the CDC began surveillance of self-reported ILI using the Behavioral Risk Factor Surveillance System (BRFSS). BRFSS conducts population-based surveillance of health conditions and health risk behaviors in persons older than 18 years of age.[61] During the pandemic, BRFSS respondents were asked additional questions pertaining to ILI, even if they did not seek healthcare for their illness.[62] BRFSS data provided the only source of information describing ILI in persons outside the healthcare system during the pandemic in the United States. The CDC also expanded its existing surveillance systems for ambulatory and hospitalized cases, and when combined with the new BRFSS data, we were able to estimate the overall burden of pH1N1 illness in the population using a simple mathematical model.[20] The CDC is now working on enhancing its modeling capacity in order to improve burden estimation for future public health crises, including pandemics.

Figure 13-11

The influenza disease burden pyramid and surveillance inputs important to overall burden estimation.

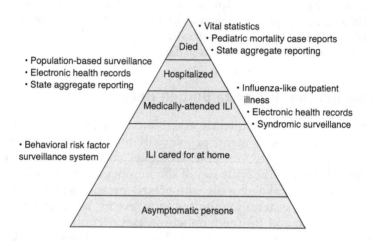

CONCLUSION

In retrospect, it seems unlikely that some of the most valuable lessons learned during the response would have been discovered in any scenario other than an actual influenza pandemic. In this respect, experience might have been the best teacher, and the modern public health community can consider itself fortunate that 2009 H1N1 was a relatively mild influenza virus. As such, the experience of responding to the 2009 pandemic may provide the best lessons for preparing to respond to future public health crises. So, to conclude, let us hear from people involved in the response at many different levels about what they would have done differently, given the opportunity.

Dr. Joe Bresee, Chief of the Influenza Epidemiology and Prevention Branch at the CDC:

I think that most of the things that the CDC did during the response were reasonable and appropriate given the information we had at the time. The quick changes to surveillance and data handling, the rapid development of critical policies, timely development of a national vaccination program, and the implementation of a broad and effective public communication campaign—all were remarkable achievements under the circumstances, and I would say that these accomplishments are typical of CDC work. For the next pandemic, we will do a better job of communicating—both to each other among the folks involved in the response, and to our partners in the public, the scientific colleagues and colleagues in public health. You can always do a better job of communicating.

Dr. Michael Shaw, Associate Director for Laboratory Science in the Influenza Division at the CDC:

Actually, not much. I think it went very well at the beginning; extremely well. It would have been nice to have had an idea of what was going on in Mexico earlier than we did. If we had been able to get specimens a little earlier, we might have had the vaccine maybe a month earlier. We couldn't decide on a good vaccine strain to use until we had more information about the circulating viruses. And that just requires data, and data requires time. And that's something you can't speed up.[7]

Toby Crafton, Chief of Staff for the 2009 H1N1 Response at the CDC:

Staffing was a huge problem, getting people. The CDC never has a problem getting people to respond to an event or to a catastrophe for about a month, and then after a month, people are like, "I got another job I have to do." To get people to give up what they're doing for three or four months is really asking a lot. But we learned early on that unless you get people for two months, then you are wasting their time and our time as well. Because by the time they get up to speed to what's going on, they're rotating off again unless they are there for a while.[7]

Joe Gregg, Deputy Team Lead for the Surveillance and Outbreak Response Team in the Influenza Division at the CDC:

The amount of data coming in and the requests for information going out both increased exponentially within a few days of the response. To process and respond, we needed a lot of personnel with very specific skill sets. At first, we resorted to asking people we had worked with before and knew had the skills we needed. That worked for about three weeks and then we ran out of people. On top of that, we often needed to interpret the same data multiple times a day to meet information requests from different agencies. In hindsight we could have planned better by having a clear information cycle and standardized reports. We finally got there, but it wasn't until several months into the response.

Dr. David Sencer, CDC Director during the last swine influenza epidemic in 1976:

> Well, the advice I gave was basically to do what's right. If you have to take an unpopular stance, do that. But you need to expect the unexpected. Things are going to happen that you could not have anticipated. Make sure of your facts. Put heavy emphasis on the surveillance and then find a way to communicate this not just to the health professionals but to the public. And I think one of the outstanding successes of CDC in H1N1 was that they were able to take the scientific information and present it in such a fashion that the public could accept it, could understand it, and could realize that the CDC was playing right flat on the table. There were no hidden things going on.[7]

DISCUSSION QUESTIONS

1. Which of the competencies described in the Appendix does this case demonstrate?
2. Dwight D. Eisenhower once said: "Plans are nothing, planning is everything." Does this case illustrate this concept? If so, how?
3. What were the benefits of opening the CDC Emergency Operations Center?
4. What are the advantages of having a national surveillance system for influenza already in place before a pandemic?
5. How should the CDC handle the assignment of personnel during an emergency response?

REFERENCES

1. Abdel-Ghafar AN, Chotpitayasunondh T, Gao Z, et al. Update on avian influenza A (H5N1) virus infection in humans. *N Engl J Med*. 2008;358:261–273.
2. Beigel JH, Farrar J, Han AM, et al. Avian influenza A (H5N1) infection in humans. *N Engl J Med*. 2005;353:1374–1385.
3. World Health Organization. Cumulative number of confirmed human cases of avian influenza A/(H5N1) reported to WHO. Available at: http://www.who.int/influenza/human_animal_interface/H5N1_cumulative_table_archives/en/. Accessed June 27, 2011.
4. Barry JM. *The Great Influenza: The Epic Story of the Deadliest Plague in History*. New York, NY: Viking; 2004.

5. Department of Health and Human Services. HHS pandemic influenza plan. Available at: http://www.hhs.gov/pandemicflu/plan/. Accessed November 5, 2010.
6. Centers for Disease Control and Prevention. Epidemic Intelligence Service. Available at: http://www.cdc.gov/eis/index.html. Accessed March 28, 2013.
7. H1N1 oral history project, David J. Sencer Museum at the Centers for Disease Control and Prevention. Taken from transcript of interview conducted as part of CDC's H1N1 Video Archive available at http://intranet.cdc.gov/ecp/video_archives.asp
8. Mandell GL, Bennett JE, Dolin R. *Mandell, Douglas, and Bennett's Principles and Practice of Infectious Diseases.* 7th ed. Philadelphia, PA: Churchill Livingstone/Elsevier; 2010.
9. Thompson WW, Shay DK, Weintraub E, et al. Influenza-associated hospitalizations in the United States. *JAMA.* 2004;292:1333–1340.
10. Estimates of deaths associated with seasonal influenza—United States, 1976–2007. *MMWR.* 2010;59(33):1057–1062.
11. Fiore AE, Uyeki TM, Broder K, et al. Prevention and control of influenza with vaccines: recommendations of the advisory committee on immunization practices (ACIP), 2010. *MMWR Recomm Rep.* 2010;59(RR-8):1–62.
12. Shinde V, Bridges CB, Uyeki TM, et al. Triple-reassortant swine influenza A (H1) in humans in the United States, 2005–2009. *N Engl J Med.* 2009;360:2616–2625.
13. Swine influenza A (H1N1) infection in two children—southern California, March–April 2009. *MMWR.* 2009;58:400–402.
14. World Health Organization. *International Health Regulations (2005).* 2nd ed. Geneva, Switzerland: Author; 2008.
15. Lessons from a Virus. In: Laboratories AoPH, ed., 2011 Available from http://www.aphl.org/AboutAPHL/publications/Documents/COM_2011Sept_FluStories_Digital.pdf.
16. Update: swine influenza A (H1N1) infections—California and Texas, April 2009. *MMWR.* 2009;58:435–437.
17. Update: infections with a swine-origin influenza A (H1N1) virus—United States and other countries, April 28, 2009. *MMWR.* 2009;58:431–433.
18. Fiore AE, Fry A, Shay D, Gubareva L, Bresee JS, Uyeki TM. Antiviral agents for the treatment and chemoprophylaxis of influenza—recommendations of the advisory committee on immunization practices (ACIP). *MMWR Recomm Rep.* 2011;60:1–24.
19. Brammer L, Postema AS, Cox N. Seasonal and pandemic influenza surveillance. In: M'Ikanatha NM, ed. *Infectious Disease Surveillance.* 1st ed. Malden, MA: Blackwell; 2007:254–264.
20. Shrestha SS, Swerdlow DL, Borse RH, Prabhu VS, Finelli L. Estimating the burden of 2009 pandemic influenza A (H1N1) in the United States (April 2009–April 2010). *Clin Infect Dis.* 2010;52(suppl 1):S75–S82.
21. Tokars JI, English R, McMurray P, Rhodes B. Summary of data reported to CDC's national automated biosurveillance system, 2008. *BMC Med Inform Decis Mak.* 2010;10:30.
22. Hales C, English R, McMurray P, Podgornik M. The biosense influenza module. International Society for Disease Surveillance Conference. Raleigh, North Carolina, 2008.

23. 2009 pandemic influenza A (H1N1) virus infections—Chicago, Illinois, April–July 2009. *MMWR*. 2009;58:913–918.
24. Janusz KB, Cortes JE, Serdarevic F. Influenza-like illness in a community surrounding a school-based outbreak of 2009 pandemic influenza A (H1N1) virus—Chicago, Illinois, 2009. *Clin Infect Dis*. 2011;52(suppl 1): S94–S101.
25. Guh A, Reed C, Gould LH. Transmission of 2009 pandemic influenza A (H1N1) at a public university—Delaware, April–May 2009. *Clin Infect Dis*. 2011;52(suppl 1):S131–S137.
26. Iuliano AD, Reed C, Guh A, et al. Notes from the field: outbreak of 2009 pandemic influenza A (H1N1) virus at a large public university in Delaware, April–May 2009. *Clin Infect Dis*. 2009;49:1811–1820.
27. Longini IM Jr, Koopman JS, Monto AS, Fox JP. Estimating household and community transmission parameters for influenza. *Am J Epidemiol*. 1982;115:736–751.
28. Morgan OW, Parks S, Shim T, et al. Household transmission of pandemic (H1N1) 2009, San Antonio, Texas, USA, April–May 2009. *Emerg Infect Dis*. 2010;16:631–637.
29. France AM, Jackson M, Schrag S, et al. Household transmission of 2009 influenza A (H1N1) virus after a school-based outbreak in New York City, April–May 2009. *J Infect Dis*. 2010;201:984–992.
30. Cauchemez S, Donnelly CA, Reed C, et al. Household transmission of 2009 pandemic influenza A (H1N1) virus in the United States. *N Engl J Med*. 2009;361:2619–2627.
31. Magill SS, Black SR, Wise ME, et al. Investigation of an outbreak of 2009 pandemic influenza A virus (H1N1) infections among healthcare personnel in a Chicago hospital. *Infect Control Hosp Epidemiol*. 2011;32:611–615.
32. Donnelly CA, Finelli L, Cauchemez S, et al. Serial intervals and the temporal distribution of secondary infections within households of 2009 pandemic influenza A (H1N1): implications for influenza control recommendations. *Clin Infect Dis*. 2011;52(suppl 1):S123–S130.
33. Iuliano DA, Dawood FS, Silk BJ. Investigating 2009 pandemic influenza A (H1N1) in U.S. schools: what have we learned? *Clin Infect Dis*. 2011;52(suppl 1): S161–S167.
34. Marchbanks TL, Bhattarai A, Fagan RP, Ostroff S. An outbreak of 2009 pandemic influenza A (H1N1) virus infection in an elementary school in Pennsylvania. *Clin Infect Dis*. 2010;52(suppl 1):S154–S160.
35. White LF, Wallinga J, Finelli L, et al. Estimation of the reproductive number and the serial interval in early phase of the 2009 influenza A/H1N1 pandemic in the USA. *Influenza Other Respi Viruses*. 2009;3:267–276.
36. Fraser C, Donnelly CA, Cauchemez S, et al. Pandemic potential of a strain of influenza A (H1N1): early findings. *Science*. 2009;324:1557–1561.
37. Yang Y, Sugimoto JD, Halloran ME, et al. The transmissibility and control of pandemic influenza A (H1N1) virus. *Science*. 2009;326:729–733.
38. Anderson RM, May RM. *Infectious Diseases of Humans: Dynamics and Control*. New York, NY: Oxford University Press; 1991.

39. Rothman KJ, Greenland S, Lash TL. *Modern Epidemiology*. 3rd ed. Philadelphia, PA: Wolters Kluwer Health/Lippincott Williams & Wilkins; 2008.

40. Cowling BJ, Fang VJ, Riley S, Malik Peiris JS, Leung GM. Estimation of the serial interval of influenza. *Epidemiology*. 2009;20:344–347.

41. White LF, Pagano M. Transmissibility of the influenza virus in the 1918 pandemic. *PloS One*. 2008;3(1):e1498. doi:10.1371/journal.pone.0001498.

42. Jain S, Kamimoto L, Bramley AM, et al. Hospitalized patients with 2009 H1N1 influenza in the United States, April–June 2009. *New Engl J Med*. 2009;361:1935–1944.

43. Skarbinski J, Jain S, Bramley A, Lee EJ. Hospitalized patients with 2009 pandemic influenza A (H1N1) virus infection in the United States—September–October 2009. *Clin Infect Dis*. 2010;52(suppl 1):S50–S59.

44. Fowlkes AL, Arguin P, Biggerstaff M, Gindler J. Epidemiology of 2009 pandemic influenza A (H1N1) deaths in the United States, April–July 2009. *Clin Infect Dis*. 2010;52(suppl 1):S60–S68.

45. Hancock K, Veguilla V, Lu X, et al. Cross-reactive antibody responses to the 2009 pandemic H1N1 influenza virus. *N Engl J Med*. 2009;361: 1945–1952.

46. Ross T, Zimmer S, Burke D, et al. Seroprevalence following the second wave of pandemic 2009 H1N1 influenza. *PLoS Curr*. 2010;2:RRN1148. doi:10.1371/currents.RRN1148.

47. Peters PJ, Skarbinski J, Louie JK, Jain S. HIV-infected hospitalized patients with 2009 pandemic influenza A (pH1N1)—United States, Spring and Summer 2009. *Clin Infect Dis*. 2010;52(suppl 1):S183–S188.

48. Deaths related to 2009 pandemic influenza A (H1N1) among American Indian/Alaska Natives—12 States, 2009. *MMWR*. 2009;58:1341–1344.

49. Wegner JD, Castrodale LJ, Bruden DL, Keck JW. 2009 pandemic influenza A H1N1 in Alaska: temporal and geographic characteristics of spread and increased risk of hospitalization among Alaska Native and Asian/Pacific Islander people. *Clin Infect Dis*. 2010;52(suppl 1):S189–S197.

50. Novel influenza A (H1N1) virus infections among health-care personnel—United States, April–May 2009. *MMWR*. 2009;58:641–645.

51. Wise ME, De Perio M, Halpin J, Jhung MA. Transmission of pandemic (H1N1) 2009 influenza to healthcare personnel in the United States. *Clin Infect Dis*. 2010;52(suppl 1):S198–S204.

52. Centers for Disease Control and Prevention. FluView. Available at: http://www.cdc.gov/flu/weekly/. Accessed April 26, 2010.

53. Molinari NA, Ortega-Sanchez IR, Messonnier ML, et al. The annual impact of seasonal influenza in the US: measuring disease burden and costs. *Vaccine*. 2007;25:5086–5096.

54. Jhung MA, Swerdlow DL, Olsen SJ. Epidemiology of 2009 pandemic influenza A (H1N1) in the United States. *Clin Infect Dis*. 2010;52(suppl 1): S13–S26.

55. Andreasen V, Viboud C, Simonsen L. Epidemiologic characterization of the 1918 influenza pandemic summer wave in Copenhagen: implications for pandemic control strategies. *J Infect Dis*. 2008;197:270–278.

56. Chowell G, Ammon CE, Hengartner NW, Hyman JM. Transmission dynamics of the great influenza pandemic of 1918 in Geneva, Switzerland: assessing the effects of hypothetical interventions. *J Theor Biol.* 2006;241:193–204.

57. Olson DR, Simonsen L, Edelson PJ, Morse SS. Epidemiological evidence of an early wave of the 1918 influenza pandemic in New York City. *Proc Natl Acad Sci USA.* 2005;102:11059–11063.

58. Update: influenza activity—United States, August 30, 2009–March 27, 2010, and composition of the 2010–11 influenza vaccine. *MMWR.* 2010;59:423–430.

59. Centers for Disease Control and Prevention (CDC). Interim Pre-Pandemic Planning Guidance: Community Strategy for Pandemic Influenza Mitigation in the United States. 2007. Available at: www.flu.gov/planning-preparedness /community/community_mitigation.pdf. Accessed May 5, 2013.

60. Lee LM. *Principles and Practice of Public Health Surveillance.* 3rd ed. Oxford, England: Oxford University Press; 2010.

61. Centers for Disease Control and Prevention. Behavioral Risk Factor Surveillance System Operational and User's Guide Version 3.0. December 12, 2006. Available at: ftp://ftp.cdc.gov/pub/Data/Brfss/userguide.pdf. Accessed December 21, 2010.

62. Self-reported influenza-like illness during the 2009 H1N1 influenza pandemic—United States, September 2009–March 2010. *MMWR.* 2011;60(2):37–41.

14

Mandatory Vaccination and H1N1: A Large Urban Hospital's Response

Doris R. Varlese and Kevin Chason

BACKGROUND

It was the summer of 2009 in New York City. An outbreak of a novel strain of the influenza virus, initially called "Swine Flu" and then renamed "H1N1," had spread from an outbreak in Mexico a few months earlier. H1N1 was first identified in New York City at a private high school after several students became ill following vacations during spring break in Mexico. H1N1 quickly spread throughout the New York City area. Several persons had fallen ill and died. Media attention was intense. A writer for the *Los Angeles Times*, reporting on the plethora of media attention, wrote "the 24-hour outlets endlessly scroll new numbers, of states and nations reporting possible cases, of schools closing, of death tolls rising."[1]

The infectiousness of H1N1 was different from that of seasonal influenza in that it disproportionately affected younger people and pregnant women. The U.S. Department of Health and Human Services (DHHS) had declared a public health emergency on April 26, 2009. Each day, the New York City Department of Health and Mental Hygiene (DOHMH) reviewed several factors at schools such as increases in influenza-like illness (ILI).[2] The New York City DOHMH defined ILI as visiting a healthcare office "with chief complaint including fever with either cough or sore throat or the mention of the word 'flu.'"[3] In an attempt to slow transmission of the virus, the DOHMH recommended to School Chancellor Joel Klein that the city close certain schools.[2] As of May 23, 2009, 40 schools in New York City had each been closed for several days.[2]

IMPACT ON HEALTHCARE SYSTEMS

On the days that schools were closed, hospital Emergency Department (ED) visits generally increased in the neighborhoods where the schools were located. During that spring, a large urban hospital (we will call this "Urban Hospital") saw its ED visits double—from a typical 250 visits per day to over 500 visits during the peak days. Administration of Urban Hospital monitored the school closings closely, expecting that if a neighborhood school was closed due to the city's concern about H1N1, ED visits would increase even more.

The increase in patients coming to the ED presented challenges for Urban Hospital. The ED experienced longer waiting times before patients were seen, periods of overcrowding, and difficulties in triaging patients with ILI. In order to handle the increased number of patients, Urban Hospital increased available medical staff by having ED physicians work additional shifts. Hospital administrators also increased the hours that the pediatric and adult clinics were open, and staff screened patients who presented to the ED with ILI at locations outside the ED. In consultation with its in-house attorneys and risk managers, Urban Hospital developed protocols to direct patients with ILI away from the ED to the outpatient clinics (alternate locations) so as not to violate the federal Emergency Treatment and Active Labor Act (EMTALA). EMTALA is a federal law requiring that EDs provide all patients who seek care with a medical screening examination, stabilizing treatment, and if necessary, hospital admission transfer to another facility. While ED visits increased at Urban Hospital during this time, hospital admissions did not. Almost all patients with ILI were treated at the ED or outpatient clinics and their condition merited being sent home.

PUBLIC HEALTH SURVEILLANCE

When tracking the rate of persons with ILI presenting to EDs throughout the city, the New York City DOHMH identified a trend of ED visits increasing, with a peak in late May (see **Figure 14-1**).[3] By July 23, 2009,

Figure 14-1

Rate of ILI syndrome visits from NYCDOHMH.

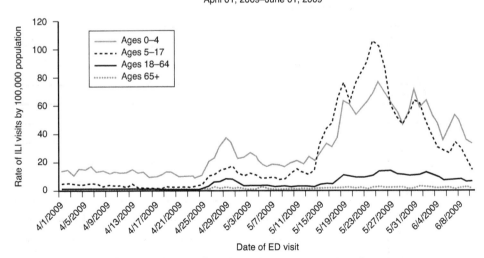

Source: New York City Department Health and Mental Hygiene. 2009. New York City Department of Health and Mental Hygiene health alert #22: Novel H1N1 influenza update June 12, 2009. http://www.nyc.gov/html/doh/downloads/pdf/cd/2009/09md22 .pdf. p. 6. Accessed August 30, 2011.

the data compiled by federal Centers for Disease Control and Prevention (CDC) showed that there were 2,738 confirmed and probable cases of H1N1 reported in New York state with 63 deaths (see **Table 14-1**).[4]

Table	
14-1	**U.S. Human Cases of H1N1 Flu Infection**

States and Territories[a]	Confirmed and Probable Cases	Deaths
States		
Alabama	477	
Alaska	272	
Arizona	947	15
Arkansas	131	
California	3,161	52
Colorado	171	
Connecticut	1,713	8
Delaware	381	
Florida	2,915	23
Georgia	222	1
Hawaii	1,424	3
Idaho	166	
Illinois	3,404	17
Indiana	291	1
Iowa	165	
Kansas	204	
Kentucky	143	
Louisiana	232	
Maine	145	
Maryland	766	4
Massachusetts	1,370	5
Michigan	515	9
Minnesota	670	3
Mississippi	252	
Missouri	76	1
Montana	94	
Nebraska	313	1

States and Territories[a]	Confirmed and Probable Cases	Deaths
States		
Nevada	467	
New Hampshire	247	
New Jersey	1,414	15
New Mexico	232	
New York	2,738	63
North Carolina	483	5
North Dakota	63	
Ohio	188	1
Oklahoma	189	1
Oregon	524	5
Pennsylvania	1,960	8
Rhode Island	192	2
South Carolina	244	
South Dakota	45	
Tennessee	283	1
Texas	5,151	27
Utah	988	16
Vermont	59	
Virginia	327	2
Washington	658	7
Washington, DC	45	
West Virginia	243	
Wisconsin	6,222	6
Wyoming	111	
Territories		
American Samoa	8	
Guam	1	
Puerto Rico	20	
U.S. Virgin Islands	49	
Total (55)*	**43,771 cases**	**302 deaths**

[a]Includes the District of Columbia, American Samoa, Guam, Puerto Rico, and the U.S. Virgin Islands.

Source: Adapted from: Centers for Disease Control and Prevention. Novel H1N1 flu situation update. July 24, 2009. Available at: http://www.cdc.gov/h1n1flu/updates /072409.htm. Accessed August 30, 2011.

A NEW VACCINE

On June 11, 2009, the World Health Organization (WHO) raised the worldwide pandemic alert level to phase 6, indicating that a global pandemic was underway.[3] Given that no vaccine existed for this novel virus, the CDC developed a vaccine against the H1N1 strain and arranged to have its contractors manufacture it. The CDC planned to make the vaccine widely available by providing it free of charge to hospitals, physician practices, clinics, health departments, and other entities. When production of the H1N1 vaccine was slower than expected while demand for the vaccine was strong, there was not enough supply to meet the vaccine demand. This shortage would later have implications for the mandatory vaccination of healthcare workers in New York State.

A NEW REGULATION

On August 6, 2009, at the request and approval of New York Health Commissioner Richard Daines, MD, the New York State Hospital Review and Planning Council (SHRPC), a body authorized to issue regulations affecting healthcare facilities, adopted an emergency regulation mandating that hospitals, diagnostic and treatment centers, home healthcare agencies, and hospices, "notify all personnel of the requirement and require that personnel be immunized against influenza virus(es) as a precondition to employment and on an annual basis."[5] *Personnel* was defined as

> all persons employed or affiliated with a healthcare facility, whether paid or unpaid, including but not limited to employees, members of the medical staff, contract staff, students, and volunteers, who either have direct contact with patients or whose activities are such that if they were infected with influenza, they could potentially expose patients, or others who have direct contact with patients, to influenza.[5]

The regulation included an exception for medical contraindications.[5] The regulation became effective a week later, and facilities subject to the regulation were required to vaccinate their workers by November 30 of each year.[5] While the rule's "Regulatory Impact Statement" indicated that outreach to affected parties, including professional organizations, was conducted prior to the adoption of the regulation,[5] many in the healthcare sector, including hospital administrators and clinical providers at Urban Hospital, were taken by surprise, not anticipating this emergency regulation. The process for implementing regulations usually required at least several months and often years, with multiple discussions at the SHRPC and the SHRPC's committee meetings before a vote to adopt.

According to this new rule, influenza vaccinations were to be provided in accordance with national recommendations in effect at the time, unless the commissioner of the New York State Department of Health (NYSDOH) determined that there was an inadequate supply of vaccine. Should it be determined that there was an insufficient supply of vaccine, the regulation provided the commissioner with the authority to suspend the regulation or change the annual deadline.[5] In an August 26, 2009, "Frequently Asked Questions" document regarding the regulation, NYSDOH stated, "if the novel H1N1 vaccine is released as a fully licensed vaccine, as expected, this regulation will also require immunization against H1N1 as well as seasonal influenza this coming season."[6]

WHY REGULATION?

Commissioner Daines and the NYSDOH viewed the regulation as the most effective way to ensure that this novel virus did not spread throughout the state. The "specific reasons underlying the finding of necessity," published with the regulation, referred to "the new threat posed to health and safety by the novel H1N1 influenza A strain that is circulating in New York State," and stated, "the sooner that the emergency regulations are in place the sooner lives will be saved and other complications of influenza disease avoided."[5] As precedent, New York, like every state, already required healthcare workers to be immunized against measles, mumps, and polio.[7]

In 1990, a New York state court had affirmed the NYSDOH's authority to require mandatory physical examinations, tuberculosis tests, and rubella vaccinations for hospital personnel.[8] Further, the CDC had recommended influenza vaccinations for healthcare providers since 1981.[5] Unlike other public health crises where infectious disease spread unabated (e.g., human immunodeficiency virus [HIV] in the 1980s), in this emergency, a vaccine was available that was effective in preventing the spread of H1N1.

In an open letter to healthcare workers issued on September 24, 2009, distributed to hospitals and providers via email and reported through the media, Commissioner Daines stated, questions about safety and claims of personal preference are understandable. Given the outstanding efficacy and safety record of approved influenza vaccines, our overriding concern then, as health care workers, should be the interests of our patients, not our own sensibilities about mandates.[9]

Dr. Daines further stated that "high rates of staff immunity . . . can only be achieved with mandatory influenza vaccination" because the historical vaccination rate for healthcare worker influenza vaccination was 40% to 50% "with even the most vigorous of voluntary programs."[9]

He went on to say:

In recognition of health care's noble tradition of putting patients' interests first and understanding the need to keep our health care system functioning optimally during this challenge, federal authorities made a remarkable decision regarding the first groups to be given access to the new H1N1 vaccine . . . authorities declared that health care workers would . . . be given earliest access to the vaccine, ahead of millions of other individuals who have roughly equal or even higher risks of contracting H1N1.[9]

URBAN HOSPITAL ACTS

Prior to the onset of H1N1, Urban Hospital's chief medical officer, epidemiologist/infection control officer, and chief of infectious diseases had discussed the establishment of a policy in order to increase rates of protection against influenza among the providers. Urban Hospital considered implementing a policy whereby influenza vaccinations would be mandatory for all physicians and other licensed practitioners (e.g., dentists, podiatrists) who were appointed to the medical staff. Physicians and those other practitioners would be required to be vaccinated against influenza in order to maintain their clinical privileges at the hospital. To do this, they would have had to amend Urban Hospital's medical staff bylaws to require the vaccinations as a condition of clinical privileges. Because Urban Hospital had been considering mandatory influenza vaccinations for its own medical staff, the new NYSDOH requirement was not unwelcome.

Activating Urban Hospital's Response

When confronted with the spread of H1N1 that spring, Urban Hospital activated its incident command system (ICS). The ICS is an organizational framework for managing emergencies that governmental agencies and most hospitals use. The ICS requires that an individual, known as the incident commander, be in charge; at Urban Hospital this was the vice president of operations. The hospital's emergency management plan included four ICS branches: operations, planning, logistics, and finance. For the period during the H1N1 crisis, the ICS team established several subgroups, including the communications workgroup, the strategic advisory group, and the policy/enforcement/regulation subgroup. High-ranking individuals in hospital leadership served on the ICS team, including the hospital epidemiologist/infection control officer, the chief medical officer, the chief nursing officer, the director of pharmacy, the director of compliance, the director of security, the director of communications, the director of human resources, the vice president of labor relations, and the director of employee health services.

Urban Hospital's strategic advisory group (which included medical experts), reviewed New York state's new mandatory vaccination requirement and advised the incident commander to add the vaccination requirement as a condition of employment. As a result, the hospital decided to require all personnel to be vaccinated (all staff, residents, students, volunteers, and medical school faculty) and not just those with direct patient contact or those who, in the words of NYSDOH, performed "duties that, if they were ill, could infect patients or staff with direct patient contact."[6] In the hospital's view, it was difficult to determine who was subject to the language of the regulation, because the regulation itself was unclear regarding which workers were or were not subject to the mandatory requirement. The hospital also knew that requiring vaccination of all personnel was compelling because, due to the nature of this public health crisis and the spread of influenza, there could be a potential shortage of workers and any worker could be assigned to duties that might require contact with patients. Thus, the hospital's interpretation regarding who required vaccination appeared broader than the NYSDOH's.

Potential Liability

Any potential concerns of Urban Hospital regarding liability for possible adverse outcomes as a result of the vaccinations were alleviated by the protections provided by the federal Public Readiness and Emergency Preparedness (PREP) Act. The PREP Act provided immunity from liability for claims relating to the administration or use of vaccinations.[10] As a result, no legal tort claim (except for claims of willful misconduct) could be successfully pursued against providers administering the H1N1 vaccine. Instead, Congress authorized a fund to pay claims such as those for medical benefits, lost wages, and death benefits. While Congress enacted the PREP Act in 2005, prior to the outbreak of H1N1, PREP Act declarations issued by the secretary of the DHHS authorized that the vaccination effort be covered by the statute. In their outreach following the issuance of the new regulations, NYSDOH provided several versions of a document entitled "PREP Act Liability Coverage Fact Sheet for Health Care Providers." The policy/enforcement/regulation subgroup of Urban Hospital's ICS team received and reviewed these fact sheets, with special attention given by Urban Hospital's compliance department.

Organizing the Vaccination Program

Urban Hospital had never been faced with establishing a mandatory vaccination requirement like this before. Prior to the H1N1 outbreak, the hospital had undertaken vaccination of its workers against seasonal influenza through its Employee Health Services (EHS) division. The EHS had previously set up vaccination sites in areas of the hospital convenient to workers (e.g., outside the hospital cafeteria). Historically, influenza vaccine had never been in high demand or short supply within Urban Hospital. Physicians had been permitted to prescribe and administer influenza vaccination for both patients and their families without restriction.

Using its ICS structure, Urban Hospital established a Point of Distribution Committee, led by its clinical director of emergency management. In accordance with its emergency management plan, the incident commander assigned the committee the task of devising a plan to set up points of distribution (PODs), which were places on the hospital campus where employees, medical staff, and volunteers could quickly receive vaccinations.

The POD model was a component of Urban Hospital's emergency management plan and had been developed based upon guidance from the CDC following the anthrax attacks of 2001. The POD model was designed with the goal of vaccinating a large number of individuals who had no contraindications or complex medical questions as rapidly as possible. The hospital had undertaken exercises of its POD model but never had to implement it for an actual event. The Point of Distribution Committee met several times over a few weeks and devised a plan to staff the PODs with hospital employees and medical students who would provide the screening and vaccinations.

In New York City, the New York City DOHMH was the agency designated to receive the vaccine from the federal government, distribute it to all hospitals and community providers, and track usage. The New York City DOHMH decided to utilize their existing system, the Citywide Immunization Registry (CIR), to account for the doses provided. Providers were required to report on each individual to whom an H1N1 vaccine was administered. This requirement contrasted with the tracking mechanism issued by NYSDOH in which providers reported the aggregate number of doses administered for the rest of the state of New York. The CIR was created in 1997 for the purpose of ensuring that New York City "residents receive all recommended immunizations to protect them from vaccine-preventable diseases."[11] Prior to the outbreak of H1N1, providers were required to report all immunizations provided to people younger than 19 years of age, and were permitted to report immunizations of those older than 19 with the patient's consent.[11] Now that the New York City DOHMH was requiring them to report individual-level patient data to the CIR, providers had to obtain consent from adult patients to affect the mandatory reporting. While the CIR had not previously been used to require reporting of any adult immunizations, the New York City DOHMH chose this system to track the distribution of vaccines it had received from the federal government.

In order to receive the vaccine, individual providers and facilities were to register with the CIR. Like pediatricians throughout New York City, Urban Hospital's pediatric providers were quite familiar with the CIR, and regularly input the required information into the hospital's electronic medical records (EMR) system, which was then sent electronically to the CIR. However, other providers and administrators at Urban Hospital and other institutions were concerned about using the CIR for this new purpose given the staff time that would be needed to report individual vaccine dosages administered. Urban Hospital's ICS team first considered inputting information from the hospital PODs into the EMR system. However, that would mean that any clinical employee who could access the EMRs would be able to view a colleague's personal health information. Therefore, due to concerns about the confidentiality of its workers' personal health information, the information technology (IT) workgroup of the ICS team developed a new internal database (a POD registration system) in order to track the doses of H1N1 vaccine administered. Information from that database would then be transferred to the CIR. Two full-time members of the hospital's IT staff were assigned the task of creating the database (which was based upon an existing database), and were able to create it in a week.

The hospital's H1N1 communications workgroup developed materials to advise its workers of both the new requirement and the scheduling of PODs. Memoranda to hospital employees from the CEO and president of the medical center, the dean of the medical school, and the president and CEO of Urban Hospital stressed that their organizations were requiring all personnel to be vaccinated against influenza. The memo announced the schedule and locations of the PODs and requested clinical and nonclinical volunteers to assist with administering the vaccine and registering personnel at the vaccination sites. "Broadcast emails" were sent to the entire staff, information was provided through the printed hospital newsletter, and departmental communications were sent to employees. In addition, the hospital posted signs about the PODs and distributed handouts about the requirements and the PODs to reach those employees who did not have hospital email accounts because they did not regularly access computers during their workday. The handouts were distributed by the Security Department to workers as they entered the hospital buildings. The handout method had never been used before and was deemed effective at getting messages out to those without email.

THE PODs BEGIN

When the hospital received its seasonal influenza vaccine in the beginning of October, prior to the availability of the H1N1 vaccine, the hospital first vaccinated workers against seasonal influenza. The hospital's Pharmacy Department worked with the New York City DOHMH to coordinate receipt of the vaccine. The supply of H1N1 vaccine began arriving at Urban Hospital later in October. Because the hospital was receiving the vaccine free of charge from the federal government, in keeping with the stringent federal requirements for recordkeeping, the hospital's Pharmacy Department tightly controlled vaccine supplies at the hospital and kept meticulous records accounting for all of the vaccine.

Because the H1N1 vaccine supply was initially limited due to slow production, the hospital first focused its efforts on workers who provided care to the patients at highest risk of contracting H1N1 and seasonal influenza or who were most likely to encounter large numbers of patients with influenza, as well as workers themselves who were considered to be part of high-risk groups (e.g., workers who were pregnant). At the PODs, workers being vaccinated completed a form with basic demographic information (e.g., name, employee ID number) and were then screened for medical contraindications to influenza vaccination (e.g., adverse reactions to influenza vaccinations in the past, allergy to eggs). The POD staff then input information regarding the vaccine to be administered (e.g., manufacturer, lot number) and the anatomical vaccine administration location (e.g., left arm) into the hospital's newly created internal database. The clinical director of emergency management and the hospital epidemiologist/infection control officer, both physicians, directed the POD efforts and provided medical advice. The majority of POD clinical team members were infection control nurses, employee health nurses, pharmacists, and first- and second-year medical students under the direct supervision of a credentialed nurse or physician. Nonclinical staff included personnel from security, IT, engineering, building services, materials management, and food services departments. All of the hospital workers who staffed the PODs did so voluntarily; no one was required to staff the PODs as part of his or her regular duties.

After the PODs, the information from the hospital database was periodically transferred to the CIR electronically. Urban Hospital devoted a large amount of staff time to the input of data at the PODs and the later electronic reporting to the New York City DOHMH through the CIR. Workers who received their vaccinations from other providers (e.g., their primary care physicians) were required to complete a form documenting that they received the vaccine from an external source. Those vaccinations were entered into the hospital's new database as well, so that Urban Hospital could keep track of which employees had been vaccinated.

DISSENTION

As part of the training of personnel who would staff the PODs, Urban Hospital instructed the workers that the goal was to vaccinate as many persons who had no contraindications or complex medical questions as rapidly as possible. POD staff were instructed to ask one of the physician directors, the clinical director of

Box 14-1

In its "Frequently Asked Questions" document,[6] NYSDOH addressed the consequences of healthcare workers refusing to be vaccinated through the following questions and answers:

Q. What if a healthcare worker refuses to be vaccinated?
A. Each organization must take whatever steps are needed to comply with this regulation. Since current public health regulation [sic] also mandate that direct care staff be immune to measles and rubella and receive annual tuberculosis screening, the organization may want to adopt a similar managerial or personnel policy for dealing with individuals without medical exemptions who refuse to be vaccinated or tested. One option for workers who refuse influenza vaccination is reassignment to duties not covered by the regulation.

Q. Can a healthcare worker who refuses to be vaccinated be fired?
A. Again, steps like reassignment to non-covered duties is suggested. Each organization must comply with this regulation, just as the organization assures that healthcare personnel must be immunized against measles and rubella.

emergency management or the hospital epidemiologist/infection control officer, to intervene if workers had questions regarding medical contraindications, vaccine safety, or the hospital's mandatory vaccination requirement. The POD staff was also instructed not to discuss the merits of the mandatory vaccination requirement with those being vaccinated.

A small number of workers at Urban Hospital expressed opposition to the vaccination requirement by presenting at the PODs but then refusing to be vaccinated. The physician POD leaders intervened, attempting to address the workers' concerns. For those workers who still questioned the hospital's mandatory vaccination policy, the physicians suggested that the workers discuss the hospital's policy with their supervisors or representatives of the hospital's EHS or Human Resources Division. While the memos previously described did not state the consequences of not being vaccinated, Urban Hospital's position was that if an employee was not vaccinated, the Human Resources Division would follow the usual process for employees who did not comply with similar requirements (e.g., annual hepatitis B vaccinations)—a warning, followed by suspension, up to and including termination.

HEALTHCARE WORKERS AND OTHERS REACT THROUGHOUT NEW YORK STATE

Some healthcare workers were resistant to being vaccinated against H1N1—their primary concern being one of infringement on personal liberty. These workers believed that they should have the right to refuse to be vaccinated, yet still remain employed. Several unions representing healthcare workers, such as the Public Employees Federation, the New York State Nurses Association, and 1199/SEIU indicated that they were not opposed to H1N1 vaccinations for healthcare workers, but that vaccination should be voluntary, not mandatory. *The New York Times* quoted Joel Shufro, the executive director of the New York Committee for Occupational Safety and Health (a coalition of 200 union locals), who described the union position, saying that the unions were not opposed to vaccination, "but we oppose a mandatory program. . . . This is: You don't get the shot, you're fired."[7]

Hundreds of healthcare workers demonstrated this at a rally protesting the regulation in Albany, New York, on September 29, 2009.[12] The New York Committee for Occupational Safety and Health sent a letter to Commissioner Daines on October 2, 2009, calling on him to withdraw the emergency regulation. In addition, the New York Civil Liberties Union called upon the commissioner to withdraw the regulation, stating:

> Mandatory vaccination violates well established principles of individual autonomy, including the right of competent adults to make decisions regarding their medical care. . . . New York is the only governmental entity in the United States that has adopted a mandatory vaccination requirement to address the threat of H1N1 . . . [The WHO and CDC] have consistently taken the position that inoculation against seasonal flu, and now the pandemic variant H1N1, is strongly recommended but always voluntary.[13]

The New York State Nurses Association (a union representing nurses) stated, "While the association agrees that nurses and other healthcare providers should be immunized for seasonal influenza, it does not agree that nurses should be required to be immunized as a condition of employment."[14]

COURT FIGHTS

Susanne Field, a member of the New York State Nurses Association, filed a lawsuit in New York State Supreme Court in Manhattan challenging the mandatory vaccination regulation. Her lawsuit argued that the regulation was "arbitrary and capricious" because no other state was requiring mandatory vaccination despite international concern about H1N1.[15] On October 14, 2009, the judge hearing the case refused to issue a temporary restraining order (TRO) in that lawsuit, and a hearing was scheduled for October 22, which meant that the regulations remained in effect until the court decided whether or not they should remain in effect.[16]

Three other lawsuits challenging the regulation were filed. They were consolidated and heard by a New York State Supreme Court judge in the state capital, Albany. One lawsuit was brought by three nurses from Albany Medical Center who asserted that the regulation violated their civil rights. The other two lawsuits were brought by the New York State Public Employees Federation (the union whose workers are mostly from public agencies) and the New York State United Teachers Union. In the consolidated case, the judge issued a TRO preventing enforcement of the regulation on October 16, and a hearing was scheduled for 2 weeks later, at which time the court planned to consider whether the regulations should be permanently blocked from being enforced.[17]

At first, NYSDOH defended the mandate. NYSDOH issued the following statement:

> In two weeks the Department is scheduled to be in court, where we will vigorously defend this lawsuit on its merits. We are confident that the regulation will be upheld. The Commissioner of Health and the State Hospital Review and Planning Council have clear legal authority to promulgate the mandatory regulation. As one court said in a 1990 ruling rejecting a challenge to regulations requiring mandatory rubella vaccinations and annual tuberculosis testing for health care workers: "Hospitals . . . exist for the benefit of their patients. They exist to cure the sick. The Legislature of this State has charged the Commissioner of Health with the responsibility of making hospitals safe places to get well. These regulations are tailored to accomplish that end."[17]

However, a little more than a week later, on October 23, 2009, Commissioner Daines sent a letter to hospital administrators regarding the regulations, stating the following:

I am writing to inform you of my determination pursuant to Section 66-3.2. . . . that supplies of seasonal and 2009 H1N1 influenza vaccines are not adequate and that such vaccines are not reasonably available. Therefore, I hereby suspend the requirement for the health care personnel to be vaccinated against both influenza viruses for the current influenza season.[18]

There was speculation, though, that the real reason behind NYSDOH's decision to suspend the regulation was not the inadequate supply of vaccine, but instead the court decision regarding the TRO.

On October 29, 2009, Urban Hospital sent a memo to its workers informing them of the suspension of the regulation and stating that the hospital strongly encouraged all personnel to receive both the seasonal influenza vaccine and the H1N1 vaccine. The hospital indicated that as of that date, about 7,000 hospital faculty, staff, students, and volunteers with patient contact, almost 50% of the total staff, and approximately 10,000 patients had received the seasonal influenza vaccine.

In the October 23, 2009, letter, NYSDOH indicated that it would advance a permanent regulation requiring mandatory vaccinations for healthcare personnel.[18] In a February 4, 2010, letter to hospital administrators, NYSDOH indicated that it anticipated "adopting as a permanent regulation the emergency amendment to 10 NYCRR Title 10, Section 66-3 last year which was suspended due to vaccine shortages."[19] However, perhaps due to the union opposition, NYSDOH never proposed a permanent regulation requiring mandatory vaccination.

ACKNOWLEDGMENTS

The authors would like to acknowledge the contributions of Whitney Gruhin, who assisted with this chapter.

DISCUSSION QUESTIONS

1. Which competencies described in the Appendix does this case demonstrate?
2. What issues were involved in NYSDOH's attempt to stem the spread of H1N1?
3. What challenges did Urban Hospital face in balancing the needs of patients against the concerns of its workforce?

4. What challenges did the hospital face in implementing the mandatory vaccination regulation?

5. Do you agree with the reaction of healthcare workers at Urban Hospital in response to the mandatory H1N1 vaccination requirement? Of healthcare workers around New York state? Why or why not?

6. What implications does NYSDOH's experience with H1N1 have for future public health outbreaks? Pandemics?

REFERENCES

1. Rainey J. Hyping swine flu isn't really healthy. *Los Angeles Times.* May 1, 2009. Available at: http://articles.latimes.com/2009/may/01/entertainment/et-onthemedia1. Accessed April 12, 2013.

2. More NYC schools closed because of flu. *ABC News.* May 23, 2009. Available at: http://abclocal.go.com/wabc/story?section=news/local&id=6828016. Accessed January 24, 2012.

3. The City of New York Department of Health and Mental Hygiene. 2009 New York City Department of Health and Mental Hygiene health alert #22: novel H1N1 influenza update. June 12, 2009. Available at: http://www.nyc.gov/html/doh/downloads/pdf/cd/2009/09md22.pdf. Accessed August 30, 2011.

4. Centers for Disease Control and Prevention. Novel H1N1 flu situation update. Available at: http://www.cdc.gov/h1n1flu/updates/072409.htm. Accessed August 30, 2011.

5. Department of Health. Emergency rule making: health care personnel influenza vaccination requirements. *New York State Register.* September 2, 2009:10–14.

6. Frequently asked questions for hospitals, diagnostic and treatment centers licensed under Article 28, home care services agencies licensed under Article 36 of the PHL and hospice programs certified under Article 40 of the PHL regarding Title 10, Subpart 66-3 regulation. Albany, NY: New York State Department of Health; August 26, 2009.

7. McNeil DG Jr, Zraick K. New York health care workers resist flu vaccine rule. *The New York Times.* September 20, 2009.

8. *Ritterband v. Axelrod,* 149 Misc 2d 135 (1990).

9. Daines RF. Mandatory flu vaccine for health care workers. September 24, 2009. Available at: http://www.health.ny.gov/press/releases/2009/2009-09-24_health_care_worker_vaccine_daines_oped.htm. Accessed August 15, 2011.

10. Public Readiness and Emergency Preparedness Act, Pub L No. 109-148, 119 Stat 2818 (2005).

11. New York City Department of Health and Mental Hygiene. Fact sheet: the citywide immunization registry (CIR) and H1N1 vaccine. Available at: http://home2.nyc.gov/html/doh/downloads/pdf/cd/cd-h1n1flu-cir-faq.pdf. Accessed February 6, 2012.

12. Newman A. NY health workers protest mandatory vaccines. *The New American.* October 2, 2009. Available at: http://www.thenewamerican .com/usnews/health-care/item/1642-ny-health-workers-protest-mandatory -vaccines. Accessed April 4, 2011.

13. New York Civil Liberties Union. Letter to Richard F. Daines, MD, Commissioner. October 13, 2009. Available at: http://www.nyclu.org/files /Flu_Letter_DOH_10.13.09.pdf. Accessed September 29, 2011.

14. New York State Nurses Association. Testimony: mandated influenza immu- nizations. July 23, 2009. Available at: http://www.nysna.org/advocacy /testimonies/mandated_shots.htm. Accessed January 24, 2012.

15. Hartocollis A. Mandatory flu vaccination for N.Y. health workers is criticized. *The New York Times.* October 13, 2009. Available at: http://www.nytimes.com /2009/10/14/health/policy/14vaccine.html?_r=0. Accessed April 4, 2013.

16. New York State Nurses Association. TRO issued preventing mandatory immu- nizations. Available at: http://www.nysna.org/news/online/2009/101609.htm. Accessed August 15, 2011.

17. Hartocollis A, Chan S. Albany judge blocks vaccination rule. *The New York Times.* October 16, 2009. Available at: http://www.nytimes.com/2009/10/17 /nyregion/17vaccine.html. Accessed April 4, 2013.

18. New York State Department of Health. (2009, October 23). "Dear Administrator" letter.

19. New York State Department of Health. (2010, February 4). "Dear Hospital Administrator" letter.

15

2009 H1N1 Influenza Epidemic in Iowa

Amy Terry, Chris Atchison,
and Michael Pentella

BACKGROUND

When any population faces an outbreak of infectious disease, the natural inclination is for people to want answers. They want to know if they have been infected or if their children are infected. People look to public health to get the information that they need.

The surveillance work that state and local public health epidemiologists do—looking for disease, tracking infection, trending the spread—is valuable information for both the general population and physicians who are treating patients. Where do epidemiologists get the data to do their work? One of the most important sources is the laboratory where testing for the disease is occurring. Public health leaders look to the laboratory to provide the information that they need to perform surveillance and to craft the message to protect the public. In short, it takes laboratory testing to know who is infected.

While there are several levels of laboratories that carry out increasingly sophisticated tests, the clinical laboratory is the first line of defense against emerging microbial threats. These types of labs are primarily responsible for running the routine tests that generate the data that is critically needed for diagnosis and management of infectious diseases. As such, clinical laboratories are the backbone of infection control in healthcare facilities.

The public health laboratory must be prepared to quickly and accurately test specimens to inform the public health epidemiologists, who will then inform the public, about the outbreak and how to prevent getting sick. For laboratories to run tests reliably, the personnel who staff them must be highly skilled, with many years of technical training, education, and experience to do the work. During a health emergency that requires laboratories to perform many tests quickly in order to inform the public health response, it is not possible to immediately hire more staff to do the testing. The personnel prepared to conduct the tests are in short supply and usually have been trained for at least 6 months to a year to develop the skills needed.

Fortunately, funding has been available through the public health emergency preparedness (PHEP) cooperative agreement, which was sponsored by the Centers for Disease Control and Prevention (CDC) to build the capacity of public health laboratories to respond to emergencies at the local and state levels. This agreement required that the states and localities build sentinel laboratory networks—partnerships of clinical labs and public health labs—to provide support to facilitate testing and enhance communication during emergencies involving biological illness such as that posed by the 2009 influenza pandemic.

The public health and medical response is further complicated because people often seek medical attention simply because they may have been exposed, whether or not they are ill. People go to their primary care physician, the emergency room, or clinics because they are concerned for themselves and for their families. Often, many of these individuals have no signs or symptoms and are called the "worried well." The worried well want to know how to protect themselves and their families. When so many worried well seek care during a time when many other people are sick, such as during the 2009 H1N1 influenza pandemic, they divert limited resources from those who are truly ill. For public health agencies to provide guidance to communities, they must be knowledgeable about the incidence of disease in each community. For an accurate representation of the incidence of disease, public health officials must turn to laboratories rather than referring to the number of patient visits for flu-like symptoms. Getting the information from the laboratories requires established partnerships and strong communication.

In order to effectively exchange information during an emergency event, there needs to be an effective communication system already in place that has been formed through the development of partnerships and is regularly used. Through regular messages, information is communicated and expectations are established such that an effective partnership emerges and grows. Then, when an emergency is faced, the partners know what is expected and act accordingly. The 2009 H1N1 epidemic provided the opportunity to demonstrate the effectiveness of the partnerships and mechanisms for communication in Iowa's state-level public health laboratory.

SEASONAL AND NOVEL INFLUENZA

Throughout history, the influenza virus has caused pandemics because the virus changes and people often lack immunity to the altered virus. There are three types of influenza virus: type A, type B, and type C. Notably, the influenza A virus changes frequently due to antigenic drift and antigenic shift.

Antigenic drift results in a new strain of virus when naturally occurring mutations in the RNA of the virus cause a change in its surface structures. In a typical influenza season, the resulting illness is likely to be mild, as humans have some preexisting immunity due to previous exposures to a related strain.

The term *novel influenza virus* is used to describe a new and unique strain of influenza that has not previously circulated in the population. Novel strains arise due to a process called antigenic shift. In antigenic shift, a recombination of the genomes of two viral strains occurs, causing a major reorganization of surface antigens and the emergence of a new viral pathogen. When an antigenic shift occurs, the new strain can be vastly different from previous exposures; thus, humans have no immunity. A novel strain of influenza is frightening because the human immune system has not yet had the ability to learn how to ward off the infection. Exposure to a novel influenza virus has resulted in illness that is widespread and severe, often associated with high morbidity and mortality rates.

The virus that circulated in 2009—H1N1—was a novel strain that affected younger people the hardest. Historically, novel strains have been responsible for three pandemics prior to 2009: in 1918, 1957, and 1968. Due to the variable and unpredictable nature of the influenza virus, it is difficult to estimate annual deaths[1] during a typical season. Statistical modeling estimates that the number of deaths associated with seasonal influenza is approximately 36,000.[1] In contrast, the death toll of the 1918 Spanish influenza pandemic was an estimated 50 million people.[2] Another outbreak of the magnitude of the 1918 pandemic would quickly overwhelm hospitals, laboratories, and community resources. When the novel 2009 H1N1 strain was first identified, the virulence of the strain, the susceptibility of the population, and the transmissibility of the virus were unknown. Consequently, public health officials prepared for the worst case scenario. In Iowa, there were no deaths attributed to the 2009–2010 H1N1 virus. This is because the 2009–2010 H1N1 strain was not as virulent as past pandemic strains. In a typical year, such as the 2007–2008 influenza season, Iowa experienced two deaths in children due to infection from the seasonal influenza virus.

NATIONAL LABORATORY SYSTEM

An effective response to any outbreak or epidemic requires a collaborative effort between public health professionals and laboratory services who work in partnership with healthcare providers and others to limit exposures and effectively treat cases. In the wake of the 2001 anthrax attacks, there was heightened concern regarding the ability of the public health system to respond to biological and chemical threats, both naturally occurring and man-made. This led to a massive national initiative to improve the infrastructure of laboratories across the United States.

Leading the effort to improve the laboratory infrastructure was the Laboratory Response Network (LRN). The LRN, primarily developed as part of a national antiterrorism policy, was established in 1999 as a collaboration among the CDC, the Association of Public Health Laboratories (APHL), and the Federal Bureau of Investigation (FBI)[3] to provide a system that could quickly respond to laboratory testing needs in the event of a biological terrorism event such as the 2001 anthrax attack. Today, the LRN links state, local, veterinary, agricultural, military, and water- and food-testing laboratories and provides a rapid nationwide laboratory response for emerging infectious diseases, toxic spills, natural disasters, and environmental emergencies. To prepare for emergencies, the LRN provides the staff working at public health laboratories with regularly scheduled education and training. In addition, these staff members participate in tabletop exercises, drills, and full-scale exercises designed to simulate real-world scenarios. These exercises are invaluable in providing hands-on training and identifying gaps in training, staff, resources, and planning that can be addressed and resolved prior to a genuine event.

IOWA'S STATE LABORATORY SYSTEM

The State Hygienic Laboratory (SHL) for the state of Iowa, a member of the national Laboratory Response Network,[3] is located at the University of Iowa and provides public health laboratory services. The responsibility of the SHL is to communicate information, provide education and training, perform essential specialized services, and provide the expertise and resources to carry out public health–related activities. By being certified as an LRN participating facility prior to the 2009 appearance of H1N1, the SHL had already enhanced its ability to respond effectively to biological emergencies when the pandemic began. Through the LRN, the SHL had received training on efficiently handling emergency situations, techniques for effective communications between the state public health laboratory and the clinical laboratories throughout the jurisdiction, equipment that would be needed to respond during the emergency, and funding for sufficient staff to implement the response.[4]

THE CLINICAL LABORATORY

To meet the PHEP cooperative agreement mandate that they build a statewide laboratory network, SHL developed the Iowa Laboratory Response Network (I-LRN). The I-LRN recognized the interdependent relationship and connectivity of all clinical labs and the SHL throughout the state. Within this network, clinical laboratories are considered *sentinel laboratories* because of the role they play in acting as the first line of defense, standing guard to detect the first cases in a biological attack. Prior to the pandemic, the SHL had established communication with all of the clinical laboratories throughout the state. In 2003, Bonnie Rubin, SHL's emergency response coordinator, personally visited all 140 clinical laboratories in the state to open the dialogue. She felt that in her role as the emergency response coordinator, she could begin the discussion of how labs could partner and communicate in preparation for an emergency. These face-to-face meetings at each clinical laboratory were followed annually by regional meetings with groups of clinical laboratories.

Throughout the year, in addition to the annual meetings, the SHL provided in-person, hands-on training and numerous opportunities for online and webinar trainings on laboratory topics related to agents of bioterrorism and other threats. Testing for the influenza virus has been one of the topics regularly covered in order to involve the clinical laboratories in the state's surveillance process. Annually, the SHL conducts a teleconference dedicated to influenza, and each clinical laboratory is invited to attend. Additionally, regional programs, tabletop exercises, drills, and functional exercises are conducted on a regular basis to maintain awareness and proficiency in responding to an emergency event that might involve a biological or chemical agent.

The I-LRN developed a Google email group as a communication tool to provide timely alerts, updates on testing protocols, and to establish a mechanism for the rapid dissemination of information. As of May 1, 2004, the I-LRN Google email group regularly began to receive information regarding influenza and other biological and chemical agents.

After tools such as the Google email group and other communication mechanisms were in place, the SHL recognized that public health labs and sentinel labs are rapidly changing environments because of changes in staff, facility ownership, and other issues, such as evolving technologies that are part of the environment that laboratories operate within. To maintain a high level of preparedness, partnerships and communication mechanisms are continually maintained to keep them strong and flexible in order to respond to the full range of emergency events. The question that the SHL faced was how to sustain a high level of preparedness and maintain relevancy for the I-LRN.

The SHL addressed this challenge by establishing the Laboratory Advisory Committee (LAC) in 2004. This committee, composed of representatives from clinical and county laboratories, meets quarterly and is dedicated to sustaining the established partnerships among laboratories that perform testing on clinical specimens, focusing especially on communication mechanisms such as regular meetings where issues are discussed. For example, during an epidemic of the mumps virus in Iowa, the LAC met to discuss specimen collection and handling issues before messages about laboratory testing of mumps were sent out to all the clinical labs in the state. This review by the LAC helped to create a clear final message. The LAC provides the SHL with knowledge of what is happening on the frontlines of clinical testing and lets them know how the SHL can assist the whole I-LRN system; this is a forum for the continued success of the I-LRN.

THE TESTING PROCESS

It is important to understand how the testing process works. A physician sees a patient with signs and symptoms of illness and he or she suspects a particular disease. Sometimes a physician needs to test a specimen from the patient to confirm the suspected diagnosis. In that case, the physician collects a specimen and submits it to a laboratory. The laboratory where the physician submits the specimen is a clinical laboratory that will either perform the test at that facility or refer the test to another laboratory. For infectious diseases of importance to public health, the specimen is most often referred to a public health laboratory. A public health laboratory performs clinical lab tests for the good of the entire population and not just the individual patient. For example, testing for tuberculosis is done in a public health lab so that the results can be used to inform the actions of public health agencies to protect others from being exposed to a highly infectious disease. In the case of influenza, once the test is performed in the public health laboratory and the results are ready to report, the test results are sent back to the clinical laboratory that submitted the specimen and also to the state and local public health departments that have responsibility for infectious disease surveillance activities. In Iowa, this is reported to both the clinical lab and public health departments electronically through a secure web-based portal that was established prior to the 2009 H1N1 epidemic. Electronic reporting allows information to be sent quickly to expedite action for both patient care and public health purposes.

TRANSPORT OF SPECIMENS

Another essential component of the emergency response system in Iowa was a courier system used to transport specimens. During the anthrax attacks of 2001, the laboratories across the state mailed suspected anthrax specimens and the SHL mailed back the results. In 2001, that was the extent of the laboratory system in Iowa. The SHL's LAC recognized that one of the limiting factors in the capacity to quickly respond to a biological emergency, a critical component of being prepared, was the ability to deliver specimens more rapidly.

In 2005, Iowa implemented a courier system for the rapid delivery of specimens to the SHL in order to expedite the testing process during emergencies. Each day, a courier travels to the clinical laboratory facilities in Iowa that have requested to have patient specimens picked up and brought to the SHL. This request is made electronically by the clinical laboratories. The courier service regularly picks up specimens from these clinical laboratories Monday through Saturday and special pickup is available at other times for emergencies. Since its launch, this service has reduced delivery time for clinical specimens by 24 to 48 hours and thereby shortened the communication of results to the providers of care. When you combine the courier capabilities with the electronic reporting, physicians are able to receive test results within 24 hours rather than the 6 to 8 days required when reporting by mail. The response time for state and local public health has been reduced from over 18 hours to 6 hours in emergency events, including outbreaks, contaminated water, white powders, and natural disasters.

THE H1N1 PANDEMIC APPEARS

First recognized in Veracruz, Mexico, in March 2009, the H1NI pandemic rapidly spread around the globe. Less than a month later, the first U.S. infections of H1N1 were confirmed in California.

When analyzed, the CDC reported that this particular strain of influenza had never before circulated in humans. Studies showed that the genes of the 2009 H1N1 virus had a unique mix of human, swine, and bird influenza type A viruses. Therefore, no one was expected to have immunity to the virus and no vaccine was initially available.

This unique influenza type A virus strain was quickly seen in other parts of the United States.[5] In Iowa, the virus arrived within a week of the first reports in California, carried into the state by travelers. A businessman who lived in Southern California brought the virus to Iowa. An Iowa resident who had vacationed in Southern California also brought the virus when he returned home. Unlike seasonal outbreaks and other pandemics where the elderly were struck hardest, those that became ill with H1N1 were mostly young adults and children. The H1N1 virus that circulated in 2009 impacted a younger age group who were more frequently infected, more likely to require hospitalization, and more likely to be admitted to an intensive care unit.[5]

IMPORTANCE OF A DEDICATED WORKFORCE

When responding to an emergency, the clinical analysts who perform the testing are a critical and essential resource. The staff who responded to the H1N1 outbreak had been previously trained. The SHL sent one staff member to training conducted by the CDC at their headquarters in Atlanta, Georgia. Through a "train-the-trainer model," that person was responsible for bringing the information back to Iowa and building the skills of others at the SHL. As a general rule, administrators who run laboratories want at least one staff person who is competent to perform a test and a minimum of one other person who has been cross-trained as a backup. As a result of the experience of exercises and drills, the SHL enhanced that model by having two alternative people with the skills necessary to conduct tests so that the SHL is "three deep" for every test. By April 2009, the SHL had four staff members with the required skills and competency to perform the testing. Those administrators planning for a possible pandemic or other emergency involving infectious disease thought that, given the population and area of Iowa, four trained technicians seemed sufficient to run the expected volume of tests.

THE SHL AND LRN DURING
THE H1N1 PANDEMIC

The arrival of the 2009 H1N1 influenza strain in Iowa required the SHL to utilize its emergency response structure to meet the communication and information needs of the event. It was a huge endeavour that took the volunteer efforts of many people over thousands of hours. From the time that the first case was diagnosed in Iowa in April 2009 into 2010, the SHL was an integral part of the international response to the influenza pandemic. The LRN infrastructure played a significant role during the H1N1 influenza pandemic through communicating critical information to state and local public health laboratories. In addition, the LAC advised the SHL on issues that were facing the clinical laboratories and suggested how the SHL could help resolve the issues. The members of the LAC from clinical laboratories provided advice on communicating to physicians about the processes for specimen collection and submission.

During the HINI response, the LRN communication network was heavily utilized. National conference calls among the LRN laboratories, the APHL, and the CDC were held on a regular basis to disseminate information and provide models for a consistent message to be communicated to the media and general public. During these conference calls, the managers at state and local public health labs learned what was occurring and what might occur in other parts of the country and around the globe. The spread of the disease and concerns about the future spread were discussed. Public health laboratories learned about the volume of testing in other states and how that volume was being handled. Most importantly, what worked and what did not work was discussed. Information from the calls was then shared with others in the lab so that everyone could be aware of the spread of the virus and necessary testing and be prepared for what might happen next. The calls provided an opportunity for laboratories to support other labs by sharing resources, such as performing testing for other states. The calls were a chance to learn what was happening firsthand instead of from email or through the news media.

From these conference calls, ideas were generated for the state and local response in Iowa. From the first call alerting that cases were found in California, Iowa took action and ordered more supplies and reagents in case there were shortages in the future. Following subsequent calls, where Iowa received more information about the virus and who was becoming ill, information was shared with other laboratories throughout the state.

When the first case of H1N1 was detected in Iowa, the SHL immediately reached out to the I-LRN to educate the laboratorians—this included laboratory directors, supervisors, and technicians—about the virus, informing the labs of what to expect, what they needed to do, and what resources the SHL could provide. Through conference calls and emails, the SHL made the clinical labs aware of what was happening in the states where the virus was actively spreading so that they would be aware that the need for testing was soon going to increase and that they would need to send specimens to the SHL for testing to confirm that the influenza cases were caused by the novel strain. In addition, some of the currently available testing techniques were unable to detect the new virus. However, because of the preparations made by the LRN, the specially trained staff at the SHL were able to quickly adapt, validate, and implement new testing protocols when such tests became available during the first 2 weeks of the epidemic.

WORK AT THE SHL

During the pandemic, the SHL laboratorians tested specimens; manned a call center, responding to questions about testing; and assembled 5,000 specimen collection kits that were distributed to hospitals and clinics. In a typical 40-hour work week during the peak influenza season, one dedicated person tests about 100 specimens. In a 2-week period during the pandemic, the SHL logged 2,654 hours solely in response to the outbreak and rapidly tested more than 1,400 specimens sent by physicians and laboratories from patients with influenza-like illness across the state. At the height of the pandemic, the SHL was processing so many more samples than anticipated that staff were brought in from other testing areas to support the four staff members who were originally trained.

The originally trained staff were assigned to work an 8-hour shift each day—either from 6:00 AM to 3:00 PM or from 12:00 PM to 9:00 PM. Having two shifts each day allowed for testing of specimens that arrived both early in the morning and in the afternoon. Staff also worked an additional day each week so that testing was performed Monday through Saturday. Incremental personnel were reassigned from other areas of the lab to answer the phone, complete routine paper work, compile testing kits, and complete tasks related to the handling of specimens, such as unpacking the samples. In addition, the courier service delivered thousands of specimens to the SHL, paring the turn-around time for the delivery of test results to less than 48 hours after the collection of the specimen. This allowed the SHL to rapidly communicate results to state and local officials, thus providing accurate data to guide timely response decisions.

MEDIA AND THE WORRIED WELL

Widespread media coverage heightened concerns of the public. The intensified concerns resulted in demands for unnecessary laboratory testing by people who sought medical attention because they were worried that they may be infected with the new strain of influenza virus. The SHL issued a press release to the media to inform the public about testing and assure them that there was capacity to respond to the emergency and perform testing on those who were suffering from influenza-like illness. The media—newspapers, television, and radio—responded by contacting the SHL to get more information and further inform the public.

Even with the extra effort made to assure the public, many healthy people sought medical attention from their physicians, emergency rooms, or clinics out of concern that they had been exposed to the virus. A resultant surge in testing occurred even when people did not have the signs and symptoms of an influenza infection. Those seeking medical attention included people exposed to another person who was suffering from a respiratory illness. The SHL quickly became overwhelmed by the number of specimens. At one point, the associate director of the SHL reviewed each specimen submitted so that only patients who exhibited the signs and symptoms of influenza-like illness had their specimens tested.

The help of the sentinel laboratories and community clinicians was sought. The goal was for the sentinel laboratories to act as gatekeepers so that the SHL was not overwhelmed with unnecessary tests. The associate director of the SHL held a teleconference and requested that sentinel labs inform physicians that only specimens from patients who exhibited the signs and symptoms of an influenza virus would be tested. Further, the associate director asked the clinical labs to screen the specimens prior to sending them to the SHL to ensure that the signs and symptoms presented by each patient were documented on the test request form that accompanied each specimen. A similar message was also sent to physicians across the state through the I-LRN Google email group.

Eventually the number of worried well seeking medical care declined, and testing of specimens from patients who truly exhibited the signs and symptoms of influenza was not slowed because of the need to perform unnecessary tests.

CONCLUSION

The Iowa Laboratory Response Network serves as an example of the dual functionality of emergency preparedness. While originally developed to respond to an event involving agents of bioterrorism, such as the anthrax events of 2001, the LRN strengthened the ability of public health laboratories to respond to an emerging biological infection. The LRN is now prepared to respond to other outbreaks of infectious disease, such as mumps or measles. This network is regularly utilized and will continue to be an asset to communicate routine information and further strengthen partnerships with clinical laboratories to meet future challenges.

The 2009 H1N1 influenza epidemic was a public health emergency that captured the nation's attention and tested the preparedness of clinical laboratories and public health agencies throughout the United States. In addition to the dedication of well-trained staff, the H1N1 response was successful in keeping deaths to a minimum due in large part to the strong communication systems formed among Iowa's public health partners, sentinel laboratories, courier systems, and emergency operations planners.

Response to new and emerging pathogens requires the action of an interactive laboratory network of the public health labs, other laboratories, corporate and academic partners, and the CDC. An effective epidemic response relies on the effective functioning of day-to-day operations and established communication systems. With preparation, labs can be mobilized into action quickly. From the H1N1 experience, laboratories learned how to improve communication and be even more successful in responding to future events.

DISCUSSION QUESTIONS

1. Which competencies described in the Appendix does this case demonstrate?
2. Why is communication important during the public health response to an epidemic?
3. Describe the testing process for biological emergencies and how it works, including the impact on the patient and public health.

4. Why is influenza virus a public health risk every year?
5. How did Iowa's State Health Laboratory leverage their prior work developing the Iowa Laboratory Response Network (I-LRN) to respond to the 2009 H1N1 influenza epidemic in Iowa?
6. How did the services provided by laboratories support the action of the epidemiologists in this epidemic?
7. How did the worried well strain the healthcare system during the H1N1 influenza epidemic? What can be done to mitigate this reaction and how might planners better prepare for future biological emergencies/epidemics?

REFERENCES

1. Thompson WW, Shay DK, Weintraub E, et al. Mortality associated with influenza and respiratory syncytial virus in the United States. *JAMA.* 2003;289(2):179–186.
2. National Archives and Records Administration. The deadly virus: the influenza epidemic of 1918. Available at: http://www.archives.gov/exhibits/influenza-epidemic/. Accessed January 2, 2012.
3. Centers for Disease Control and Prevention. Facts about the Laboratory Response Network (LRN). Available at: http://emergency.cdc.gov/lrn/factsheet.asp. Accessed January 2, 2012.
4. Centers for Disease Control and Prevention. The Laboratory Response Network: partners in preparedness. Available at: http://emergency.cdc.gov/lrn/. Accessed December 14, 2011.
5. Centers for Disease Control and Prevention. 2009 H1N1: overview of a pandemic. Available at: http://www.cdc.gov/h1n1flu/yearinreview/yir5.htm. Accessed January 2, 2012.

16

The Martha's Vineyard Public Health System Responds to 2009 H1N1

Melissa A. Higdon and Michael A. Stoto

INTRODUCTION

Influenza is respiratory infection that occurs seasonally, mostly in the winter, and although many are infected, the consequences are mostly mild. In early 2009, however, a new strain of the influenza virus emerged in Mexico and the United States. Because no one had previously been exposed to the new virus—created through a process called an antigenic shift—neither natural immunities nor the existing influenza vaccine provided protection. And because the virus was similar to the 1918 "Swine Flu" pandemic, which killed millions around the world, the World Health Organization (WHO) declared a pandemic as the virus spread around the globe in April. Although it was ultimately mild, the 2009 H1N1 pandemic required a concerted effort from the entire U.S. Public Health Emergency Preparedness (PHEP) system, from the federal government down to local areas such as the island of Martha's Vineyard in Massachusetts.

The Institute of Medicine has defined the public health system as the "complex network of individuals and organizations that have the potential to play critical roles in creating the conditions for health."[1] The PHEP system includes not only federal, state, and local health departments, but also hospitals and healthcare providers, fire departments, schools, the media, and many other public and private organizations.[2]

THE MARTHA'S VINEYARD PUBLIC HEALTH SYSTEM

Martha's Vineyard is a 90-square-mile island in Massachusetts with a year-round population of approximately 16,000. The island is composed of six towns that, together with the town of Gosnold (population 75) on a separate group of islands, make up the entirety of Dukes County, Massachusetts (see **Figure 16-1**). Although the Vineyard has a reputation based on its wealthy summer visitors, the year-round population is composed of mostly agricultural and service workers, with relatively low income and education in comparison to the rest of the state. A substantial number of the year-round residents are Brazilian and speak Portuguese as their primary language, and there is also a Native American community on the island known as the Wampanoag Tribe of Gay Head, located predominately in Aquinnah, the island's smallest and most rural town.

Figure 16-1

Map of Martha's Vineyard.

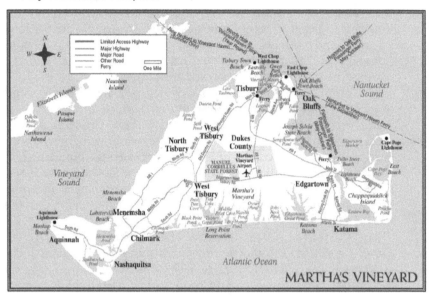

Source: Reproduced from Martha's Vineyard Tourism. Map of Martha's Vineyard. 2012. Available at: http://www.capecodtravelguide.com/marthas-vineyard. Accessed June 16, 2012.

The local public health system on the island is composed of both formal and informal structures. Unlike in many other parts of the United States, Massachusetts counties have no role in public health or most administrative matters, meaning the six town boards of health have the primary responsibility for public health matters. The largest towns have a full-time health agent and up to two other staff members, and the smallest towns have less than one full-time equivalent worker.

The 19-bed Martha's Vineyard Hospital (MVH), which is affiliated with Massachusetts General Hospital (MGH) in Boston, is the only hospital on the island. Housing several hospital-owned physician practices (including the only obstetrics practice on the island) as well as one independent practice (Vineyard Pediatrics) and the Windemere nursing home, MVH is a major part of the island's public health system. There is also a small Federally Qualified Health Center (FQHC) on the Vineyard, which is not officially affiliated with the hospital but is supervised by a MVH physician. The

Vineyard Nursing Association (VNA) also plays a role in the local public health system, contracting individually with each town, with the exception of Aquinnah, for standard public health nursing services, including immunizations and epidemiology. In addition, the Vineyard Affordable Access provides access to health care for low-income island residents, and is overseen by the Dukes County Health Council, consisting of representatives from the hospital and the schools, the town health agents, and consumers.

The Wampanoag Health Service, which provides programs and services to members of the federally recognized Indian tribe, is another part of the island's public health system. The service's contract health program provides assistance to tribal members with purchasing comprehensive health services such as inpatient and outpatient care, hospital medical office visits, pharmaceutical services, and mental health counseling through members' personal healthcare providers. In 2009, Mr. Ron MacLaren managed the tribe's health affairs.

The Martha's Vineyard Regional High School (MVRHS) serves the entire island, together with one charter school that includes kindergarten through 12th grade. Five elementary schools exist on the island, ranging in size and composition. Tisbury, Edgartown, Chilmark, and Oak Bluffs each have one school and there is a regional elementary school in West Tisbury for children from West Tisbury, Aquinnah, and Chilmark that choose not to attend the small Chilmark elementary school. Each town school within the Martha's Vineyard public school system had a limited amount of funds allocated for consultation with a physician. Anticipating the second wave of H1N1 in the fall of 2009, the school superintendent, Dr. James Weiss, appointed Dr. Michael Goldfein from Vineyard Pediatrics as the school system physician on a consulting basis.

Emergency preparedness efforts on the Vineyard have been both formal and informal. In 2002, the Massachusetts Department of Public Health (MDPH) established 7 regions and 15 subregions to coordinate emergency preparedness efforts.[3] The Cape and the Islands Emergency Preparedness Coalition, part of region 5, encompasses Barnstable County (Cape Cod), Martha's Vineyard, and Nantucket (see **Figure 16-2**). In addition to the six town health departments, MVH was represented in the coalition's hospital preparedness efforts mainly through Carol Bardwell, the chief nurse executive. The coalition has been the primary vehicle for Vineyard health departments and the hospital to access federal public health and hospital preparedness funds.

Figure 16-2

Massachusetts Department of Public Health Emergency Preparedness Regional Coalitions.

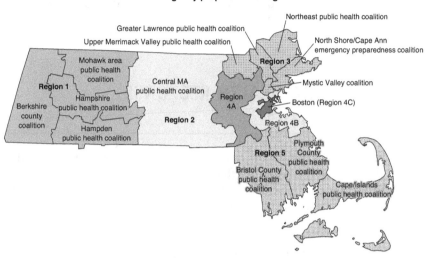

MDPH emergency preparedness regions

Source: Modified from Massachusetts Executive Office of Health and Human Services. Massachusetts Department of Public Health Bioterrorism Regions and Regional Coalitions. 2012. Available at: www.mass.gov/eohhs/docs/dph/emergency-prep/map -bt-regions-by-coalitions.pdf. Accessed June 16, 2012.

In addition, around 2005, the six towns and the Wampanoag Health Service formed the informal Martha's Vineyard Public Health Coalition (MVPHC) to strengthen communication among the six towns on the Vineyard and the Wampanoag tribe. In addition to regular meetings, the MVPHC's major activity has been to organize an annual island-wide seasonal influenza vaccine clinic, usually on Veterans Day (November 11). In addition to providing a needed preventive service, the coalition has used these clinics to test and drill approaches to mass dispensing that would be useful in an emergency. MVH, VNA, and town emergency management agencies are brought into the MVPHC's activities as needed. For example, town police departments were asked to develop a traffic plan for island-wide flu clinics.

The Vineyard's public health system is characterized by the many informal connections that one finds on a small island. For instance, in addition to participating in the Cape and Islands Emergency Preparedness Coalition efforts, MVH chief nurse executive Carol Bardwell is also a member of the island's Medical Reserve Corps (MRC) board, as are representatives of each of the six towns. Dr. Michael Goldfein, the leading practitioner at Vineyard Pediatrics, also serves as the school system physician. And Mr. David Caron, the MVH director of pharmacy, also serves as a member of the Oak Bluffs board of health.

THE PUBLIC HEALTH RESPONSE TO 2009 H1N1

The first Massachusetts cases of H1N1 were seen in early May 2009 in Boston, shortly after the pandemic emerged in Mexico, California, and New York City in April.[4] Because children seemed to be particularly at risk for infection, these and subsequent cases triggered a wave of school closings in Massachusetts and throughout the United States.

A second wave of the H1N1 epidemic was predicted for the fall, with children, young adults, and pregnant women to be most affected by the virus, triggering a national vaccination campaign. Production of the H1N1 vaccine began in May shortly after the virus surfaced. Vaccine deliveries were expected by late September or early October. In July, the Centers for Disease Control and Prevention's (CDC) Advisory Committee on Immunization Practices (ACIP) identified the following priority groups for the vaccine: pregnant women, children aged 6 months through 24 years, caregivers of children aged less than 6 months, and high risk/chronically ill individuals.[5]

As the summer progressed, the CDC encouraged the state health departments to develop plans for administering vaccines at the local level in their states.[6] In late August, MDPH expanded its vaccine distribution program by building on the existing Vaccine for Children (VFC) program for pediatric vaccines and urged hospitals and other healthcare providers not already in the system to register to be able to receive H1N1 vaccine.[7] In the registration process, MDPH asked for the number of individuals that would be vaccinated, but not more specific details such as the number of children. MDPH also alerted local health departments to prepare mass dispensing plans at this time.

Delays in vaccine production announced in late August and early September 2009 prompted MDPH to announce more specific tiers within the CDC priority groups.[8] The first tier included pregnant women, children aged 6 months to 5 years old, caregivers of children aged less than 6 months, and healthcare workers.[8] The second tier covered the remainder of the CDC's priority groups: children aged 5 years old to 24 years old, emergency medical technicians, paramedics, and adults aged 25 to 65 years in poor health.[8]

ON THE VINEYARD

In early August, a 26-year-old Vineyard man of Brazilian descent developed severe flu-like symptoms and was treated at Martha's Vineyard Hospital. MVH initiated a webcast medical discussion with physicians at their affiliate, Massachusetts General Hospital; H1N1 was confirmed, and as the patient's conditioned worsened, he was transferred to MGH, where he ultimately died on August 14.

In September, in response to MDPH's recommendations, the Vineyard health agents collaborated with the VNA to register as one entity for five of the six towns on the island, and the Wampanoag Health Service registered for the tribe and the town of Aquinnah, where most tribal members live. MVH registered for its staff as well as the physician offices owned by the hospital. Vineyard Pediatrics, an independent physician practice co-located at the hospital, was separately registered as part of the preexisting childhood immunization system to receive vaccine.

In addition, the town health agents and the VNA chose a single island-wide vaccination clinic at the regional high school, where previous seasonal flu clinics had been held, to administer both H1N1 and seasonal vaccine. Given the urgency of the situation and the understanding that vaccine would be available, the clinic was planned for September 26 rather than November 11 as in previous years. As the planned date for the island-wide clinic neared, however, vaccine production delays were announced, and the clinic was postponed first until October 24 and eventually November 11, when only the seasonal vaccine was administered.

In the last week of October, students at Martha's Vineyard Regional High School started to come down with flu-like symptoms. According to the *Martha's Vineyard Times*, for example, on Wednesday, October 29, 2009, more than 100 MVRHS students were out sick.[9] Because MDPH did not recommend laboratory testing or require case reporting, these were presumed to be H1N1 cases and the students were sent home. Absenteeism increased throughout that week and the next, and health officials assumed that this reflected students with influenza or students kept home by their parents out of concern they would be infected. According to the *Martha's Vineyard Gazette*, the worst day for student absences was on Friday, October 30, 2009, when approximately 140 MVRHS students of the 800 total MVRHS students were out sick.[10]

H1N1 vaccine started arriving on the island in late October, but only in small batches. Faced with a very different vaccine availability situation than had been expected, the Vineyard Public Health Coalition switched tactics. In a series of meetings in October with school superintendent Dr. James Weiss and the school system physician Dr. Michael Goldfein, a school-based approach was adopted. School officials did not think that parents would bring their children to a mass vaccination clinic on a Saturday; they chose to vaccinate students at their own school when it was in session. Because the school did not have enough staff to vaccinate every student in a day, the MVPHC assembled "shooter teams" consisting of health officials and Emergency Medical Services (EMS) staff from every town on the island as well as from the VNA that would go from school to school. Every Vineyard school has a full-time nurse, and because they know the children well, the school nurses were assigned the administrative paperwork and follow-up work with the students' parents as necessary. The smaller schools—the Chilmark School and the Public Charter School—were done first, beginning November 9, when 100 dose batches of vaccine first arrived. The larger schools were done later, when more vaccine became available.

Martha's Vineyard Hospital, meanwhile, had used its first doses of vaccine at a hospital-wide flu clinic on October 29, at which 209 hospital and Windemere nursing home staff were vaccinated. Rather than waste vaccine in multidose vials that had been opened, MVH also vaccinated emergency medical technicians and paramedics at this time. Having observed a fatal case at close range in August, the hospital CEO, Mr. Tim Walsh, wanted to be sure that the vaccine was used as soon as it became available. Because he assumed (incorrectly, as it turns out) that the towns were waiting to assemble enough vaccine to hold the island-wide clinic, MVH also took on the responsibility of vaccinating the pregnant women on the island (as the only obstetrics practice on the island was based at the hospital) and pre-school children. On Saturday, October 31, 2009, MVH brought on

Portuguese translators to assist with the large population of Brazilian residents on the island and hosted a flu clinic for pregnant women. On the same day, MVH held a separate clinic at which 206 preschool-age children were vaccinated.

Despite the concerted efforts of the towns and schools, the hospital and its providers, and the tribe, there were a number of problems that emerged as more vaccine became available in November. MVH, for instance, originally assumed that because it housed the island's only obstetrics practice, all pregnant women were covered in the hospital's October 31 clinic. Town health officials pointed out that some women received their prenatal care off the island or were not covered at all. Vineyard Pediatrics, which had registered to receive vaccine separate from the hospital and the towns, committed to vaccinating its own patients. Confusion arose, however, about whether this should include the patients of Dr. Melanie Miller, who worked at Vineyard Pediatrics but was a hospital employee. Although these problems were quickly resolved, they created confusion and frustration.

AFTER ACTION ANALYSIS

Overall, there were notable successes in how the Vineyard handled the H1N1 epidemic, especially with regard to mass dispensing. The decision to share personnel and resources across towns to constitute the shooter teams was essential in vaccinating school children in a timely manner. Moreover, the decision to vaccinate the children attending smaller schools first and the children at larger schools as vaccine became available was easy to explain to the general public and was well accepted. It also represents an adroitly flexible response to uncertainty about when vaccine would arrive.

Perhaps the most important achievement was the way the towns, the hospital, the tribe, the schools, and others came together in a "public health system" and shared personnel and other resources across towns to protect the health of those on the island. MVH, for instance, stepped up to vaccinate not only its employees, but also pregnant women and preschool children on the island. The Martha's Vineyard Public Health Coalition developed and tested an effective system of off-site staging areas within the hospital, which are likely to be useful in future events. The traditional "fierce independence" of the Vineyard towns, as one of those involved put it, with their own schools and health agents, makes this even more remarkable.

One important lesson from this experience relates to communication within the public health system: Do not assume that informal communication channels are either accurate or complete. For instance, despite best intentions across the board, there were a number of missed cues. MVH apparently believed that MVPHC was still planning a single island-wide H1N1 clinic, even after the focus had switched to school-based plan. And as mentioned previously, the hospital assumed that its obstetrics practice covered all pregnant women on the island. In addition, the complicated arrangement between Vineyard Pediatrics (owned by Dr. Goldfein but located at the hospital) and MVH (which employs Dr. Miller, who works with Vineyard Pediatrics) caused trouble when Vineyard Pediatrics received its own supply of vaccine. Parents were confused about whether their children should be immunized at school, at the hospital's preschool clinic, or by Vineyard Pediatrics (and if it mattered whether they were Dr. Goldfein's or Dr. Miller's patient). Some officials and parents apparently assumed that the effort to vaccinate children through Vineyard Pediatrics was coordinated with the hospital, given Vineyard Pediatrics' location on hospital property, but the effort was separate and uncoordinated.

Many of these problems were the result of incomplete knowledge of the scope of the outbreak and who had received vaccine supplies, as well as making assumptions about what others were planning to do with the vaccine they had. Despite the best efforts of the MVPHC and its informal connections to the hospital and many community health partners, communication and coordination within the local public health system located on the Vineyard did not always run smoothly. Throughout the fall, some of those involved felt that the hospital maintained a level of independence from the MVPHC. Town health agents, the VNA, the tribe, the schools, and public safety officers were generally represented at coalition meetings, but a hospital representative was less consistently present. Some health agents and school representatives felt there was a one-way relationship with the hospital and the coalition. For instance, coalition members were frustrated when the hospital would ask the coalition for information about the location and number of H1N1 cases that they came into contact with, but would not provide information from their records to the coalition. The hospital sometimes cited the Health Insurance Portability and Accountability Act (HIPAA) privacy rule as a barrier to discussing the number and locations of cases of confirmed H1N1.

One coalition member thought that the hospital was "standoffish" in general. In the future, the coalition should seek to include both MVH and Vineyard Pediatrics formally in their planning and response efforts. More generally, this experience highlights the need to build trust within the public health system.

More generally, this experience reflects the MDPH's inability to recognize informal regional public health systems,[3] even if they were "natural" like the Vineyard. For instance, Vineyard officials could have coordinated their efforts better if they knew how much and what kinds of vaccine were coming to the island. Even though Ron MacLaren, director of the Wampanoag Health Service, became known as the voice of the Vineyard, the state health department was not able to report on the amount of vaccine that had been delivered to the island. Rather, the MDPH vaccine distribution system produced reports only for the formally designated emergency preparedness regions such as the Cape and the Islands Coalition.

Communication between the state and the Vineyard was further complicated by the nature of the vaccination registration process. Faced with an urgent need to rapidly increase the number of potential vaccinators, the MDPH chose to adapt an existing registration system designed for the federal Vaccines for Children program. The resulting ad hoc system did not adequately account for the diversity of the sites to which the vaccine was being distributed. Dealing with approximately 4,500 registered sites, it was difficult for the MDPH to know that the VNA had contracted to vaccinate children in the Vineyard schools rather than the elders that are typically served by visiting nursing associations. In addition, given that the hospital and Vineyard Pediatrics were also registered, it also may not have been clear that the VNA was responsible for all of the island's school children because most Massachusetts towns registered individually. This became an issue when vaccine was in short supply and available in batches of 100. If the five towns had registered separately they might have received one batch each, whereas the VNA only received one. It is ironic that the coalition's effort to simplify the process by having the VNA register for the towns may have resulted in fewer doses being available.

Thus, another lesson from this experience is that more clarity is needed about the purpose of the registration process, as well as the implications for the amount of vaccine supplied to each registered site. Moreover, in the future, more detailed demographic information on the population served by the registered site should be collected from the point of registration.

DISCUSSION QUESTIONS

1. Which of the competencies described in the Appendix does this case demonstrate?
2. Imagine that it is Wednesday, November 4, 2009, and you are Ron McLaren, the informal leader of the Martha's Vineyard Public Health Coalition, who is about to convene the coalition's weekly meeting. At this point, flu-related absenteeism at the regional high school is peaking, various vaccine clinics are planned or underway, and the Vineyard Nursing Association (VNA) has received 300 doses of pediatric vaccine.
   a. What are the immediate decisions that have to be made? Consider the island-wide clinic (scheduled for November 11), how school-based clinics should be conducted, and how to deal with the hospital-based clinics.
   b. What do you know, and what do you need to find out? How can you get the needed information?
   c. What authority/influence do you have to accomplish what needs to be done?
3. It is February, 2010, after the action is complete, and you have been asked to prepare an After Action Report/Improvement Plan (AAR/IP) for the Vineyard's public health emergency preparedness system. Prepare a list of "lessons learned" addressing both issues that the Vineyard public health system can resolve on its own as well as issues that require changes at MDPH. The focus should go beyond specific problems that arose in the context of the case to the root causes of the problems in order to improve the system for whatever public health emergency should occur in the future. Consider:
   a. The challenges of managing under uncertainty
   b. The importance of more "local" involvement in decision making and program management
   c. The need to balance clear and precise policies with flexible implementation
   d. Increasing transparency and clarity of communications
   e. The importance of trusting relationships

ACKNOWLEDGMENTS

Interviews with local public health and hospital officials including:
Maura Valley, Assistant Health Agent, Tisbury
Marina Lent, Health Administrator and Health Inspector, Chilmark

Carol Bardwell, Chief Nurse Executive, Martha's Vineyard Hospital
Newspaper articles (various dates)
The Martha's Vineyard Gazette
The Martha's Vineyard Times
The Boston Globe

Figure 16-3

2009 H1N1 timeline.

April 21–27	CDC and Mexico issue alerts regarding novel influenza virus strain, WHO raises pandemic threat level
May 1	First Massachusetts H1N1 cases diagnosed in Boston
May	Vaccine production begins, CDC announces that the first doses are expected to be delivered in late September or early October
June 2	First case of H1N1 confirmed on Martha's Vineyard
July 29	CDC ACIP issues priority groups for 2009 H1N1 vaccine
August 14	26-year-old Vineyard man dies of H1N1
August 27	MDPH encourages as many sites as possible to register to receive H1N1 vaccine, alerts local health departments to prepare mass dispensing plans
September 14	MDPH issues guidance identifying two tiers within the ACIP high priority group
September 26	Planned island-wide seasonal and H1N1 vaccine clinic postponed
October 24	Planned island-wide seasonal and H1N1 vaccine clinic postponed
October 28	First noticeable H1N1-related school absenteeism on Martha's Vineyard
October 29	MVH and VNA vaccine staff and EMS workers with direct patient contact
October 31	MVH hold vaccine clinics for pregnant women and preschool children
November 9	H1N1 vaccine clinics held at the Chilmark, West Tisbury, and Martha's Vineyard Public Charter Schools
November 11	Island-wide vaccine clinic conducted with seasonal vaccine only
November 20	H1N1 vaccine clinic held at Tisbury School

REFERENCES

1. Committee on Assuring the Health of the Public in the 21st Century. *The Future of the Public's Health in the 21st Century.* Washington, DC: National Academies Press; 2003.
2. Altevogt BM, Pope AM, Hill MN, Shrine KI, eds. *Research Priorities in Emergency Preparedness and Response for Public Health Systems.* Washington, DC: National Academies Press; 2008.
3. Koh HK, Elqura LJ, Judge CM, Stoto MA. Regionalization of local public health systems in the era of preparedness. *Annu Rev Public Health.* 2008;29:205–218.
4. Massachusetts Department of Health and Human Services. H1N1 (swine) flu. Available at: http://www.mass.gov/eohhs/docs/dph/cdc/flu/influenza-lab-faq-101008.rtf. Accessed May 15, 2013.
5. National Center for Immunization and Respiratory Diseases (NCIRD). Use of influenza A (H1N1) 2009 monovalent vaccine—recommendations of the advisory committee on immunization practices (ACIP). August 21, 2009. Available at: http://www.cdc.gov/mmwr/preview/mmwrhtml/rr58e0821a1.htm/. Accessed June 16, 2012.
6. Centers for Disease Control and Prevention (CDC). H1N1 meeting the challenge: a new virus. Available at: http://www.flu.gov/blog/2010/01/timeline.html#. Accessed April 22, 2013.
7. Centers for Disease Control and Prevention (CDC). 2009 H1N1 vaccination recommendations. Available at: http://www.cdc.gov/h1n1flu/vaccination/acip.htm. Accessed June 16, 2012.
8. Massachusetts Department of Health and Human Services Guidelines for the vaccination of employees of licensed clinics, dialysis centers, hospitals and long term care facilities against seasonal influenza and pandemic influenza H1N1. Available at: http://www.mass.gov/eohhs/docs/dph/quality/hcq-circular-letters/2009/dhcq-0908521-attachment.pdf. Accessed April 22, 2013.
9. Steward, R. Superintendent confirms H1N1 cases in Island schools, October 29, 2009, Martha's Vineyard Times. Available at: http://www.mvtimes.com/marthas-vineyard/news/2009/10/29/h1n1-school-cases.php?page=2. Accessed April 22, 2013.
10. Seccombe, M. Flu Hits High School Hard; - Clinic Nov. 11. November 5, 2009, Martha's Vineyard Gazette. Available at: http://mvgazette.com/news/2009/11/06/flu-hits-high-school-hard-clinic-nov-11. Accessed April 22, 2013.

Public Health Preparedness and Response Core Competency Model

Elizabeth McGean Weist, Kristine M. Gebbie, Elizabeth Ablah, Audrey R. Gotsch, C. William Keck, Laura A. Biesiadecki, and John E. McElligott

RATIONALE FOR DEVELOPMENT OF THE MODEL

The Public Health Preparedness and Response Core Competency Model Version 1.0 (see *www.asph.org/userfiles/PreparednessCompet encyModelWorkforce-Version1.0.pdf*), as mandated in the Pandemic and All-Hazards Preparedness Act of 2006,[1] was developed in 2009–2010 by the Association of Schools of Public Health (ASPH) and sponsoring organization, the Centers for Disease Control and Prevention (CDC). The competency model was created to provide a current benchmark for the competencies that the public health workforce needs to perform assigned prevention, preparedness, response, and recovery roles in accordance with established national, state, and local health security and public health policies, laws, and systems.

The competencies apply to *all* hazards that have potentially negative health consequences. In keeping with the National Response Framework and Target Capabilities List, all-hazards incidents covered by the model include terrorist attacks; natural disasters; emerging infectious diseases; health emergencies; environmental threats; other major events such as the use of chemical, biological, radiological, nuclear, high-yield explosives (CBRNE) agents; and food and agriculture incidents. This approach is supported by research demonstrating that worker competence in responding to one type of disaster or emergency translates to competence in related situations.[2,3] The all-hazards approach taken in creating the Public Health Preparedness and Response Core Competency Model spans the continuum of the U.S. Department of Homeland Security mission areas—namely, to prevent, protect, respond to, and recover from incidents.

TARGET AUDIENCE

The Public Health Preparedness and Response Core Competency Model represents individual competencies that midlevel workers, *regardless of their employment setting*, are expected to demonstrate to ensure readiness for all-hazards events. The model applies both to workers in public health organizations and workers with public health functions in nonpublic health entities.

Model developers defined a midlevel public health worker targeted for this competency model as an individual with either:

- 5 years of experience with masters in public health equivalent or higher *degree in public health*, or
- 10 years of experience and a high school diploma, bachelors, or *non-public health graduate degree.*

These midlevel public health workers who play public health–specific roles represent the backbone of the public health workforce, numbering an estimated 300,000 or more individuals. The staff included among the target audience who lack public health education or population-based experience and who work in other roles (e.g., in administration, human resources, technical and clinical areas) within public health organizations are among those considered essential to all-hazards preparedness and response. Rationale is that in the event of an all-hands-on-deck emergency, such staff are necessary contributors to the overall effort.

MODEL DEVELOPMENT PROCESS

Working within a 29-year-old cooperative agreement mechanism, ASPH and CDC staff, along with consultants (the project team), interacted closely to craft and launch the competency development initiative. The project team assembled a leadership group (see *www .asph.org/UserFiles/LeadershipGroupMembers8.pdf*), populated by representatives from both public health academe and practice, to help guide the process.

In brief, the project team conducted three rounds of a modified Delphi-type process in which they presented slates of competencies, and/or their domains, to vested stakeholders, refining the model after each round. Round 1 presented 11 preliminary domains that were suggested by the leadership group. Between rounds 1 and 2, staff gathered nearly 60 resources (see *www.asph.org/document .cfm?page=1126*) that included competencies, competency-like statements, learning outcomes, job actions, performance indicators, and skill lists that were aligned with the 9 refined domains that emerged from round 1. From these resources, staff populated a "starter slate" that included more than 1,100 competencies and competency-like statements. A consultant distilled this starter slate to 201 competencies among the 9 domains for review and comment by expert workgroups (one for each of the 9 domains). The workgroup members whittled down the candidates so that in round 2, stakeholders were invited to comment on a list of 29 draft competencies in 9 domains. In round 3, stakeholders provided input on an even more refined slate of 21 draft competencies (listed without domain titles). After a three-month vetting period with the public health preparedness community and consultation with the leadership group on suggested changes, the project team reassembled the remaining 18 competencies into 4 new overarching domains: model leadership, communicate and manage information, plan for and improve practice, and protect worker health and safety. The resulting competency set was presented to the public in December 2010.

THE MODEL

The model delineates the performance goal of proficiency for the target audience—midlevel public health workers. To a great extent, an individual worker's ability to meet this performance goal is grounded in competencies acquired from three other sources, as applicable to the worker's level of training and position/role:

1. *Foundational public health competencies*, such as the Council on Linkages Between Academia and Public Health Practice Core Competencies for Public Health Professionals (see *www.phf.org/ resourcestools/Documents/Core_Public_Health_Competencies_III .pdf*), which are applicable to public health professionals in governmental public health organizations; the ASPH Master's Degree in Public Health Core Competency Model (see *www .asph.org/publication/MPH_Core_Competency_Model/index.html*), for those in the target group with master of public health (MPH) degrees; and the competencies from the Interprofessional Education Collaborative (IPEC), representing the professions of medicine (both allopathic and osteopathic), nursing, pharmacy, dentistry and public health (see *www.asph.org/userfiles /CoreCompetenciesforInterprofessionalCollaborativePractice.pdf*).

2. *Generic health security or emergency core competencies*, such as those that may stem from NIMS courses (see *http://training.fema.gov/IS /NIMS.asp*), and the new core competencies for disaster medicine and public health recommended for all health professionals (see *www.dmphp.org/cgi/content/abstract/6/1/44*).[4]

3. *Position-specific or professional competencies*, such as those developed for public health nursing (see *http://www.achne.org/files/Quad% 20Council/QuadCouncilCompetenciesforPublicHealthNurses.pdf*),

environmental health (see *www.apha.org/programs/standards /healthcompproject/corenontechnicalcompetencies.htm)*, health education (see *www.nchec.org/credentialing/credential/*), public health law (see *www.publichealthlaw.net/Training/TrainingPDFs/PHLCompetencies .pdf*), applied epidemiology (see *http://www.cste.org/dnn/Portals/0 /AppliedEpiCompwcover.pdf*), administrative support (see *http://nsdta .aphsa.org/PDF/CompetencyGuides/Administrative_Support.pdf*), and informatics (see *http://www.nwcphp.org/docs/phi/comps/phi_print.pdf*).

Beyond these competency sets, the 18 competencies in the 4 domains of the model listed in the following section are critical to building and sustaining the capacity of midlevel public health workers to fulfill their responsibilities in emergencies.

PUBLIC HEALTH PREPAREDNESS AND RESPONSE CORE COMPETENCY MODEL

1. Model Leadership

1.1 Solve problems under emergency conditions.
1.2 Manage behaviors associated with emotional responses in self and others.
1.3 Facilitate collaboration with internal and external emergency response partners.
1.4 Maintain situational awareness.
1.5 Demonstrate respect for all persons and cultures.
1.6 Act within the scope of one's legal authority.

2. Communicate and Manage Information

2.1 Manage information related to an emergency.
2.2 Use principles of crisis and risk communication.
2.3 Report information potentially relevant to the identification and control of an emergency through the chain of command.
2.4 Collect data according to protocol.
2.5 Manage the recording and/or transcription of data according to protocol.

3. Plan for and Improve Practice

3.1 Contribute expertise to a community hazard vulnerability analysis (HVA).

3.2 Contribute expertise to the development of emergency plans.

3.3 Participate in improving the organization's capacities (including, but not limited to, programs, plans, policies, laws, and workforce training).

3.4 Refer matters outside of one's scope of legal authority through the chain of command.

4. Protect Worker Health and Safety

4.1 Maintain personal/family emergency preparedness plans.

4.2 Employ protective behaviors according to changing conditions, personal limitations, and threats.

4.3 Report unresolved threats to physical and mental health through the chain of command.

Use of the Model

The model was designed for immediate use by CDC-funded Preparedness and Emergency Response Learning Centers (PERLC), formerly titled the Centers for Public Health Preparedness (see *http://preparedness.asph .org/perlc/index.cfm*), as mandated in congressional legislation.

The PERLC responded to Model Version 1.0 by considering the unique workforce development needs in their approved service areas (as identified by prior needs assessments) and delivering trainings that they consider aligned with the core competencies. PERLC grantees also created a listing of knowledge, skills, and attitudes (KSAs) that further expands upon the competencies and, thus, provides more specificity to individuals and groups that aim to refine existing trainings and develop new ones (see *http://www.asph.org/userfiles /KSA.pdf*). To locate trainings aligned with the core competencies and/or Public Health Emergency Preparedness (PHEP) capabilities, see the Public Health Training Center Database (*http://bhpr .hrsa.gov/grants/publichealth/trainingcenters/search.html*), a gateway catalogue of distance-accessible training and train-the-trainer tools developed by the CDC-funded Preparedness and Emergency Response Learning Centers and the HRSA-funded Public Health Training Centers. Courses are available in many formats such as podcasts, DVD, video, web-based, and self-study guides.

Other public or private entities are invited to examine the model and apply it in whole or part, as well as use it to supplement existing competency models, as appropriate, for their own workforce development programs and policies.

Other users of the model are expected to include the following:

- *National, regional, tribal, state, and local health policy makers and program planners,* such as individuals working to fulfill the new preparedness objective in HP2020 (see *www.healthypeople. gov/2020/topicsobjectives2020/overview.aspx?topicid=34*), to assist in maintaining and enhancing the workforce needed for national health security
- *Employers,* such as supervisors and human resources managers, to shape hiring, performance appraisals, and succession planning
- *Educators and trainers of individuals who perform essential public health services,* such as public health learning institutes and centers as well as those involved with the PERLC and Project Public Health Ready (see *www.naccho.org/topics/emergency/pphr /index.cfm*), to assess worker skills, determine the need for additional training, and conduct periodic drills and exercises that reinforce the competencies and refresh readiness
- *Fellow response and incident command system partners,* so that non-public-health professionals who contribute to protecting and securing the nation's health and safety can better understand public health roles and integrate such staff to reach their full potential in command center teams and in interdisciplinary planning, field work, and other mitigation, response, and recovery activities
- *Employees,* to undertake self-appraisals and determine where additional training may be needed to support one's role and/ or to fill functional gaps within an organization preparing for all-hazards situations
- *Evaluators,* to develop performance metrics and structure performance reviews of exercises, drills, or actual emergencies
- *National accrediting bodies,* such as the Public Health Accreditation Board (PHAB; see *www.phaboard.org/*), to aid in advancing the quality and performance of public health organizations, upgrading standards for preparedness and response-specific functions, and enhancing preparedness and response roles of disciplines that interact with the public's health
- *Researchers,* to assist in studying the impact of training upon performance as well as the long-term influences of workforce readiness upon health outcomes[5]
- *Students,* including those contemplating entrance into the field of public health emergency preparedness and response (to preview the knowledge, skills, and abilities they would be expected not only to demonstrate but to have oversight over, if not at first, then eventually as they rise to managerial roles), those engaged within educational and training programs (to track

their learning progress), and those returning after many years in the field (to gauge how their less-experienced colleagues are likely to perform and, thus, to reflect upon their own learning needs in light of the listed expected behaviors).

NOTE

More information about this competency model is available online at *www.asph.org/document.cfm?page=1081*. Feedback, particularly from personnel using this model at the local, state, and national levels, is encouraged and can be submitted to *competency@asph.org*.

ACKNOWLEDGMENTS

This competency development project was supported under a cooperative agreement from the Centers for Disease Control and Prevention (CDC) through the Association of Schools of Public Health (ASPH) grant number U36/CCU300430-28. Its contents are solely the responsibility of the authors and do not necessarily represent the official views of the Centers for Disease Control and Prevention, the Department of Health and Human Services, or the U.S. government. The authors are grateful for the partnership with Dr. Andrea Young and Dr. Robyn Sobelson, who worked closely with ASPH on this project through the Office of Public Health Preparedness and Response at the Centers for Disease Control and Prevention during the competency model development process.

REFERENCES

1. Pandemic and All-Hazards Preparedness Act, S 3678, 109th Cong, 152 Congressional Record S11220 (2006) (enacted).
2. Ablah E, Tinius AM, Konda K. Collective lessons learned. *J Public Health Manag Pract*. 2009 March;15(suppl):S31–S35.
3. Fowkes V, Ablah E, Oberle M, et al. Emergency preparedness education and training for health professionals: a blueprint for future action. *Biosecur Bioterror*. 2010 March;8(1):79–83.
4. Walsh L, Subbarao I, Gebbie K, et al. Core competencies for disaster medicine and public health. *Disaster Med Public Health Prep*. 2012 Mar;6(1):44–52.
5. Gebbie KM, Weist EM, McElligott JE, et al. Implications of preparedness and response core competencies for public health. *J Public Health Manag Pract*. 2013, 19, 3, 224–230, doi: 10.1097/PHH.0b013e318254cc72.1–7.

Index

Note: Page numbers followed by "*f*" and "*t*" indicate figures and tables, respectively.

CPSIA information can be obtained
at www.ICGtesting.com
Printed in the USA
FSHW020635031019
62556FS